A
Darker
Ribbon

A Darker Ribbon

Breast Cancer, Women, and Their Doctors in the Twentieth Century

Ellen Leopold

BEACON PRESS
BOSTON

BEACON PRESS
25 Beacon Street
Boston, Massachusetts 02108-2892
www.beacon.org

BEACON PRESS BOOKS
are published under the auspices of
the Unitarian Universalist Association of Congregations.

05 04 03 02 01 00 99   8 7 6 5 4 3 2 1

This book is printed on recycled acid-free paper that contains at least
20 percent postconsumer waste and meets the uncoated paper
ANSI/NISO specifications for permanence as revised in 1992.

Text design by Anne Chalmers
Composition by Wilsted & Taylor Publishing Services

Library of Congress Cataloging-in-Publication Data
    Leopold, Ellen
        A darker ribbon : breast cancer, women, and their doctors
    in the twentieth century / Ellen Leopold.
            p.   cm.
        Includes bibliographical references.
        ISBN 0-8070-6512-9
        1. Breast—Cancer—History—20th century.   2. Breast—Cancer—
    Social aspects.   I. Title.
        RC280.B8   L37   1999
        616.99'449'00904—dc21
                                                        99-27201

FOR LILY AND CATHERINE

To die—takes just a little while—
They say it doesn't hurt—
It's only fainter—by degrees—
And then—it's out of sight—

A darker Ribbon—for a day—
A Crape upon the Hat—
And then the pretty sunshine comes—
And helps us to forget—

The absent—mystic—creature—
That but for love of us—
Had gone to sleep—that soundest time—
Without the weariness—

—Emily Dickinson

Contents

Acknowledgments

IN CARRYING OUT the research for this book, I spent time immersed in medical books and archives that are of little surviving interest to anyone but historians. But interleaved in this material was a body of evidence I always found shocking, no matter how many hours of dutiful note-taking had dulled my concentration. What never failed to electrify me were the photographs of women, shown naked to the waist, revealing breast tumors of truly monstrous sizes and shapes arrayed across their chests. For whatever reasons, their physicians had determined that their tumors were inoperable; they had been left to suffer the unmitigated pain of cancer in the breast itself as well as the insidious but invisible spread of disease throughout their bodies. These photographs are, then, a record of a wholesale medical surrender.

And yet, the women they portray had agreed to sit for the camera. Despite their nakedness and the desperate condition of their bodies, they seem, at least to me, to stare back, not with shame or anger, but with a kind of dignified resignation. The upright heads and shoulders facing the lens head-on evoke the candor of a buttoned-up Victorian portrait. The image is grotesquely at odds with the fulminating disease on display below.

Why did these women agree to be photographed? Were they flattered into believing that their tumors were rare enough to "excite" the interests of other surgeons? Or were they already in a dissociated state, inducing in themselves the protective numbing effect that medicine had failed to supply? Did it ever occur to any of them to say no? Try as I might to comfort myself with speculative answers, I can never have even the remotest idea of what these women were really feeling. I do know that there will never be any more subjects like them, nor photographs of them. We now see in them the abuse of women as medical specimens. "What determines the possibility of being affected morally by photographs," Susan Sontag has written, "is the existence of a relevant political consciousness." The feminist consciousness that has emerged in the decades since most of these photographs were taken now finds these images offensive as well as disturbing.

But the photographs are also medically, as well as morally, obsolete. It is now rare for signs of disease in the breast to go untreated long enough for it to flaunt its deadliness in such a profusion of demonic shapes. In any case, it is representation of disease at the microscopic rather than macroscopic level that interests medical science today.

The photographs nonetheless survive, a dark album of images that record the death-in-life so characteristic of this disease. Their subjects remain unnamed, the suffering they recall undocumented. And there are thousands of them. Over the past few decades, feminist historians have written about the accumulation of unrecorded life lived by unknown women: This book is an acknowledgment of their unrecorded suffering and deaths.

Of course, I have many more immediate obligations to the living. The brief and formal acknowledgment I can offer them here is, I know, a very poor substitute for the abundant prose they deserve. So, as a stand-in for much more, I say thank you, most especially, to Martha Matzke, Lynne Walker, Sarah Flynn, and the trio @way.com—Raymond Eisenstark, John J. Simon, and Ernie Eban. Their all-purpose support (humor, hand-holding, and practical advice) have been invaluable. I am also indebted to David Birnbaum, John Breitner, Linda Falstein, Hulda Flynn, Jean Hardisty, Ann Klefstad, Kurt Kuss, Lynne Lane, Catherine Leopold, Dene Leopold, Eunice Leopold, Alan J. Lieberman, Charles C. Mann, John Mason, Lynn Phillips, Patricia Potts, Lily Saint, Max Saint, Judith Vichniac, and Susan Woll. Thank you all.

It has been a pleasure to work with Deanne Urmy, my editor at Beacon Press. She entered into the spirit of this book with great enthusiasm and with an equally great sensitivity to the issues involved—and managed to keep these qualities alive and productive for the duration of the project.

For permission to reproduce archival material, I would like to thank the Alan Mason Chesney Medical Archives of the Johns Hopkins Medical Institutions; Papers of George Crile, Jr., M.D., The Cleveland Clinic Foundation Archives, Cleveland, Ohio; Rachel Carson Papers, Beinecke Rare Book and Manuscript Library, Yale University. I am grateful to Frances Collin, literary executor of the Rachel Carson Estate, for her permission to reproduce Carson's letters; to Helga Sandburg Crile, for granting me access to the correspondence between her late husband and Rachel Carson and for allowing me to include her husband's letters in this book; and to Elizabeth N. Shor for permission to cite material from the Sim Family correspondence at the Nebraska State Historical Society. I am also grateful to *The Nation* and to *Sojourner: The Women's Forum,* where some of the material and the ideas I have developed here first appeared.

For their expert advice I would like to thank Dr. Steven Come and Dr. Paul Busse, both at the Beth Israel Deaconess Medical Center, Boston (who are, of course, not responsible for the use I have made of their medical wisdom); Jonathan Rosenthal at the Museum of Television and Radio, New York; and Linda Lear, for her gracious help with the Rachel Carson material.

Finally, I would like to thank the staff at the many libraries who made access to much of the material I needed to write this book miraculously straightforward. I would particularly like to thank those working at the Schlesinger Library, Radcliffe College, the Harvard/Radcliffe College Libraries, and the Countway Library of the Harvard Medical School.

Introduction

FIGURATIVELY SPEAKING, the breast has probably been the most overworked organ of a woman's body since time began. As Marilyn Yalom demonstrates in her wide-ranging survey, *A History of the Breast*, everyone seems to have a claim on it. Men and women are aroused by it, artists represent it, poets apostrophize it, babies are nourished by it, fashion and commerce fetishize it—and disease afflicts it. All of these responses to the breast, including the last one, are conditioned, if not wholly determined, by the culture in which they operate. The breast attracts so much attention and is a site of conflict for so many of society's values and beliefs that it often seems not to belong to a woman at all.

Writing on the subject reinforces this sense of a woman's alienation from her own breasts. It ranges from the obvious to the obscure, from the history of breastfeeding and wet nursing in different countries and different centuries to the use of the breast in political propaganda. All of the recent writing has brought to the fore the contributing role of culture, highlighting the impact of the dynamic but elusive set of values governing society at any one moment. This has given us a richer, if less determinate, view of human history. Society, we have discovered, is too intricate and too dynamic to reconstruct with anything approaching a sense of closure. There are simply too many forces at work for anyone ever to have the "last word."

Breast cancer, however, as a subject for social historians, has not been part of this burgeoning literature. The liberating effects of Susan Sontag's *Illness as Metaphor,* published in 1978, and of James Patterson's *The Dread Disease,* published a decade later, have not completely lifted the embargo on the disease (or on cancer of the lung or prostate, for that matter). These are cancers whose deadliness has, if anything, increased over the course of the century (lung cancer was virtually unknown in 1900). Yet the histories of these diseases remain unwritten.

In the case of breast cancer, the void in the literature stands in stark contrast to the extremely visible and voluble presence of the disease in contemporary culture. Breast cancer may not yet have a well-documented past but it certainly has a vibrant present. There is no public forum now in which breast cancer is not at home. It has been taken up as a cause by celebrities of all stripes (politicians, entertainers, sports figures) and its problems are thoroughly and regularly aired in all media. Pink ribbons adorn the chests of thousands of Americans, a measure of the success of the breast cancer activism of the 1990s. There is hardly a community in the United States that has not participated directly in some fund-raising or consciousness-raising event organized by groups of women at the local, regional, or national level.

At the heart of this success are the two million American women who live with breast cancer today (including myself). For many of us, breast cancer is no longer a medical emergency but a chronic condition, one we may live with for the rest of our lives. Our interest in the disease may remain as intense as ever but it is no longer so urgent. We can now afford to broaden our outlook, to consider the social and political dimensions of the disease alongside its immediate impact on our individual lives. But if breast cancer activism has provided an outlet for our concern for the future of the disease, the available literature on the subject has made no attempt to gratify our curiosity about its past.

How is it that a subject so utterly taboo, for so long, has become so commonplace so quickly, taking up residence in every cultural medium, from soap operas to sculpture? And what made the stigma surrounding the disease so powerful to begin with? These are questions that have not yet been addressed. But it may be that the cumulative impact of two million women and the repercussions of their experiences, whether as private individuals or as activists, has finally generated a critical mass of interest in a longer perspective on the disease. As a de-mobilized army in reserve, restored to normal life (at least for the time being), these women provide an impressive counterweight to the more traditional image of women stricken with this illness, succumbing without demur to a deadly enemy. Their active and often committed lives are a reminder that death from breast cancer, although it still cannot be dismissed, may now at least be delayed.

This small shift in the balance of power may be just what was needed to make a social history of the disease finally possible. Of course whatever is written today, before the end of the story is known, will soon reveal its limitations. This makes its bias very different from those evident in the histories of vanquished killers like typhoid and polio. There can be no triumphalism here, no retrospective selection and highlighting of just the right set of clues that, quietly gathering momentum despite false starts and setbacks, lead the story to its elegant conclusion. A history of breast cancer told today will, on the contrary, betray a clear lack of a unifying thread. But the open-endedness it offers instead has some advantages as well. The tangled and inconclusive story lines can be more closely investigated, not for their contribution to the ultimate cure but for their contribution to the evolution of modern breast cancer "culture." Lacking the narrative drive of a history of disease that is racing forward to meet its appointment with destiny, the story of breast cancer can afford to move at a slower pace, taking the time to linger in some unproductive cul-de-sacs, to gain in texture what it loses in plot. Its story, in other words, cannot be rushed or compromised by the so-called benefits of hindsight. Its indeterminate status also provides an opportunity and an open invitation, as the writers of literature on AIDS have demonstrated, to readers themselves to play a role in determining the final outcome.

Until now, breast cancer as a subject has been orphaned, separated from the mainstream literature of history and sociology, just as the experience of the disease itself has been cordoned off from society, a private experience suffered by women individually, at the margins of public consciousness. Outside of medical journals, writing on the subject has been limited, both in its output and in its scope. Before the 1970s, it could be found in the pages of medical histories, primarily. Written largely by medical men, these histories made no concessions to culture whatsoever but traced the changing odds between men and mortality as though they arose from one extended experiment carried out under laboratory conditions. Since women, in these renderings, were no more than carriers of disease, they rarely appeared as actors in the drama.

Over the past few decades, two newer genres have arisen that have turned these histories upside down, not only introducing women into the story but placing them at the center. These are the personal narratives of illness written by breast cancer survivors (like Betty Rollin's *First You Cry*) and the self-help manuals written largely by medical professionals (with Susan Love's *Breast Book*, first published in 1990, perhaps the best-known example). Many of these books are hybrids, combining both approaches. Almost all of them focus, for the most part, on the immediate needs, practical and emotional, of the recently diagnosed woman.[1]

The sharp discontinuity between the earlier medical commentaries on disease and the current outpouring of memoirs is jarring. The first are written exclusively by men and largely for men; the second almost exclusively by women and largely for women. The first takes a very long perspective on history; the second, none at all. In one it is disease itself that provides the thread of continuity; in the other it is the individual consciousness of the writer. But if there seems to be little to connect the genres, they do share one critical attribute: a complete disregard for the determining influences of society and culture.

This book is an attempt to supply that missing perspective. Stepping back for a moment from current controversies and taking a longer, retrospective look reveals a great deal about the derivation of contemporary attitudes toward the disease. These, it turns out, can be traced back to ideas and habits of mind that have been around for decades, if not for centuries. We have no conscious connection to any of this past, of course, because until recently the history of breast cancer has been subject to the same unconditional prohibition as has the discussion of most other aspects of the disease. Personal narratives have been more acceptable, not just because they provide immediate comfort to the newly diagnosed woman but also because they pose no challenge to the status quo. Cut off from both history and politics, they make no effort to explain the long-term failure of medical science to prevent or cure the disease. Their goals are short-term, immediate, and aimed at individual readers, not at society at large.[2]

Written history, on the other hand, may be less immediately instrumental but its long-term implications are just as significant. Contemporary beliefs about and attitudes toward breast cancer do not simply mirror contemporary cultural themes or medical views. They reflect instead the markings characteristic of any disease of great antiquity, the scarred remains of earlier attempts to rationalize, pacify, or deny an enemy that could not be subdued. As long as the disease survives, traces of all the myths or superstitions it ever conjured up will cling to it, however discredited they may be. Only a cure or, ultimately, prevention, can ever really lay them to rest, once and for all. Until then, our response to breast cancer will continue to reflect the defeat of every strategy—offensive or defensive—that has ever been put up to contend with its perennial deadliness.

The unequal contest to date between clinical medicine and virulent pathology has, in the case of breast cancer, been aggravated by the dynamics of inequality between men and women, expressed primarily through the doctor/patient relationship. Echoes of nineteenth-century beliefs still hover over this pairing as well, despite the solid efforts of feminism to dispel them. Here too, as long as breast cancer retains its power to kill, every encounter between a male doctor and a newly diagnosed woman re-creates the necessary conditions for inequality, no matter how enlightened either or both partners in the drama may be.

It is the interaction between these two struggles—the first between medical science and the biology of breast cancer, the second between the men who, for most of history, have dictated the terms of this struggle and the women whose disease has occasioned it—that gives this history its distinctive features. Breast cancer has inevitably brought the two historical strands into close proximity, with variable results. At times, their joint impact has been a regressive one, paralyzing or prejudicing scientific research, medical treatment, and public awareness. At other times, it has been more innovative, opening up some new perspective on either the behavior of the disease or the behavior of the women who are vulnerable to it. Catalysts for change in one sphere have indirectly spurred change in the other, although sometimes after considerable time lags and with unexpected effects. In the pages that follow, I have attempted to pull apart and examine the dynamics of these two themes, at least partly in the hope that a closer inspection might help to broaden our understanding of current controversies, whether among activists, historians, or interested noncombatants.

The book uses a combination of case studies, correspondence, and commentary to document both the continuity and the complexity of the changes that have led to a public candor in the handling of the subject. The groundwork for this approach has been laid over the past two decades by important work on the impact of nineteenth-century medical theory and practice on the lives of women. Feminist revisions of the history of the doctor/patient relationship have also played an important role. I have been fortunate in being able to apply this scholarship to the early history of breast cancer and, with this foundation, to move the story forward into the uncharted waters of the twentieth century.

Although a great deal of medical history does appear in these pages, the book does not set out to provide a thoroughgoing social history of treatment in the twentieth century. There is little coverage, for instance, of the long-term pattern of access to medical care among different groups of women, nor of the history of the medical institutions (hospitals and clinics) providing that care. Although women physicians have obviously had an impact on breast cancer treatment, this is mentioned only briefly. The possibility of being treated by an all-women team of physicians—surgeon, radiologist, oncologist—has only quite recently become a reality and remains an exceptional rather than a common occurrence. For most of the period covered in this book, women physicians constituted a significant if quite small minority of doctors (about 5 percent up to the 1970s). The history of government intervention in the fight against cancer is also given little space.

Rather, the story told here is based on a selective analysis of those aspects of the social history of the disease that have, in my opinion, contributed most over the past 100 years to *the patient*'s understanding of and response to it. So although this book proceeds in a loosely chronological order, it is organized thematically rather than along a straight narrative path.

This means that the 100-year career of the radical mastectomy, which remained the primary treatment for breast cancer for most of a century, plays a prominent role in the pages that follow, while chemotherapy, a relative newcomer in the treatment arsenal, does not. It also means that more attention has been paid to the role of sexual politics in shaping the perspective of the medical profession as a whole than to the unquestionable skills and compassion of thousands of individual practitioners. The prejudices of society may have a powerful impact on the practice of medicine but it would be hard to argue that physicians have consciously contrived to do harm rather than good. They have not. The generations of surgeons who strove to "perfect" the radical mastectomy were operating in good faith on scientific principles as they understood them. The history of breast cancer treatment, therefore, cannot be portrayed as a conspiracy against women, although women have often been poorly served by it. Their responses, after all, have been shaped just as much by their cultural milieu as have those of the physicians who treat them. The intention here is not to cast blame but to identify the underlying cultural ideas at work, in order to understand why they have had such different consequences for men and for women.

I should also add that I do not want to minimize the benefits of the treatments that medicine in the first 75 years of the century made available. Undoubtedly, they kept a great many women alive. My criticism of radical surgery in this book is directed more toward those factors (not, strictly speaking, either medical or scientific) that served to prolong clinical dependence on a misguided model of disease. Resistance to change unquestionably slowed the pace of progress while continuing to subject thousands of women every year to unnecessarily disabling surgery. My retrospective impatience with this loss of momentum is perhaps more excusable in the context of a search for a cure that is, alas, still ongoing.

Every disease has its own history.[3] What makes each one unique is the particular way in which, as the writer David B. Morris has expressed it, the biology of a disease intersects with the culture in which it appears. The biology in this case has turned out to be fiendishly complex, compared with, for example, the biology of polio or of smallpox. Breast cancer is a cluster of intractable, adaptable, and unpredictable diseases that originate in human breast tissue (male and female).[4] Their furtive biology has marked the nature of scientific and clinical responses to the disease every bit as much as it has influenced the interactions between physicians and patients. But this fact tends to get lost because the "science" of breast cancer is simply too esoteric, requiring a grasp of a body of knowledge that lay beyond the reach of most "students" of the disease. Although this book emphasizes the social rather than the scientific response to breast cancer, it does try to examine some of the ways in which medical science and practice have accommodated the peculiarities of its biology.

For a variety of reasons, breast cancer, as a disease within American culture, has seemed to pose much less of a threat to society than many other diseases, such as polio or AIDS. It is a disease of women (rather than of men or of children) and also a disease of women who are, typically, past their childbearing years (the risk of getting the disease at 60 is more than 100 times greater than it is at 30). It is not contagious. It is not, properly speaking, an epidemic, felling masses of people at once; it is more a disease of individuals. Also unlike an epidemic, it does not suddenly appear and just as suddenly depart but remains steadily, relentlessly present. It does not, in fact, appear at all but remains offstage, hidden away from public view.

All of these characteristics tend to deprive the disease of the high drama evoked by epidemics. Epidemics mobilize an immediate and widespread public response, summoning all the skills, practical and precautionary, that can be made available through agencies of public health. Everyone is caught up in them. Inevitably, they are attention-grabbing and make headlines. The opportunities they offer for both tragedy and heroism make media coverage of them irresistable. Not surprisingly, the paper trail they leave behind has made them popular with medical historians. But, as the historian of medicine Charles Rosenberg has written, chronic diseases, those that take up permanent residence in the culture, may play "a more fundamental social role . . . than the dramatic but episodic epidemics of infectious disease that have so influenced the historian's perception of medicine; we have paid too much attention to plague and cholera, too little to 'dropsies' and consumption."[5] I would add breast cancer to the list of historical wallflowers. As a disease that sets off powerful if poorly understood reactions to female sexuality, its history has much to tell us about American society's long-term accommodations to the physical and emotional needs of women.

The book is divided thematically into three parts and moves forward in loosely chronological order, from the end of the nineteenth century to the end of the twentieth. Chapter 1 thus begins by examining the sexual politics of the disease at the end of the nineteenth century. The views then current on the role of women within the traditional American family play an important part in shaping the social response to breast cancer. Particularly relevant are society's changing expectations of women as they age and as their relationship to reproduction alters. Medical attention in the late nineteenth century, reflecting the imperatives of society at large, concentrated almost exclusively on the preparation of girls and young women for the consuming roles of motherhood. Because symptoms of disease in postmenopausal women played no role in the dynamic of social reproduction, they attracted much less attention.

Symptoms of disease in younger women were another matter. Any who chose to deviate from the prescribed path of marriage and motherhood, who hoped to be educated or employed or even to experience the pleasure of exercise or dancing, would suffer bodily punishment for their transgressions. This would be meted out to them, not in the form of a whipping or any other form of physical torture but in the form of disease, brought on by their own disobedience, according to the wisdom of prevailing medical authority. Breast cancer in a young woman was only one of many such expressions of disfavor.

But breast cancer was not a manufactured disability, unlike so many of the "female ailments" dreamed up by nineteenth-century doctors to preserve women's inferior status. It was a real killer, and one that compromised the very femininity that Victorian culture worked so hard to preserve. The failure of existing medical science to cure or even to "manage" the disease led eventually to its disappearance from family physicians' areas of competence. Its corresponding absence from the popular medical literature of the time documents the lack of enthusiasm for treating the disease among family physicians charged with the care of female patients.

But the decline in the involvement of family physicians (and early gynecologists) just before the turn of the century was met and no doubt abetted by the corresponding rise of surgery to a position of undisputed authority in the treatment of breast cancer. Chapter 2 discusses the wide implications of this change. The increasing availability of surgery was a mixed blessing. It meant that many more women suffering from painful symptoms of disease in the breast could now be treated. But it also meant that more women submitted to treatment that exacted a terrible toll on their bodies. By the turn of the century, the radical mastectomy, as refined by William Stewart Halsted, first professor of surgery at Johns Hopkins, had become the "gold standard," and survival rates following surgery appeared to improve. But the apparent success of radical treatment had as much to do with the benefits of earlier detection, a more careful selection of surgical candidates, and improvements in anaesthetic and pre- and postoperative care as with any curative powers of the surgery itself.

Part Two illustrates the standard treatment at work. It reproduces two correspondences, each between a breast cancer patient and her surgeon, each running from diagnosis to death. The shift down in scale from the abstract discussion of Part One allows a more intimate look at the individual experience of breast cancer and at some of the smaller-scale consequences of the ordeal that are inevitably lost in the broader historical narrative.

Both women in these correspondences underwent Halsted mastectomies, the first performed by Halsted himself in 1917, the second more than forty years later. Their letters, covering the periods 1917–22 and 1960–64, represent, both chronologically and thematically, a dead center in the history of breast cancer as I have construed it. The half-century spanning the years from the beginning of the first correspondence to the end of the second marks a kind of steady-state in the social and medical management of the disease, a static plateau in which few new ideas or expressions of dissatisfaction were allowed to disturb the prevailing dogma. The treatment of breast cancer set in place by Halsted and his students remained fundamentally unchanged throughout this period.

The two women patients were educated and articulate and both were determined to play an active role in the management of their disease. The first, a woman we will call Barbara Mueller, had been born in 1867 and was in paid employment at the time of her diagnosis. The second woman was the scientist and writer Rachel Carson (author of *Silent Spring*), who was exceptionally well qualified to participate in such a correspondence. The two surgeons, William Stewart Halsted and George Crile, Jr., were equally prominent in their own field. Born about fifty years apart (Halsted in 1852 and Crile in 1907), their working lives spanned a century of breast cancer treatment (1880s to 1980s) that was dominated by the radical mastectomy. Halsted was the surgeon most responsible in the United States for the almost universal use of this procedure. Crile, after the mid-1950s, became one of its most vociferous detractors. (Halsted practiced medicine at a time when surgery constituted the only treatment for breast cancer. By the end of Crile's working life, radiation and chemotherapy, including hormone therapies, had reduced surgery to only one among many alternatives.)

Whatever improvements had taken place in the refinement of existing therapies between the 1920s and the 1960s had not reduced the death rates from metastatic disease. On the contrary, breast cancer deaths continued to rise. Barbara Mueller may have thought that the radiation treatment she sought but failed to obtain could have kept her alive. But the more powerful and more accurate radiation available to Carson decades later did not save her either. How was it possible that so little progress had been made, that scientific research and clinical practice seemed to have lost their forward momentum during all these years?

Part Three begins to answer this question. The evolution of the medical response to the disease, which lay at the heart of Part One, is now joined by the history of women's participation in the disease experience. The story of breast cancer in the twentieth century is as much about the assimilation of women into the establishment culture as it is about the pace of medical progress. Once the basic treatment paradigm (radical surgery) had been put in place and became more readily available, its position could only be consolidated with the active support of the population it was designed to serve. The battle for the hearts and minds of women, as it turned out, was far easier to win than any battle against biology.

Physicians realized early on that women had to be educated to accept treatment for breast cancer. In particular, they had to be rescued from the paralyzing fatalism that cancer often evoked. They had to become patients, to demonstrate, by their willing submission to treatment, their absolute faith in the therapeutic value of surgery. In 1913, the American Society for the Control of Cancer, the precursor to the American Cancer Society, was set up by physicians to achieve just this transformation.

With no mandate (or funds) to undertake research, the fledgling society was neither well placed nor encouraged to evaluate the effectiveness of the treatment it advocated. What it *was* set up to do was to influence public opinion. This it achieved through massive public relations campaigns that sought to bring women to treatment as expeditiously as possible, by reassuring them, in the words of a much-used slogan, that "in the early treatment of cancer lies the hope of cure." The fact that women continued to die even after being treated was never addressed. Surgeons were cast as heroic lifesavers, rescuing women from the brink of death; women were profoundly dependent upon their intervention and grateful for it.

As Chapter 5 documents at some length, the combination of early detection and early treatment, first set in place by the education campaigns of the cancer charity, has been this century's stand-in for genuine cure or prevention. It has been kept alive, over most of the period, by regular transfusions of new technology. The steady improvement of diagnostic techniques has repeatedly given it a new lease on life as incidence and death rates from breast cancer continued to rise. The American Cancer Society, the original mastermind of this strategy, has never faltered, over three-quarters of a century, in its promotion of early detection. Their unwavering support has had a disproportionate influence on the public's awareness and understanding of the disease as well as on the strategies adopted by smaller, local organizations committed to similar goals.

From its beginnings, women themselves became the primary purveyors of this message as well as its beneficiaries. First mobilized by the American Society for the Control of Cancer in the late 1920s, the high point of their voluntary participation occurred ten years later when they were recruited on a national basis into the ASCC's newly formed Women's Field Army. Enlisted in their thousands, these women raised the operating income for the parent organization while they leafleted, broadcast, and delivered the message of early detection to American womanhood. In other words, the campaigns traded on and reinforced all of society's sexist expectations of woman: that she take responsibility for her own health without forgetting her responsibilities for others and that she carry out, on an unpaid basis, the labor-intensive strategies that were drawn up by medical men but packaged as serving not *their* "best interests" but her own. The dilemma set in place by this dynamic would prove to be a hard one for feminism to crack.

Feminism may not have been ready to resolve this impasse but, by the time of Rachel Carson's death in the mid-1960s, it was poised to make its presence felt in other areas of American society. Chapter 6 returns to the sexual politics described in Part One but this time reexamines them in the context of the women's health movements of the 1960s and 1970s. The strategies pursued by the early birth control and abortion campaigns were centered on health issues dominated by society's obsessive concern with control over reproduction. For better or for worse, breast cancer fell outside that magic circle. Of course, there were important aspects of the earlier health campaigns that provided essential underpinning for the later development of breast cancer awareness (primary among them, the rise of feminist consciousness with its insistence on a woman's right to control her own body).

But the objectives of the earlier campaigns, and the strategies pursued to advance them, differed widely from those the breast cancer movement would adopt years later. The earlier emphasis, for example, on legislative change and legal doctrine were of little use to women seeking to alter the outcome of a disease, not a debate. The involvement of the courts in defining access to abortion also created alliances between feminists and reform-minded professionals (legal and medical) that were not available to breast cancer activists. A closer look at some of these discrepancies may help to explain the apparent head start that the crusades for birth control and abortion enjoyed and the long interval that elapsed between their coming to maturity and the first stirrings of breast cancer awareness.

Chapter 7 documents, at a more detailed level, the actual emergence of breast cancer within the culture over the past fifty years. It interweaves changes in the way the disease has been portrayed in various media with changes in the biomedical approach to it. Although it is impossible to pin down with any precision the way these two interact, it is clear that increasing attention paid to both the culture and the science of breast cancer has had the synergistic effect of raising the visibility of both. By the early 1970s, there is sufficient interest for the disease to establish a beachhead within the culture.

Its arrival at this juncture is documented by tracing, primarily in print media, the gradual loosening of male control over the representation of the disease. It begins with the first testaments in women's magazines in the 1930s, 1940s, and 1950s, where women's stories, often told by male doctors, served primarily as a cover for public health warnings promoting early detection and early treatment. When women finally begin to tell their own stories, they are still heavily chaperoned by medically credentialled men (sometimes their husbands, sometimes their doctors). Women's magazines played an important role in this history. They provided not just an opportunity for women to describe their own ordeals but a platform for those few pioneer doctors with "hereti-cal" ideas about treatment. These ideas may have reflected their pa-tients' preferences (for less extensive surgery), but they were anathema to the rest of the medical profession and so failed to gain admittance to the pages of prestigious medical journals.

By the time Betty Ford's breast cancer was announced in 1974, Americans had been well prepared for the sudden burst of interest in the disease. The concurrent emergence of the first breast cancer activ-ist, Rose Kushner, points the way to the mass movement of the future but, in the 1970s, it remains at a distance. Rose Kushner's work, chal-lenging the authority of surgeons and the wisdom of standard prac-tices, did not fit the prevailing notions of cultural acceptability. The lack of widespread political or even feminist endorsement for many of her initiatives inevitably delayed their entry into the mainstream. As an introduction to what was still a controversial subject, the personal narratives of women with experience of the disease were preferred by American women over the wide-ranging political program—and the anger—of Kushner.

Part Three ends with a discussion that steps back from the detailed history of the earlier chapters to evaluate the overall shift in conscious-ness since the early 1970s and its implications for the future. It argues that the mainstream perspective we now bring to the subject did not originate in any feminist or progressive program for social change but grew instead out of the time-honored tradition of female volunteerism. This has meant that the radical aspects of breast cancer activism have had to be grafted onto an inherently conservative tradition, one that passively accepted unequal roles for women and men. As a result, the sexual politics of breast cancer have been until recently poorly under-stood.

We have had little incentive to understand the disease as an ex-pression of the culture (including politics and the economy) at large. We have not been encouraged to think of breast cancer as an integral part of the history of twentieth-century medicine and its institutions. Rather, in keeping with its origins, contemporary awareness of the dis-ease has been defined more by the accumulation of individual life stories than by any wider understanding. This bias toward the individual experience has, in turn, influenced the nature of contemporary debate on the subject, defining both its scope and its point of view.

If the experience of breast cancer through most of the century could be characterized as wholly "private," it could now more aptly be described as "privatized." If the disease has not yet lost its stigma, it has certainly shed the secrecy that once isolated every woman caught in its web. But open recognition of the disease has not been accompanied by any sense of social responsibility for it. Yes, women have mobilized in the thousands in breast cancer coalitions across the country to increase the level of research funding at the national level. And, yes, they have effectively broadcast their dissatisfaction with the scarcity and quality of research into women's diseases. But the burden still falls largely on their shoulders. Every one of the 180,000 American women diagnosed each year is still individually responsible for getting herself screened, biopsied, treated, and monitored. And those lucky enough to escape a positive diagnosis (this time) are, equally, burdened with the responsibility to maintain their disease-free state (through so-called lifestyle modifications like diet and exercise). These are the symptoms of an implied social policy that, in the absence of an effective cure, emphasizes the individual rather than the social control of disease.

The sense that progress toward prevention has stalled is neatly conveyed by the recent transformation of the role of surgery. Once the universal treatment for this disease, the therapeutic role of surgery has now been surpassed by its cosmetic potential for women undergoing a mastectomy. Over the past quarter century, the refinement of surgical techniques using the patient's own skin and muscle to reconstruct a breast have produced astonishing results. So adept has plastic surgery now become that the local control of disease by mastectomy not only paves the way for the return of the sacrificed breast, but also provides open-ended opportunities for cosmetic enhancements that extend to the other breast as well. The lure of cosmetic makeovers, coming at a time when a newly diagnosed woman is most vulnerable, is understandably powerful. But the decision to go down that path postpones recovery for months. The succession of operative procedures that follow keep a woman "medicalized," adding further layers of risks and complications to those already associated with the disease. And all without improving her odds for survival one bit.

Any improvement in the survival rates that can be squeezed out of existing therapies is more likely to come from chemotherapies than from surgery. But the ultimate source of breast cancer prevention remains unknown. There is still little sense that society as a whole has thrown its weight behind the eradication of the disease, as it did in the 1950s in the national assault on polio. Instead, there is, as there has always been, pressure on women themselves to play a more active role in cancer control. There is, for example, discussion of personal responsibility for breast cancer (through so-called lifestyle modification) but not of public or corporate accountability (through the control of toxic substances), of cures for the disease but not of prevention, of public dollars allocated to research but not to health care services.

These limitations reflect the concerns and priorities of contemporary culture. But they also reflect the failure of breast cancer to make common cause with broader political interests, either in theory or in practice. Perhaps a greater understanding of the influences that have shaped contemporary awareness of the disease (as developed in this book) can help to deepen its connections in the next generation with other movements for social change.

The nineteenth century's response to breast cancer may have had a powerful impact on the handling of the disease in the twentieth century but the picture drawn in this book of the actual experience of breast cancer a hundred years ago will be unfamiliar if not absolutely foreign to many women afflicted with the disease today. What has been outlined here is the experience that might have been familiar, at least in part, to white middle-class and upper-middle-class women living any time between the 1850s and 1950s. But for many others—self-supporting women or women who lived without men, poor women, single mothers, many minority and working-class women—the experience of breast cancer bore little resemblance to the story told here. Most of these women never had the luxury of a decline into semi-invalidism. For all of the twentieth century, for instance, a much greater proportion of Black than of white women in the United States were employed (both married and unmarried) and they were working for lower wages. The same was true for other ethnic groups (Japanese- and Chinese-Americans among them). Many of these women never had any medical treatment for their breast cancers at all simply because they couldn't afford to pay for it. But many others stayed away because they feared or distrusted the mainstream medical establishment. The practice of medicine did, after all, incorporate all of society's prejudices, elitist, racist, and homophobic, as well as sexist. Women whose race or sexuality or poverty was deemed by prevailing medical opinion to be deviant or pathological were hardly likely to expose themselves to the scrutiny of a white male doctor.

But despite the discrepancy between the lived experience of many women and the prescribed cultural response, there are still grounds to justify the centrality of the white middle-class experience. First of all, middle-class cultural values may not have monopolized society's response to the disease but they exercised a disproportionate influence over those giving and receiving treatment for it. By the end of the nineteenth century, most doctors in the medical mainstream were largely middle-class husbands and fathers. Middle-class wives and daughters constituted their clientele. This doubling of domestic and professional roles provided endless opportunities for the crossover of sexual politics between home and office. In both locations, the oppression of women expressed itself in a bodily submission to male authority. In both contexts women were considered to be physically at risk if not overtly ill. Encounters in one sphere simply reinforced those in the other, strengthening the impression that the paternalism underlying both was part of the natural order of things. A middle-class doctor could not fail to bring his prejudices to bear on any encounter with a woman patient, whether educated, indigent, or self-supporting.

An even more important rationale for the dominance of the white middle-class perspective is that breast cancer, perhaps uniquely among women's diseases, struck most often among just this group of women. Having children at a later age and having fewer children increased a woman's overall lifetime risk for the disease. And the image of the cosseted unproductive wife was, statistically, not inaccurate. At the turn of the century, when almost 40 percent of African American women were already employed outside the home, only 3 percent of white married women had jobs of any kind.

White women also enjoyed a significant advantage in life expectancy. Black women in both the north and the south died at younger ages than white women.[6] If the life expectancy for American white women at the turn of the century was around 49, just the age when women began to enter a high-risk zone for breast cancer, then many Black women were simply not living to be old enough to contract the disease.[7] The life expectancy for white women at birth (just under 80 years) still remains significantly higher than for African American women (just under 74).

In any case, breast cancer as a recognized disease of its own was hardly noticeable at the turn of the century. The estimated number of breast cancer deaths in the United States in 1900, based on the census, was about 3,780, roughly 3,330 deaths among white women, 380 among Black women, and 80 among white men. Recognized and recorded cancer of the breast among white women was still a rarity; among Black women it was, statistically, almost insignificant (among white men, it was totally invisible).[8]

White women continued to account for the vast majority of breast cancer deaths through most of the century. As late as 1950, the death rate for African American women was still about 22 percent lower than for white women. It was not, in fact, until the early 1980s that mortality among African Americans first outstripped that for white women.[9] So the view of the illness as a predominantly white middle-class experience in the early decades of the century when the modern medical response to it was put in place, though it needs to be qualified, does seem to have some justification in historical fact. There was, in any case, little recognition before the 1970s or 1980s that the actual experience of breast (and other) cancers might be significantly different for minority women; for the most part, they have had to face the same set of attitudes and the same options confronting the majority population. The prominence given to the white middle-class experience in this book does not excuse the lack of attention paid to the Black or any other minority experience of breast cancer, then or now. The dearth of sufficient evidence—records, narratives, statistics—is the illustration of yet another social and institutional failure for which redress needs urgently to be made.

Part
One

1 ?•

The Prehistory of Breast Cancer

BREAST CANCER is an ancient disease. There has been no period of recorded history in which it cannot be found. One of the earliest known scientific documents, written over three thousand years ago by an Egyptian physician, describes it in detail.[1] The Greeks and Romans followed suit. Everyone had something to say about it because everyone could see it. Unlike cancer of the liver or prostate, the symptoms of breast cancer were visible and palpable, as well as fatal.

The diagnosis of cancer in the breast may be almost as ancient as the disease itself. In this respect, it is unlike other diseases where a progressive change in diagnosis over time appears to accompany parallel changes in medical science. Kidney disease, for example, was diagnosed as "dropsy," then as Bright's disease, and most recently as end-stage renal disease. Every "upgrade" in diagnosis signals a change in prognosis and in treatment that alters the outlook of both patient and physician. By comparison, the constant appearance of the word "cancer" in every diagnosis, no matter how much it may be qualified by other defining attributes, suggests the presence of a hard and stony core of disease, of almost geological antiquity, that remains impervious to human intervention.

In the case of breast cancer, the failure of intervention has been much more conspicuous because it has been attempted much more often. The easy access to the disease *on* rather than *in* the body prompted early and sustained attempts to cure it; any treatment seemed worth trying when death was the only alternative. And almost every conceivable treatment was tried, at one time or another, including purging and bleeding, the compression of the breast with lead plates, the direct application of calamine, goat's dung, arsenic and zinc chloride pastes. None of these treatments (some of which were used for centuries) had any curative power. All were highly visible failures.

The prehistory of breast cancer—that is, its cumulative history before the end of the nineteenth century—has been totally lost to modern consciousness. We don't normally relate any feature of the disease in its modern form to a distant memory of its past. If anything, we disown that past, even if we do so unconsciously, by concentrating our attention exclusively on the disease as it exists now. When confronting treatment today, no one wants to be reminded of the millennium of failure behind us. But even without conscious awareness, our habits of mind still betray the presence of age-old impressions and representations of the disease. These half-remembered accusations and old wives' tales are the camp followers of breast cancer, cropping up wherever the disease shows itself. Brought back into view by every new diagnosis, they open a window on the very long legacy of terror that has always accompanied the disease. And as long as breast cancer remains an active killer, these atavistic responses will continue to reverberate.

At their heart is some dimly perceived suggestion of personal responsibility, some sense that disease is a manifestation of sin. Many religions, of course, have exploited this imputed relationship in one way or another. Both the Old and New Testaments of the Bible make an explicit connection between the wrath of God and disease. The Christian church takes a very broad approach to the theology of sin and sickness. There is not one privileged set of beliefs governing doctrine in this area, but many, and they are often contradictory. Some emphasize the body as the temple of God and encourage men and women to care for it accordingly. For them, disease would be considered an affliction. Others deny any value to corporeal reality. Emphasizing spiritual health at the expense of the health of the body, they might welcome disease as a test of faith. Equally incongruous have been the varied practices of Christian healers and miracle-workers. Throughout the centuries they have relied upon a curious mix of secular and spiritual ideas. Miraculous cures—the casting out of demons associated with disease, the raising of the dead—combine religious faith and conjuring practices in equal measure. This close interweaving of the sacred and the profane has been described as "Christian magic."[2]

The belief in disease as a divine punishment for sin (or for any form of moral "uncleanliness") opened the door to extreme forms of human punishment as well. The aggressive response of humans to incurable disease illustrates the unholy alliance between magical and spiritual thinking that has often passed for religious fervor. Evoking repugnance and terror, the deformed and the diseased became perfect scapegoats. Arguably, the more visible the signs of disease, the more defenseless its victims. Leprosy, whose disfiguring symptoms could not easily be hidden away, was considered to be retribution for the sin of lust. Lepers were literally banished from society. Already marked as sinners by their evident symptoms, they could be blamed for whatever social ills stalked their communities. As both carriers and victims of malevolent spirits, they had to be cast out, as by a spell. So the ill and the infirm would be punished several times over, first, for displeasing God; second, for reminding others of God's awful power; and third, for bringing the contagion of evil into human society. Martin Luther is said to have believed that deformed children had been fathered by the Devil so that killing them was no sin. Disease, in other words, could be life-threatening in many ways.

These ideas and many others like them have been woven in and out of the literature and mythology of Western culture for centuries. Even now, they have not lost their sting. Although they have been formally abandoned by modern medical science, the inheritance of a millennium is not so easily dislodged.[3] Modern ideas that enable us to identify bacteria, viruses, and damaged genes are relative newcomers compared to the venerable explanations of causality enshrined, among other places, in the Bible. There are, of course, those who still accept these ideas in their original form, who cannot wholly dismiss the idea that breast cancer may be a sign of sin. And there are many others who have adapted the idea by redefining "sin" to include, for instance, derelictions from medically approved "lifestyles." The success of so many current victim-blaming theories—that, for instance, breast cancer is caused by high-fat diets or by unresolved emotional trauma—shows how well the ground had already been prepared by ancient arguments we are now reluctant to acknowledge. We seem to tolerate them in modern dress and we don't ask too closely about their pedigree. Their mixed parentage—their fusion of the pious and the pagan—is something we clearly shy away from.

Given this inheritance, it's not surprising to find that newly diagnosed women still have a fear of being stigmatized by their cancers. Even if society no longer has easy answers to the question, "Why me?", public exposure remains risky. Every new diagnosis stirs up all our primitive responses to the disease. Whether expressed or not, the continuing eruption of fear and its backlash in scapegoating are reminders of how unresolved these reactions still are. How much more dangerous, then, the revelation of breast cancer must have been 100 years ago, before modern medicine or modern psychology had even begun to challenge religion as the moral arbiter of disease. In this framework, the decision to maintain secrecy would seem a wise course of action.

Whatever its original impulse, the progressive exclusion of the disease from social intercourse was intensified over time by the continuing failure of medical treatment to influence the outcome of the disease. The wholesale denial of breast cancer, the determination to force it underground and render it invisible, must surely reflect the shame of the medical profession as well as that of the patient. If the disease remained implacable, despite the best efforts of doctors to restrain it, wasn't this a sign of divine retribution at work? Surely, the best response to this display of almighty displeasure was a respectful silence?

The imposition of a taboo probably derives from many sources. Although a detailed investigation of its origins lies beyond the scope of this book, it's clear that the long-lived status of breast cancer as a forbidden subject—a taboo relaxed only within the past thirty years—was a socially conditioned response to the continued presence of disease. Denial was an implicit recognition of the fear and helplessness of both doctors and patients. Although it may in the end have served the interests of the former more than those of the latter, it would not begin to disappear until both parties to the disease began to see possibilities for changing the odds for survival.

This change of perspective is, of course, a very new development. For most of the past century, the embargo on the public acknowledgment of breast cancer remained firmly in place. But banishing the disease from society did not make it go away. Paradoxically, it allowed all the beliefs and superstitions associated with breast cancer to flourish, since they were given a free reign in the netherworld they inhabited. Among women particularly, who naturally had more reason to fear the disease, curious notions of sin and sickness from every source mingled freely with one another, mixing angels and demons, stigmatas and evil eyes.

As a basis for a rational understanding of a serious disease, this was clearly inadequate. It left women at the mercy of every quack and unprincipled practitioner in business. Before the end of the nineteenth century, there were still many different schools or "sects" to choose from, each offering its own medical philosophy and its own remedies. There was little incentive, from any quarter, to enlighten women. Doctors knew that there was little they could do to influence the outcome of disease, once it had announced itself. If a patient believed she was possessed by demons or being punished by God, what could she expect from medical intervention? Very little indeed. She might be just as likely to seek help from a spiritual healer as from a doctor. The multiplicity of touted remedies and cures—all useless—helped to camouflage the failure of allopathic medicine.

Before women could respond more effectively to the disease, they needed to be educated. Education could enlighten them, substituting a rational foundation for the myths and superstitions they had been fed and sharpening their powers of discrimination. Many women understood this but their efforts to promote the idea met with the active resistance of men. If female ignorance was the price of patriarchal stability, it was a sacrifice that men were willing to make.

The need to preserve the patriarchy interfered with a doctor's understanding of disease as much as a woman's. As I will describe below in more detail, many erroneous scientific ideas about women's bodies were based on irrational fears that were sanctioned by scripture as well as by popular custom. All of them played a role in defining the scope and the substance of medical theories, influencing the physician's approach to his subject as well as his treatment of individual patients. The hierarchies the doctor imposed on the female frame, that is, his implicit ranking of body parts and their symptoms, obviously had a hand in guiding the selection and interpretation of clinical evidence that formed the basis of his working hypotheses.

The historical relationship between the practice of medicine and concurrent scientific beliefs is not a straightforward one. But it is crucial to any understanding of the history of breast cancer. Over the past century, the evolution of the modern medical response to the disease has depended on a great deal more than the validity of underlying scientific principles. As the longevity of our notions of sin and sickness demonstrates, the survival of ideas (whether religious, moral, or medical) depends on the strength of the social infrastructure supporting them. Belief systems do not fall away simply because the premises on which they were founded are unproven, or even demonstrated to be false. Scientific beliefs are no more immune to pressures from the nonscientific world than are spiritual beliefs from the nonreligious. Although scientific beliefs all fly under the flag of a higher authority, citing scientific objectivity, the laws of nature, or divine wisdom, they serve other, more worldly masters as well. Discredited ideas, if sufficiently protected, can, in fact, discourage or withstand competition for long periods of time.

The cultural history of breast cancer, and particularly of radical surgery, uncovers the complexity of support structures that keep an idea in place. Taking a more oblique look at the disease through the lens of culture opens a wider perspective on the way society impinges upon science and vice versa. It's perhaps easier to see the nature of this relationship in the context of a disease that itself incorporates so many of society's attitudes to women, in both theory and practice. (The history of, say, kidney disease would be less revealing in this context.) The failure of the twentieth century to abolish breast cancer, to relegate it to the status of historical curiosity rather than allowing it to become an even more compelling medical concern, is not simply a scientific failure. It is one that clearly implicates society at large rather than just the esoteric branch of it we call medical science.

As an approach to medical history, the decision to place culture and society in the foreground could hardly be more of a challenge to the traditional approach to the subject. The standard historical texts on breast cancer, written almost universally by medical men, tend to distill the story they are telling into a pitched battle between a hero (surgeon or scientist) and a deadly enemy (pathogen or virus). They dispense with complicating details (like the patient) and lead inexorably to the control if not to the eradication of disease.

Authors of these histories have often been mentored by the men whose life work they are recording; their work is an homage to the work of the Master. The hagiographic tone is hard to miss. As one representative history, written in 1953, expresses it: "The epic of breast surgery is a pageant of time rich in the biography of many men of medical eminence . . ."[4] There is no parallel pageant of patients; they appear primarily as carriers of disease. The story line sticks close to the essentials; each surgeon or scientist adds a piece or two to the puzzle before passing on the baton to the next in the line of succession. The gaps between one advance and the next are closed or at least compressed, minimizing the long stretches of inertia in which progress has stalled or researchers have turned down blind alleys.

We now realize just how much has to be sacrificed in this kind of history to force the story into its teleological framework. Patients (their attitudes toward their own bodies and toward the medical profession, their concepts of disease, expectations of treatment, and so on) are not the only missing ingredients. The changing dialectic between medicine and society (its institutions, economic organization, belief systems) is equally absent from the earlier generations of medical histories.

The alternative frameworks currently in favor have opened up the subject to an astonishing range of perspectives, each adding new contours to the largely one-dimensional official histories. And although they may produce versions of history that are untidy and inconclusive, they at least broaden our outlook. At the same time, they deter us from making futile attempts to encircle the past. They urge us, in other words, both to exploit and to respect its inevitable open-endedness. This, at least, has been the presumption behind the history that follows.

The sexual politics of disease: "a whole sex of patients"

The breast itself carries so many of the culture's expectations of women, particularly of their nurturing and sexual obligations, that any symptoms of disease or disorder it manifests can have disproportionately powerful reverberations. In this context, it is clearly a part of the body that stands for the whole. Assaults to women's breasts—either by disease or by medical treatment—have come to express, in a most concentrated form, the more generalized violence to women sanctioned by society as a whole. Every loss of a breast inevitably reawakens this primitive response, reviving earlier dramas of self-abasement, sacrifice, and submission to punishment.

The martyrdom of Saint Agatha shows how intertwined these associations inevitably are. In third-century Sicily, the Christian Agatha lost her breasts, not to disease, but as punishment for rejecting the sexual advances of a governor of the Roman Empire, engaged in a campaign to persecute Christians. Miraculously, her breasts healed, but she died days later after being rolled over hot coals. Agatha's later adoption as the patron saint of breast diseases emphasized the sanctity of suffering, highlighting the inevitable martyrdom of women, to whatever cause. Few other forms of amputation carried this indiscriminate endorsement of passivity.[5]

Agatha was not the only saint to have her breasts cut off. Baring-Gould's *Lives of the Saints* includes at least ten others. Most of them, according to legend, were stripped naked and comprehensively assaulted, having some combination of eyes, teeth, tongue, and nails pulled out as well. Representations of these women either portray them with pincers at the breast just before the moment of amputation or else show them carrying their own breasts on a plate or a book. All of these images send the message that breasts are not inalienable parts of a woman's body at all but more provisional appendages, allowed to remain in place only as long as she remains available and tractable.

It's easy to see how useful this lesson would be in a society like that prevailing at the end of the nineteenth century, which still discouraged women from promoting their own interests rather than those of others.

In this context, the loss of a breast to disease would symbolize, first and foremost, the loss of a woman's availability, as sexual partner, mother, and household manager.

Hovering behind this loss would be the imputation of blame; symptoms of disease would be incriminating evidence in themselves. However irreproachable the life of a woman had been, the sense of divine retribution implied by the disease kept attention fixed on its social consequences rather than its personal ones. The potential life-support, physical pleasure, and reassuring comfort linked to breasts were bodily expressions of a woman's role at the heart of her family. All were reminders that she put the needs of others before her own. Any pleasure a woman might take in her own body or her own life was deemed to be inconsequential to the culture, a secondary effect, derived from the pleasure she gave to others. What did matter was the preservation of family life. Inescapably, breast cancer put this at risk.

Unlike many other fatal diseases (heart conditions and most other cancers), cancer of the breast announced itself in a tangible fashion. Both the symptoms of disease and the results of treatment were apparent. Women were either consumed by grotesque tumors or visibly diminished by radical surgery. In either case, it would be hard for immediate family members to miss the connection between a woman's compromised physical state and her ultimate decline to invalidism and eventually death. As her illness worsened and she began to relinquish domestic responsibilities, the family would begin to experience an inversion of the expected hierarchy of roles. A terminally ill woman could no longer maintain even the fiction of managing or caring for her household. Those traditionally dependent upon her were now called upon to serve. Unlike a woman dying in childbirth (a much more common death for women before the turn of the century), a woman with late-stage breast cancer might linger for months, in a state of pain that could only reinforce the helplessness of those attending her. And her death left no compensating new life in its wake.

The literally unspeakable horror once associated with breast cancer may owe something to this destabilizing aftermath, which does such violence to the traditional image of the nuclear family. The idea that a family, if it had to, could function without a presiding female presence was unthinkable for nineteenth-century culture. Fortunately, breast cancer was rare enough before the turn of the century not to threaten the stability of the traditional family. But it could be made rarer still by suppressing any evidence of it where it did erupt. If there was no way to escape the terrible void it created, there was at least a way to disguise it. Once the loss of a breast came to be understood as a harbinger of this larger family tragedy, it was almost inevitable that the disease would be concealed. A woman might be ill within her own home without arousing suspicion. It was not hard to disguise both the source of her illness and eventually even the cause of her death. This might inflict terrible emotional conflict on those left behind, but it left the underlying patriarchal arrangements untainted by any sign of divine disfavor. If a wife's illness carried even the suggestion of a sexual failure, no husband, especially one now in a position to remarry, would want this to become generally known. Secrecy worked in his favor.[6]

Breast cancer, exiled from society, became a topic as unfit for the parlor as for the pulpit. Within middle-class society, it descended into the black hole of social taboos, where, joining other female conditions (including menstruation and menopause), it fell prey to superstition and magical thinking. But unlike these other complaints, it was not just a normal process with sexual implications simply too embarrassing to countenance. It was a lethal disease.

The tension that arose from the contradiction between its status as a taboo topic and its continuing deadliness inside the home tranformed breast cancer into a killer by stealth, adding greatly to its capacity to terrify. Under the spell of this socially sanctioned witchcraft, individual families suffered in silence. They became the sacrificial victims of the culture at large, offered up to buy immunity for and to protect the innocence of the wider community. As long as the charm held, the underlying family structures would remain intact.

Sadly, the evil eye, once in place, proved very resistant to change. The positively Victorian behavior it continued to elicit throughout much of the twentieth century (prudery and morbidity as well as sexism and superstition) attests to the immobilizing effects of terror, whether manufactured or not. But to keep the breast cancer taboo alive required propping up aspects of family life that were already under threat from other quarters. These antiquated coping mechanisms would eventually capitulate, but this was more the result of external pressures forcing their way into the family from outside it than of any internally generated opposition set in motion by the appearance of breast cancer.

Breast cancer, in other words, did not fundamentally disturb the status quo. Its sexual politics were, if anything, regressive. Most women, by the time they became ill, had already fulfilled their primary function within the nuclear family: childbearing. Whatever acts of reproductive resistance a wife had engaged in to prevent or to terminate an(other) unwanted pregnancy came to an end at the end of her childbearing years. If these could be construed as acts of self-determination that challenged a husband's authority, they at least had a finite lifespan within a marriage. By the time breast cancer usually arrived on the scene, the battles for autonomy were over. So were most of the other battles for independence. By the time most middle-class women reached middle age, they had given up any struggle they might earlier have waged for education or employment. Breast cancer, in this sense, confirmed the end of their social as well as sexual usefulness.[7] And its onset often coincided with the arrival of menopause, adding further weight to the idea of cancer as just another symptom of female decline. Finally, at the turn of the century women were not expected to live much beyond their early 50s, and so the connection between breast cancer, menopause, and death could actually be quite close, all occurring within a very short period of time.

Where society's interest in the dynamics of marriage was driven by the imperatives of reproduction, the practice of medicine inevitably followed suit. The concern with the ability of women to produce healthy children was everywhere evident in the medical literature. And though it was most nakedly expressed in the nineteenth century, the underlying belief system that it reflected survived well into the twentieth. So central was childbearing to the medical understanding of women that any complaint anywhere in the body was understood as either the cause or the effect of some reproductive disorder. All roads led back to the womb, confirming the conviction, as one nineteenth-century doctor put it, that "the Almighty, in creating the female sex, had taken the uterus and built up a woman around it." This meant that "any imbalance, exhaustion, infection or other disorder of the reproductive organs could cause pathological reactions in parts of the body seemingly remote."[8]

Breast cancer was one of those pathological reactions. It was not defined by its own symptoms or its own behavior but by its peripheral relationship to the central drama of childbearing. Its appearance signaled a delayed response to an earlier reproductive failure of some kind.[9] A Victorian health manual describes cancers as "especially liable to arise in those women who have suffered several abortions or unnatural labors. Undoubtedly they are more frequent in the married than the unmarried, and they evidently bear some relation to the amount of disturbance which the system has suffered since childbirth and the grief and mental pain experienced."[10] Another nineteenth-century medical textbook stated that tumors were caused by "a derangement in the uterine functions producing a vascular determination which extends to the breast."[11] The initiating "derangement" could be almost anything from "great mental grief" to "disturbed rest, exposure to cold, late hours, fatigue." Any of these irregularities could force a tumor "to extend to a malignant state, and advance very rapidly."[12] Additionally, cancer was also linked to women who had used birth control,[13] and, as late as 1925, to women who had worn tightly fitted corsets that restricted the blood flow to their breasts and womb.[14] As a warning of the consequences of sexual impropriety, negligence, or a wayward lifestyle, the threat of breast cancer served as a stick to beat women into reproductive submission.

Whatever its place in the reproductive firmament, the disease certainly helped to reinforce the belief in a woman's innate constitutional inferiority. It was another confirmation of gender-based infirmities that justified her designation as the "weaker sex," at least in middle-class homes where wives were not expected to do the heavy lifting. The ability to keep a wife in semi-retirement as an invalid was in itself a status symbol among the upper and middle classes, evidence that the husband's finances were secure enough to support unproductive household members besides his children. How could women ever be suited to regular employment if they were so vulnerable to chronic illnesses, especially those from which they failed to recover? As long as breast cancer was perceived as another "female malady" confirming women's unfit state for productive labor (mental or physical), there was little incentive to intervene and interrupt its course.

Even at the time (the last quarter of the nineteenth century), not all women accepted the common explanation given for "feminine invalidism." One contemporary, the Anglo-Irish feminist Frances Power Cobbe (1822–1904), interpreted women's "seizures" as "Bad-Husband Headaches" arising "from nothing but the depressing influences of an unhappy home." She derided the idea "that the Creator should have planned a whole sex of Patients" and pointed to the lingering influence of an outmoded idea that had been current at the beginning of the century: "The very word 'delicacy,' " she wrote, "properly a term of praise, being applied vulgarly to a valetudinary condition, is evidence that the impression of the 'dandies' of sixty years ago that refinement and sickliness were convertible terms is not yet wholly exploded."[15] One may ask, more than a hundred years later, whether these prejudices are even now "wholly exploded" or whether some traces of the meaning they carried in the early 1800s still remains in circulation almost two centuries later.

If women like Frances Power Cobbe could escape the descent into invalidism by avoiding marriage altogether, those who took the more conventional path found it harder to evade its consequences. Once on the inside, it would be more adaptive to make an accommodation with what Cobbe called the " 'delicacy' delusion" than to kick against it. Over time, a woman would come to lose whatever confidence she might have had in interpreting her body's natural functions herself and to substitute instead the perspective of her husband or physician. With this renunciation would come the loss of her discriminating powers as well, those that might once have helped her distinguish between regular monthly changes and more serious or unusual signs. All symptoms now became equally suspect.

Relegating breast cancer to the status of a female malady took it out of the limelight. There were, in fact, many benign diseases of the breast (mastitis, fibroids, cysts, and so on) whose symptoms mimicked those of cancer. It was easy to mistake one for the other, especially before the use of biopsies. The similarity in their symptoms and short-term behaviors made it easy to lump them all together, to view them all as evidence of the "natural" tendency of women's bodies to break down, to show the expected signs of what Emily Martin refers to as "failed production."[16] As she points out, medical science had already recast menstruation and menopause as pathological rather than physiological conditions, so adding breast cancer to the bundle would not be much of a stretch.

But breast cancer differed from chronic invalidism; its victims did not lie about in a state of perpetual ornamental languor; they became seriously ill and died. Its inclusion within this larger rank of female complaints was therefore doubly harmful. First, grouping it with what were essentially normal conditions may have camouflaged its seriousness and so contributed to a woman's delay in seeking treatment or advice. But equally unfortunate, the mistaken association between breast cancer and reproductive processes inadvertently lent support to medical arguments that treated them *all* as diseases. In other words, the confounding of biologically defined pathology with culturally defined illness had detrimental effects on both. Playing up the dangers of menstrual irregularities justified ever more radical medical interventions to control them; playing down the potential dangers of breast cancer let doctors off the hook. They could not, after all, be expected to "cure" but only to "manage" ills inhering in the female condition itself. By submerging the disease within the broader context of reproduction, family doctors essentially abandoned it and delayed by several decades the arrival of better informed clinical scrutiny.

The apparent randomness of breast cancer was particularly problematic. Only a small minority was afflicted. Some became ill well before the end of their childbearing years. Some even showed symptoms of the disease while pregnant. In a culture that relied so heavily on notions of responsibility and blame, there was no easy way to accommodate an essentially blameless death. But reconceived as a "female malady" rather than a disease, breast cancer could attract the same moral censure that accompanied reproductive failures. Based on a presumed direct link between the uterus and the central nervous system, all women's ailments were thought to be diseases of the nerves. This made it possible to consider breast cancer, like menstrual irregularities, the product of a diseased mind. "The cases are so frequent," wrote one physician, "in which deep anxiety, deferred hope, and disappointment, are quickly followed by the growth or increase of cancer, that we can hardly doubt that mental depression is a weighty addition to the other influences that favour the development of the cancerous constitution."[17]

Whatever the consequences of women's "deep anxiety, deferred hope, and disappointment," their sources clearly lie in lives that were unbearably constricted, in every sense. Corseted in uncomfortable, even painful clothes; forbidden the diversions of sports, dancing, exercise of any kind; denied education and access to employment; women's lives were inert, physically and socially. Any attempts to break out of this mold, to exercise their minds, or their arms and legs, met with the disapproval of a society that largely represented the interests of men. But rather than punishing women directly (and forcing men to show their hands), society would allow them to punish themselves, bringing harm to their own bodies.

Here was a visible demonstration of early victim-blaming that has survived to become even more prominent today.[18] When a woman began to change from being what Ehrenreich and English called a "uterine woman" to a "mental woman," her body would pay for it. "First," according to one male pundit, "she loses her mammary function," since, as Ehrenreich and English put it, "lactation seemed to represent woman's natural unselfishness."[19] A threat to the established male order is, in this way, transformed into a threat to a woman's unborn children. Any symptom of mammary dysfunction, then, becomes confirmation of a woman's impropriety, her violation of what is permissible. Once blame has been established, there is no longer much incentive to disentangle imagined from organic causes of disease.

And passing on responsibility to women serves to relieve the consciences of men. First, by allowing society to express their hostility for them, men as husbands and fathers escape the burden of guilt imposed by the conflict between their need to discourage women's emancipation on the one hand, and their wish to remain concerned for the well-being of their wives and children on the other. Second, as physicians, men cannot be held responsible for their failure to cure or prevent a disease that women have brought upon themselves.

Of course, it would have been impossible until quite recently to articulate these responses at all. In the nineteenth century, they were literally unthinkable, suggesting as they did that men's loyalties to their wives or to their patients were divided, that acting in the "best interests" of one did not necessarily promote the "best interests" of the other. (Virginia Woolf, who knew quite a lot about the damage caused by the oppression of women, did not herself become familiar with the concept of "ambivalence" until shortly before her death in 1941.) As long as society continued to evade these difficult contradictions, first denying and then tolerating the gross inequalities that they gave rise to, there would be little impetus to look more deeply into the causes of a disease that drew so much attention to the sources of this very conflict.

The medical message: the written word

Because most women left little or no written trace of their disease, we are forced to rely more heavily on the written evidence of breast disease supplied by medical men. In the last quarter of the nineteenth century, this mostly took the form of textbooks written by doctors for their medical colleagues and manuals written for their women patients (some of which were cited in the previous section of this chapter). Our reliance on this material, once again, strengthens the bias of history toward the upper-middle-class perspective, since the doctors who took up this task represented the more literate end of the medical spectrum. Their books were aimed at audiences that reflected a comparable level of literacy, if not of education (still largely denied to middle-class women).

Most of these texts were written decades before the emergence of recognized medical specialties. There were, for example, no governing bodies of gynecologists that made available to would-be practitioners a single treatise summarizing all the diseases and conditions that they could be expected to treat as well as the procedures they might be called upon to perform. Medicine was still an overcrowded and unregulated field, as full of quacks as of competent men and, increasingly, women. There was little consensus about any aspect of it.

Medical texts and manuals themselves reflect this state of flux. They should be viewed less as challenges to a well-organized status quo and more as documents hoping to construct one. They were part public relations documents, whipping up support for particular theories of disease or forms of treatment, part testimonials to the skills of the authors' mentors (now handed on to the authors themselves), and part genuine textbooks disseminating state-of-the-art information. Inevitably, they also played a role in the struggle undertaken by some doctors to differentiate themselves and their practices from the herd. The books that focused on women's diseases represent one such effort to establish a medical specialty with its own interests and clientele. Collectively, they reveal an attempt to stake out a territorial claim for those female conditions that, well down the road into the twentieth century, will set formal limits to the emerging specialties of obstetrics and gynecology.

What is most peculiar about this progressive demarcation of "female" conditions is its persistent exclusion of the breast. Understandably, the rich commentary on these textbooks that has emerged over the past 25 years has been less concerned with questions of inclusion than with the medical profession's preoccupation with reproduction as the determining factor and governing metaphor of women's health.[20] The perspective adopted here reveals a different bias.

Comprehensive manuals written by doctors for their students, colleagues, or their female patients included every female ailment that might conceivably have a bearing on the health of a woman before, during, or after pregnancy but none that might afflict her outside this context.[21] Healthy breasts might sometimes be considered an adjunct to childbearing but even this did not always qualify them for inclusion.

After all, in the event of a woman suffering from serious postpartum breast disease, a wet nurse could supply a substitute for the mother's breast; but there was no substitute for her uterus.

There are almost no references either to breasts or to breast cancer in medical manuals that address "women's diseases" at the turn of the century.[22] This is just as true for textbooks aimed at medical practitioners as it was for those aimed at women themselves. A standard textbook, *Diseases of Women*, first introduced in 1907 and re-issued at regular intervals over the next several decades, does not even mention breasts until its ninth edition, published in 1941.[23] Many others, spanning shorter periods, never get there at all. They include the most popular gynecological textbook of the late nineteenth century, which appeared in six editions between 1868 and 1891.[24] The complete absence of the breast from all these texts attests to its falling outside the commonly held definition of female reproductive anatomy.

Even if breast cancer was a relatively rare event a century ago, benign breast disease was not. And the behaviors of many breast conditions clearly connected them to the hormonal cycles that governed reproduction. What contributed to their exclusion was not primarily a fear of cancer. Many manuals included detailed descriptions of cancers of the vulva and vagina; these were considerably rarer than cancers of the breast. The exclusion of the breast reveals less a fear of pathology than a probable fear of female sexuality, one aggravated by the inability of medicine to make any headway against the more aggressive forms of the disease.

The breast, unlike the other female organs, was a visible reminder of a woman's sexual capacities and, as a result of its relative physical prominence, highly eroticized. A woman taking a breast complaint to her doctor might describe it to him but never undress to reveal it. Many doctors never touched their patients at all. But if a woman agreed to have her breast examined, she could not be hidden away behind the sheets that all but obliterated her when undergoing a pelvic exam. She and the doctor had to face each other directly. This made it much harder for a physician to preserve his physical and professional distance and for the patient to protect her sense of privacy.

The medical reluctance to acknowledge this difficulty in practice is

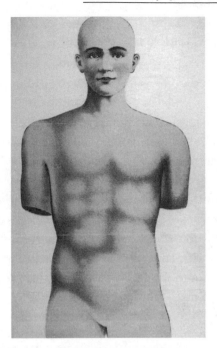

From J. H. Kellogg, *Ladies Guide in Health and Disease*, 1882. *Permission of Harvard College Library. Photograph by David Caras.*

indirectly expressed in the avoidance of the subject in print. One of the late nineteenth-century textbooks expresses this evasion in visual terms. The frontispiece to the *Ladies Guide in Health and Disease* (published 1882)[25] depicts an utterly sexless torso with no breasts, no hips, no waist, no private parts, and no body hair (pubic or otherwise). Yet the accompanying diagram that offers an inside view of that body reveals it to be female, at least in part. Even inside the body, however, only the uterus, ovaries, and fallopian tubes are illustrated, not the breasts or genitals. To the modern reader, there could hardly be a clearer expression of the belief in the male body as the norm and the female as deviant from the standard issue. Late twentieth-century sensibility is disturbed by this image of a neutered female body. But a contemporary woman reader of the 1880s would be less likely even to notice its distortions, since they were consistent with the denial of female sexuality that was endemic in the culture.

The absence of breast cancer from published health manuals was another clear illustration of the unspecified and unresolved "difficulties" posed by the disease. These difficulties did not exist on paper only. Breast cancer could be as unwelcome in hospital wards as it was in the formative medical literature (the body of knowledge that would become gynecology). According to a recent history of American gynecology, in the 1870s, the women supervisors of New York's newly established Women's Hospital began to complain about the increasing numbers of breast cancer patients that were being treated in the wards and "argued against admitting them. . . . [They] saw breast cancer as *separate* and not fitting under the rubric of female disorders that originally defined the hospital" (my italics).[26] This "separate" status of the disease in theory—its lying beyond the reproductive concerns of women of childbearing age—encouraged its actual separation from the treatment of other gynecological disorders in practice. In the semipublic arena of the hospital ward, the appearance of breast cancer revived disturbing and unwelcome echoes of sexuality in women deemed to be no longer sexually active. It also intimated a direct link between these uncomfortable sexual overtones and death.

The same unspoken malaise had the effect of discouraging women with symptoms from seeking medical help in a timely manner. The lack of correspondence in the available literature between their own experience and any medically recognized syndrome would inevitably be discouraging. Either their symptoms were too insignificant to warrant inclusion or they pointed to a condition that was so deadly that it could not be named. Neither possibility offered an incentive to further action.

The ambivalence that women experienced about whether to present symptoms to their doctors and, if they did, how to do it, was an accurate reflection of the doctor's own conflicted response to a patient's narration of "complaints." According to one practitioner, some women demonstrated

a tendency to exaggerate their symptoms (so that) an occasional pain becomes a constant agony and profuse menstruation a dangerous flooding. The most marked instances of this type will bring with them a carefully compiled record of their ailments, which they propose to read through to their medical adviser. . . . (others) may keep their maladies long to themselves, for fear they should be pronounced to be cancer or tumour.[27]

As long as physicians remained innocent of their own prejudices, a medical consultation would carry a double risk for any woman patient. A doctor's patronizing or infantilizing response was probably accepted by most women as normal. But where a doctor's unexamined misogyny overwhelmed his clinical judgment altogether, it might literally put a woman's life at risk. After all, some monthly irregularities are in fact signs of cancer and need to be further investigated. A woman's careful monitoring of the frequency and duration of any discharge from a nipple, for example, would clearly provide useful information to any open-minded clinician. The possibility of a physician's disregarding her data and dismissing her symptoms as signs of neurasthenia might easily discourage a woman from ever entering a doctor's office.

Many late Victorian manuals were written explicitly for women. These books represented an extension of medical "knowledge" from the doctor's office into the home. And for many women they did, no doubt, offer new concepts that, however laden with sexist misconceptions, at least helped them to interpret the physiological processes of their own bodies. But for women with breast cancer, these manuals brought home the culture's wholesale rejection of the disease. Their refusal to mention the female breast served only to strengthen the prevailing social taboo. They were more guides to self-denial than to self-help, with an unwritten instruction to suffer in silence.

Those medical men whose practices were increasingly confined to women and women's ailments came in time to establish the medical specialties of obstetrics and gynecology. What had once been an informal rejection of the breast in all its manifestations (benign and malignant) eventually became a formalized exclusion. What had begun as fear or repugnance in handling breast disease became, through repeated lack of practice and experience, genuine ignorance. Eventually, women's doctors lost their qualification to diagnose breast conditions at all.

Meanwhile, the women they treated remained in ignorance of this process. They continued to take their problems to the same kind of doctor, often one specializing in women's diseases. And while they inevitably absorbed their doctors' prejudices, it is probable that they also retained some understanding of their bodies, either intuitively or based on medical lore passed down to them by their mothers and grandmothers. This would naturally, if unconsciously, resist the partitioning of one set of organs from another. It would, in other words, be as natural for women to bring a worrying breast lump to the attention of their doctors as it would be to mention irregular menstrual bleeding. But as time went on and specialist medical education narrowed the focus of women's diseases, the doctor's ability to evaluate breast complaints would fall well below his or her capacity to judge signs of serious disease in the uterus or cervix. Few medical doctors, of course, would be willing to admit this shift in the focus of their expertise, but even fewer patients would ever expect them to.

Breast cancer, then, may be seen as something of a casualty of late nineteenth-century theories of disease. Viewed as a delayed reproductive failure, it commanded less urgent attention than the more exigent problems of women who were about to become or still were fertile. Furthermore, the continuing failure of family doctors to control the deadliness of the disease must have aggravated whatever sexual reticence or fear was already there to begin with. Medical treatments seemed to have exhausted the possibilities of nineteenth-century chemistry. The impotence of medicine—the failure of all the caustic pastes, live or dead animals, lead plates, bleeding—to make any headway at all against the disease may have helped to keep alive the idea that breasts were dangerous. The high mortality of breast cancer cases certainly provided a disincentive to treat them. Losing patients to disease did not, after all, enhance a doctor's reputation. Whatever the mixture of motives that informed medical theory and practice, their cumulative impact was clear. The emerging field of medicine that would evolve into gynecology treated the breast as a cuckoo in the nest.

2

The Dominance of Surgery

IF FAMILY MEDICINE failed to show much enthusiasm for breast disease, there was no lack of interest coming from another quarter. Surgery had no qualms whatsoever about treating the breast. On the contrary, general surgeons had been amputating women's breasts for centuries. Treatment for breast cancer, in other words, was already part of the surgical repertoire. It was also part of the canon of surgical literature. Stretching back to the early nineteenth-century monographs of Sir Astley Paston Cooper in England,[1] surgeons had laid claim to the body of knowledge that defined medical understanding of the breast. They wrote all the standard texts that specified its conditions, benign and malignant, as well as establishing the criteria for what was considered normal and what was considered operable.[2] These were written for professional audiences, not for lay readers.

Surgery carried out before the advent of anesthesia, asepsis, or blood transfusions was necessarily limited to emergency operations on parts of the body that were easily accessible. Used primarily for the treatment of gunshot wounds, fractures, and abscesses, and to remove diseased limbs, operations were inevitably bloody and brief, often requiring physical strength as well as finesse. They were also dangerous. Deaths from wound infection, hemorrhage, or shock were common. No one would willingly submit to surgery as anything other than a last resort. Amputations for late-stage breast disease were, like amputations for gangrene or septicemia, attempts at crisis management.

In reality, before the last quarter of the nineteenth century, these operations were as much experiments as bona fide treatments. They were performed primarily on indigent women in charity hospitals by surgeons who had often had little prior experience with live patients (but occasional practice on corpses). Many of these women were already close to death by the time their "cases" reached the attention of an interested surgeon. In extremis, they were willing guinea pigs. Middle-class women, on the other hand, kept well away from surgery— and from hospitals, known to them as the place where the poor went to die.[3]

Before the end of the nineteenth century, there were few standards governing either surgical education or surgical practice. The possession of medical credentials signified no common body of knowledge and guaranteed no particular expertise. Surgery was still just one of many "medical" approaches to treatment. It had to compete with a dizzying array of therapies associated with many different medical "sects." These included the practice of homeopathy, based on the administering of minute doses of substances producing similar symptoms to those already present, that is, "curing like with like"; botany, offering plant and herbal remedies; and hydropathy, promoting water cures. An astonishing number of charlatans added to the confusion, peddling quack remedies and engendering false hopes.

In the days before cancer institutions had the reputations to attract customers themselves (in the way that Memorial Sloan Kettering or the M. D. Anderson Cancer Center might do today), middle-class patients had to rely on a personal referral to an individual physician, with a family doctor or friend serving as intermediary. Many of these physicians enjoyed widespread public acclaim; royal patronage or knighthoods bestowed in Europe were the ultimate guarantee of competence. But despite physicians' occasional celebrity, the public had little real knowledge of their accomplishments and few means of finding out.

Once established, the reputations of these public figures were rarely subject to correction by either disgruntled former patients or their grieving relatives. The thread of social or family connection that linked the physician to his or her patient served as a powerful inhibitor. More important, women treated for breast cancer were perhaps the least likely of patients to complain of their experiences to friends, let alone to outsiders. They would not, in any case, have known where to draw the line between medical incompetence and treatment failure. The very concept of medical *mal*practice can only have meaning in relation to a preexisting consensus of *practice*. Without any formal agreements specifying reasonable expectations of treatment, it was impossible to hold individual physicians responsible for treatment failures. Whatever their nominal allegiance to the Hippocratic oath ("first do no harm"), doctors—the honorable and dishonorable alike—set their own ethical standards, and patients, in accepting treatment from them, unwittingly agreed to these standards.

The experience of Emily Gosse, an educated middle-class English woman diagnosed with breast cancer in 1856, illustrates the desperate plight of the cancer patient.[4] Gosse had first consulted her own doctor, Henry Salter, who was her husband's cousin. He recommended that she go to see Sir James Paget, then considered the preeminent cancer authority in London. Paget recommended immediate surgery, which Gosse rejected.[5] Salter then drew her attention to a rather controversial American doctor, Jesse Fell, who was then in London promoting a "new and fantastic cure" for breast cancer. Although the secret ingredients of this alleged cure were never disclosed to her, Gosse put herself in Fell's hands. His treatment, which proved to be agonizing, involved the repeated application of toxic ointments to the breast together with plasters inserted directly through incisions into the tumor itself. When this failed to stop the spread of the disease, Gosse turned for relief to a well-known homeopath. She died shortly afterwards.

There were no clear boundaries between any of these three practitioners, no set roster of medical conditions or diseases which each was authorized to treat. Nor was there any agreement about the human physiology underwriting each therapy that purported to explain the body's response to treatment. So little was known about the biological behavior of disease that inconsistencies between one medical approach and another would not have been apparent to the patient. But she would certainly have had some sense that the serial treatments she had undergone were less complementary (in the way that radiation and surgery are deemed to be today) than competitive.

The move from one doctor to another signaled a defeat, and must certainly have been accompanied by a discouraging sense of discontinuity, of starting all over again from scratch. Doctors from different medical sects did not confer with one another about a patient's prognosis; they hardly spoke the same language. It was the patient herself (or some male relative representing her) who kept track of her own symptoms and carried her medical history along with her from one doctor to the next. The fact that breast cancer was a chronic rather than an acute disease facilitated this peripatetic search for a cure and, no doubt, provided additional opportunities for unscrupulous practitioners.

Toward the end of the nineteenth century, the unregulated scramble of the medical marketplace began to give way to a more cooperative and orderly approach. The outlines of a medical infrastructure began to emerge as informal groups of practitioners with shared interests set standards for both medical education and practice which would eventually transform them into modern professionals. At the same time, advocates of allopathic medicine rose to dominance, outflanking homeopathic, hydropathic, and all other competing therapies.

Proprietary disputes over boundaries played a central role in the transformation of the medical professions. The results of these conflicts, in which the ills of the body were subjected to a complex process of gerrymandering, determined the territorial realms of medical specialties. The twentieth century would come to formalize them, through an increasingly sophisticated elaboration of institutions governing training, professional development, and research in each area. In the struggle for the control of women's bodies, the primary battles were first, between male and female midwives, then between obstetricians and gynecologists, and, finally, between gynecologists and abdominal surgeons. In none of these battles was breast disease a contested issue.

Medical treatments for breast diseases (bloodletting, leeching, caustic pastes of one kind or another) may have been largely discredited by the middle of the nineteenth century, but they did not immediately disappear. Their survival, like that of radical surgery a century later, had as much to do with the treatment vacuum around them as with any demonstration of their therapeutic value. Eventually, some form of therapeutic nihilism must have set in, as physicians despaired of finding any more promising alternatives. Of course, the decision to pursue no treatment at all had been an option all along, a choice with a respected pedigree going all the way back to Hippocrates (400 B.C.) and surviving intact through the Middle Ages. Some medieval healers believed that any treatment would only accelerate the disease; some, in fact, called it " 'touch-me-not' because the more one applies to it the worse it gets."[6]

Increasingly orphaned from the care of all other "female" conditions, breast disease seems to have fallen without much controversy into the lap of surgery. In letting go of it, gynecology lost an opportunity to develop an integrated specialty that would have taken responsibility for *all* the medical conditions of women, normal and pathological. However limited the possibilities might have been for a more "holistic" approach to women's health, they were surely weakened by the severing of breast complaints from the "body" of gynecological practice.

That the break between gynecological and breast surgery occurred early is evident from the story of the American Charlotte Cushman (1816–76), an internationally popular Shakespearean actress, who was diagnosed with breast cancer in 1869. She too, like Emily Gosse, first consulted with James Paget. When he told her that surgery was her only option, she sought a second opinion from the equally renowned American surgeon Marion Sims, then living in Paris. Sims was a controversial figure, considered by many to be the father of modern gynecology (he established the first women's hospital in New York in 1855). Earlier, he had developed a procedure for the repair of vaginal tissue damage caused by mismanaged childbirths that left women hopelessly incontinent. To develop his surgical techniques he practiced on black female slaves, many of whom he purchased expressly to use as subjects in his experiments. He was not squeamish about sur-

gery, performing more than thirty procedures on the same patient, until he finally succeeded in correcting her condition. Yet when called
upon to confirm Charlotte Cushman's diagnosis of breast cancer, he
recommended no treatment at all, advising her "to do nothing, to live
well, take care of her general health, amuse herself, and forget her trouble if possible."[7]

That Cushman should choose to consult Sims at all shows the absence, at the time, of clear demarcations between one surgical specialty
and another. That he should respond with such apparent disregard for
the seriousness of her situation shows either an ignorance of the prevailing medical responses to breast disease or, possibly, indifference or
hostility to them. Cushman in the end took Paget's rather than Sims's
advice, undergoing not just one but two rounds of surgery, and dying
seven years later.

This defection of gynecological practice from an active engagement
with breast disease coincided with the emergence of general surgery in
the United States as a respected and well-organized field in itself. For
most of the nineteenth century, American surgeons had looked to Europe for innovations in both theory and practice. Techniques introduced by the British surgeon Joseph Lister to promote antiseptic and
aseptic conditions in the operating theater were in common use in Europe well before they were adopted in the United States. It was not unusual for ambitious young surgeons to travel to Europe (particularly to
Germany) to complete their medical training, bringing back with them
the latest in scientific theory and surgical practice.

Toward the close of the century, the nature of this relationship began to change. For a start, the reputation of American surgery (and
medical practice in general) had been greatly enhanced in the eyes of
Europeans by the official medical history of the Civil War.[8] Published
in three volumes between 1870 and 1888, its well-organized and detailed documentation of the wartime surgical experience (which included over 26,000 amputations) was much admired by European
critics.

More important, the last decade of the century witnessed several
mutually reinforcing innovations both in the organization of surgical

training and in surgical techniques. So, although it might be an over-simplification to suggest that at the end of the nineteenth century surgeons rushed in where mere doctors had feared to tread, it is not entirely false. The career of William Stewart Halsted (1852–1922), who was to play a critical role in the development of breast cancer surgery, exemplified the transformation of the surgical profession.

What Halsted added to an operation that had been performed in one form or another for centuries was the routine removal of the breast together with the overlying skin, the underlying pectoral muscles, and the axillary lymph nodes, all taken in one piece (*en bloc*). What justified such radical intervention was Halsted's belief that the disease spread outward from the breast in an orderly, predictable fashion along specific lymphatic pathways. Such a process, he believed, could only be halted by the exacting and uncompromising extraction of all tissue, muscle, and lymph nodes that might otherwise become channels for dissemination to other organs in the body. In this paradigm, wholesale clearance of the chest area provided the only hope of survival. If it failed to stop the disease, then surgical intervention had come too late or had been inadequate. The only remedial course of action consistent with the theory was to undertake more surgery, eliminating tissue and lymph nodes further along the suspected pathways in the hopes that there was still a chance of reaching the outermost areas of disease before it reached vital organs.

Halsted was never able to prove this theory, but he didn't have to. The success of his operation and its extraordinary influence over American surgical practice really owed more to a fortuitous combination of circumstances than to any rigorous evaluation of the evidence. Halsted was in exactly the right place at the right time. As the first professor of surgery at Johns Hopkins Medical School in the 1890s, he developed the nation's first surgical residency program. Until then, surgeons had been largely self-taught and, for the most part, practiced in hospitals that had no affiliations with either medical schools or research labs. Halsted brought all of these interests together, encouraging the joint pursuit of scientific investigation and surgical practice among those he trained. Eleven of his residents went on to set up residency programs of their own,[9] in new departments of surgery at new medical schools. They took with them and transplanted all the basic features of the "Halsted tradition"—its surgical principles and practices, including the radical mastectomy. Within a few decades, surgeons all across the country had been trained to perform the operation. The radical mastectomy quickly established itself as the "gold standard" of treatment; it remained in this unchallenged position for three-quarters of a century.

The procedure itself called up images of heroic rescue, with the surgeon intervening at the last moment to perform a life-saving operation. In its early days, it could provide immediate and visible relief from often painful and distressing symptoms. Unlike many of today's patients, whose tumors are often picked up by mammography while they are in otherwise perfect health, earlier generations of women knew very little about the disease until they began to suffer its symptoms. Shrouded in secrecy, women had to endure what was often excruciating discomfort or pain from very large tumors, ulcerating skin, bleeding nipples, and other signs of disease. What the surgeon promised them was immediate relief from these symptoms and, down the road, rescue from local recurrence.

This provision of relief, which we would now consider a palliative measure, was for Halsted the cornerstone of treatment, one he confounded with "cure." The surgeon and the mastectomy rose to prominence together at a time when medical science believed that breast cancer was a local or a regional disease which could be cured by local intervention. Surgery had the advantage of conceptual simplicity, with a logic that could be easily grasped by the patient as well as the physician. The breast was visible as an organ lying outside the body; disease of the breast could therefore also be viewed as in some sense originating *outside* the body. Removing the breast could be seen as sparing the patient, since it was presumed to halt the spread of disease to more vital organs within the body.

Analogies with the mechanics of the visible, physical world reinforced this view. Diseased tissue was thought to be "rotten," like part of an apple or the branch of a tree. The apple or tree could be saved by chopping off the unwholesome part. However painful the pruning, the outlook was optimistic. The surgeon and his patient believed that diseased tissue could be surrounded and severed, cordoned off from the healthy body, both physically and emotionally.

Now that breast cancer is recognized as a systemic rather than a local disease, it is no longer possible to take comfort from these metaphors. But, like his contemporaries, Halsted could no more imagine cancer cells passing into the bloodstream before a tumor in the breast was large enough to be palpable than he could understand that a local recurrence was not life-threatening in itself but a pointer to the likelihood of metastasis elsewhere in the body.[10] And so he clung to his belief in local control and set about improving the techniques that made it feasible.

The more extensive procedure that Halsted advocated required innovations in surgical techniques to allow the surgeon to carry out longer operations without putting the patient at risk from hemorrhaging or infection. Halsted devised several of these improvements himself, contributing significantly to the development of safer surgery. For example, he introduced the sterile rubber glove and designed surgical tools that could be used to stop bleeding without causing major damage to the tissues involved. He used fine silk to suture wounds because he found that it could be more completely sterilized and would cause less inflammatory reaction than catgut. He improved the delivery of anesthesia to the patient. The control of hemorrhage, the gentle handling of tissues, and the painstaking attention to detail became hallmarks of the "Halsted School of Surgery."[11]

Halsted's own innovations were part of a rapid series of changes enlarging the scope of surgery from the 1890s on. The introduction of diagnostic x-rays in 1895 made it possible to intervene much earlier in the disease process. Advances in the histological analysis of tissue samples (in biopsies) also facilitated earlier diagnosis. Improved anesthetic techniques enhanced the safety of operative procedures while the steam sterilization of instruments enhanced the safety of the operating environment. The discovery of blood groups and of effective techniques for blood transfusion reduced the risks of hemorrhaging. The application of all these new techniques rapidly transformed the reputation of surgery and made it a more attractive option for the middle classes, who had always been able—but now might also be willing—to pay for surgical treatment.

Halsted made good use of all these surgical improvements. Above all, they allowed him to slow down the process of surgery, stretching out the time in the operating theater from a matter of minutes to one of hours. Ironically, it was the very fastidiousness of his approach that enabled him to "perfect" his mastectomy, facilitating its rise to dominance.

For the next three-quarters of a century, thanks in part to his contributions, radical surgery would monopolize the treatment of breast cancer in the United States. But while American surgeons were slow to abandon it, many other countries—Canada, England, Sweden, France—moved quickly after the Second World War to introduce less radical surgery used in conjunction with other treatment modes, primarily radiation.[12] By 1950, when radiation oncology was thriving in Europe, there were still less than fifty board-certified radiotherapists in the United States.[13]

Between 1889 and 1931, Halsted and his students carried out radical mastectomies on 878 patients. Fifty-six of these women died from complications of the surgery itself, from shock, wound infection, hemorrhage, and so on, a mortality rate of 6.4 percent.[14] This was a higher rate of death than that achieved by some of Halsted's contemporaries. Arpad Gerster, a surgeon at New York's Mount Sinai Hospital, was an important champion in the United States of Lister's principles of antiseptic surgery. In carefully assessing his own experience of radical mastectomies in the 1880s, he noted that of "sixty-seven cases, two died directly in consequence of the operation; none, however, on account of septic processes established in the wound. Thus the author's rate of mortality from accidental wound infection . . . would be 0; from other causes beyond the influence of the surgeon, a trifle less than 3 per cent."[15] Surgeons carrying out radical mastectomies at Massachusetts General Hospital between 1894 and 1904 achieved similar results, an operative mortality of 3.6.[16]

Since Halsted himself had introduced many of the innovations in antiseptic methods and was known to be an exceptionally careful technician, the higher death rates associated with his procedures may seem an unexpected result. But Halsted may have been a more fastidious and painstaking surgeon than many of those he trained. And, perhaps more important, the cases under review included 119 patients (about one in seven) who were subject to even more heroic surgery than that included in the standard Halsted procedure. In an operation that pointed the way to what became known as the superradical mastectomy, these women also had lymph nodes removed from the base of their necks, putting their bodies under even greater stress and at greater risk for postoperative complications.[17]

Of the Halsted patients who survived their surgery and who could be traced, only 12 percent were still alive after 10 years.[18] All were grossly disfigured. So extensive was the operation that a medical jingle that circulated through the hospital had an orderly ask Dr. Halsted at the end of the procedure, "Which half goes back to the ward?"[19] Many suffered permanent loss of the use of the arm on the side of the operation, or intermittent painful swelling of the hand and arm. Some complained of itching or infection at the site of skin grafts on the breast or on the thigh where the skin for the graft had been taken.

Since radical surgery was the *only* primary treatment available to these women, it's impossible to compare their survival rates with those arising from some alternative form of treatment. But it is possible to get some idea of the relative effectiveness of radical mastectomies by looking at the fate of women who had no treatment at all, who let the disease follow its natural course. Before the advent of mammography, there were many women whose tumors were deemed to be inoperable by the time they saw a doctor, whether because their disease was too far advanced or because they were considered to be at too great a risk for the procedure (too old or too sick). Adding to their numbers were women who simply refused treatment altogether.

The progression of the disease in these untreated women gives us a glimpse of the natural history of breast cancer. Modern studies attempting to assess its impact did not begin to appear until just after

Halsted's death.[20] However diverse their study methods, the results of these surveys are remarkably similar. Almost all of them show an average survival period after the onset of symptoms of about three years. A study investigating the case histories of 250 untreated women diagnosed before the mid-1930s revealed that 44 percent of them (109) were still alive after three years, 18 percent after five years, and 4 percent after ten.[21] While these results are not comparable to Halsted's or to any other surgeon's long-term patient follow-up, they do at least suggest both the variability of breast cancer and the difficulty involved in attempting to disentangle the "curative" effect of treatment from other underlying factors at work keeping the patient alive.[22] Researchers still face this problem today.

Keen to improve upon his results, Halsted periodically attempted follow-up surveys of his patients. Here too he was an innovator. The same meticulous attention to detail that characterized his surgical technique helped him to piece together the beginnings of a more comprehensive case study approach that would eventually become common practice. Even though his focus remained on local control, Halsted's interest in follow-up may also reflect a suspicion that breast cancer, unlike other conditions treated by amputation, might be more of a chronic disease, and therefore one that would benefit from a longer perspective.

A form letter dispatched to discharged patients in June 1914 invited them to revisit the hospital where they would be "seen together or within a few minutes of each other"; i.e., they were not to expect a private consultation with the doctor. Their surgeon, according to the letter, was "greatly interested in perfecting the operation which was performed for you on _____. It must still be improved in certain particulars; for example, we desire to obtain absolutely perfect motion and power and to eliminate entirely the swelling of the arm which formerly was occasionally sufficient to be annoying to the patient." Note that there was no expression of interest in the participants' current state of health, apart from symptoms connected with the surgery.

This was not a check-up to examine the patient for possible recurrence but an invitation to take part in ongoing research. Voluntary participation in the follow-up was intended to benefit the next generation of patients (in the tradition of clinical trials today). Of course, Halsted's rather ad hoc efforts preceded the introduction of methodological and statistical rigor in the design of clinical trials. Patient follow-up was also a bit of a hit-and-miss affair. Replies to these group summons often provided Halsted with his only means of discovering the fate of many of his patients. Those who did not recover typically died at home, beyond the reach of institutional record-keeping. Many family members did respond to his form letters to inform him of his patient's death, an event that had sometimes taken place years before. Many probably did not. Others responding to his invitation complained that their suffering was too great to permit them to leave home. Some did agree to come and welcomed the opportunity.

Consequences for the doctor-patient relationship

The move away from the medical to the surgical management of breast cancer involved much more than just a shift in the mode of treatment. Surgery introduced a radical new protocol between physician and patient that emphasized not their shared concerns but the inequities between them.

A surgeon was almost certainly male and almost certainly a stranger to a newly diagnosed woman and to her family. As a generalist rather than a specialist, he would have had little experience with and certainly no training in handling the special needs of breast cancer patients. He may, in any case, have had little interest in the interpersonal aspects of medical care. A woman, responding to this, would have had no reason to feel comfortable in his presence or to trust him. With no prior experience of surgery herself, she would be as unaccustomed to the conventions of hospital life as she would be to the bedside manner of her doctor. Yet, arriving in what was often a desperate state, she would be expected to submit utterly to his authority, placing her life entirely in his hands.

By comparison, the open-ended association between a family or general physician and patient had been low-key indeed. In the doctor's office or the home, the fear of breast cancer was often shared equally by the patient and her physician, even if it was never directly acknowledged by either. They may well have already known one another. Each, therefore, would already have some idea of what to expect from the other and would know how to interpret what was said and, perhaps, what was left unsaid. The sense of fatalism that intensified with time as the disease spread through the body may have established a kind of unspoken partnership between them, as both came ever closer to an admission of failure.

Halsted was certainly familiar with this expression of therapeutic nihilism that distinguished the response of physicians from that of surgeons:

> I sometimes ask physicians who regularly consult us why they never send us cancers of the breast. They reply, as a rule, that they see many such cases but supposed that they were incurable. . . . The conscientious physician could not under the circumstances advise his patient to be operated upon, and he was justified in treating her with salves and internal remedies.[23]

Even if these treatments were ineffectual, the familiarity of the established medical routine of which they were a part could also be an important source of comfort. If the doctor had been a regular visitor to the home, he or she would be accustomed to the patient's family circumstances and would be able to call upon relatives for consultation and support. Even if there was little to offer except palliative care, arrangements could be made to minimize the disruption of domestic routines and to maximize the comfort of the patient (at least in the homes of married women, or in middle-class homes where some help was available). If there was no medical treatment that could allay a woman's symptoms for long, there were also few that would be likely to kill her outright. The patient's condition may have been chronic and ultimately fatal, but treatment, although often painful, was rarely violent or immediately life-threatening. When death approached, the presence of the doctor would be consoling to a woman's family and perhaps also to her.

Surgeons were not the social inferiors of their patients; they were not asked, as were many family physicians, to ring at the tradesman's entrance. They did not stoop to make house calls at all. Instead they quickly became medicine's heroes, larger than life, called upon when all other treatments had been exhausted, to perform kill-or-cure procedures that required skill, stamina, and courage. The same symptoms that signaled defeat to the family doctor gave the surgeon a license to operate. Surgeons understood their procedures as measures of last resort. The elevation of any medical condition from "chronic" to "life-threatening" raised the stakes in the confrontation between man and microbe; the permissible risks rose accordingly. The violence of surgery was an inevitable consequence of a battle that was now perceived as staving off death rather than disease.

Nowhere is this larger-than-life view of the surgeon clearer than in the case of Halsted. The surgeon's authority was unassailable, his judgments never challenged. So great was his stature, in fact, that his apparent failure to establish effective relationships either with his patients or his students was, during his lifetime, entirely overlooked. History has tended to disregard this aspect of Halsted's career as it has forgiven his addiction to cocaine because of his overriding accomplishments as a clinician and educator.[24] But his formidable scientific achievements stand in marked contrast to an equally formidable personal ineptitude. As one of his former students put it, Halsted "spent his medical life avoiding patients—even students when this was possible. . . . A bed-to-bed ward visit was almost an impossibility for him."[25] Although he approached his patients with unfailing courtesy, his impeccable good manners almost certainly masked a deep discomfort. "Women came to regard Halsted," wrote another medical historian citing one of Halsted's residents, "as always a little distant and not to be treated with familiarity."[26]

If this was fairly typical behavior for a physician of his time, his relations with his residents were not. These were known to be strained. If he felt that his residents performed unsatisfactorily, his "look and silence could be worse than a verbal reprimand. When he did express his anger his words were so bitingly sarcastic as to 'shrivel completely' those at whom they were directed. . . . One of Halsted's closest surgical associates observed that in more than 30 years he never heard Halsted publicly compliment a resident."[27]

What would now be recognized as a dissociation of the medical and emotional aspects of medical care was beyond the comprehension of most practitioners of Halsted's generation. Nevertheless, it seems likely that Halsted's own uncomfortable relations with both his residents and his patients manifested itself in a way that was not typical, even for the time. How much of this was attributable to his lifelong addiction to cocaine and how much to temperament is impossible to say. But it is a question worth asking, because his importance as a role model for the rising surgical profession cannot be overestimated, either in its scope or its duration. So important has been his contribution to modern surgery that some more modern practitioners have asked whether "his remarkable character and influence . . . were a substantial reason why so much attention was paid to his operation."[28]

No family doctor had ever wielded such authority over patients, or over the long-term practice of medicine. Of course none had the weight of institutional authority behind them, or the same capacity to make or break the careers of those they helped to train. Institutional affiliation and support must certainly have helped to embolden the surgeon, prodding him to take risks that were unimaginable to the family doctor. Lacking the incentive or the resources to innovate left local physicians with more modest options at their disposal. But this limited their capacity to do harm as well as their capacity to cure. Where a family doctor had prescribed or directly administered treatment for breast cancer in the form of pills or pastes, he or she remained more a mediator of the disease process than a direct actor in the drama of treatment. The medical (as opposed to surgical) management of illness was, typically if not universally, more indirect. It rarely involved penetration of the body,[29] preserving some distance between doctor and patient.

In closing this gap and making a much more direct assault on a woman's body, surgery inadvertently ignored the capacity of the immune system to play any kind of independent role on its own. The surgeon, naturally enough, wanted to believe in the exclusive curative power of his craft and so had little incentive to investigate the "host" response to disease. The imagery that surrounded the performance of radical surgery encouraged this misreading of the behavior of breast cancer, suppressing the more complex reality of the tumor biology involved. The enactment of surgery as a rescue mission to capture an enemy kept alive the idea of a cancer as an encapsulated malignancy, something essentially alien to a woman's body. It was approached as a thing to be physically grasped and extirpated, enabling the patient to be "snatched from the jaws of death," and leaving her free of disease.

There was no room for subtlety here. The heroism that was ascribed to radical surgery depended upon the starkness of the contrast between good and evil and the gravity of the contest between them. The female body had to be recast as both inert (lacking any capacity of its own to respond) and dangerous (harboring an enemy). Some might argue that these beliefs about women were already well established in a society where the fear of women's sexuality was still completely repressed. In this reading, the aggressive behavior of surgeons would reflect no greater misogyny than was already present in the culture at large.

It certainly was already present in surgical practice. Well before mastectomies became routine, gynecologists had been castrating young women by removing their healthy ovaries, in the name of treatment for epilepsy, nymphomania, and insanity, as well as for a variety of menstrual irregularities like "pelvic neurosis." The abuse of power suggested by this "fashion in surgery" is a vivid demonstration of the absolute power still granted to men over women's bodies.[30]

Breast cancer surgery expresses the sexual tensions of patriarchy more starkly. Unlike reproductive organs hidden away within the body, the breast has always had a visible presence in the culture. As the most tangible sign of female sexuality, it attracts a great deal of erotic as well as aesthetic interest. Both are renewed on a daily basis, evoked in every exchange between a man and a woman. Surgery on the breast, therefore, does not occur in a social vacuum. How it is handled (literally and figuratively) inevitably invites comparison with other more familiar approaches to the breast.

In this context, the surgical removal of the breast has to be seen as a violent act. The apparent barbarity of the procedure raises the question of male intent. The breast is, after all, a source of conflicting responses: a place where erotic attraction mixes with a fear of dependency. It is not much of a stretch to view surgery as yet another opportunity to punish a woman for the ambivalent feelings she provokes. The fact that it is acted out under the guise of healing only intensifies the ambiguity of this relationship. The procedure, in other words, calls out both the best and the worst impulses of men toward women. But this tension remains wholly unacknowledged. The words say one thing, the gestures another. The contradiction between the apparent purpose of the procedure and the contrary passions it seems to enact elevates mastectomy to the level of high drama.

Not surprisingly, the performance of surgery came to govern every other aspect of the doctor/patient relationship, both pre- and postoperatively. The role scripted for the patient—the formalities exchanged in the doctor's office beforehand and in the surgical ward afterward—maintained a rigid separation between the socially approved interpretation of events and the darker undercurrents of meaning. There was little risk of a woman's crossing the line between the two. The terror of that knife held her in thrall.

The emotional charge of this central act contributed powerfully to a woman's panic in the face of a cancer diagnosis. It signaled a clear break in the nature of her relationship with the medical profession. What had sometimes been an exchange between equals (when breast cancer had been in the hands of the family doctor) now became a most unequal partnership. At its most reductive, the aura surrounding breast surgery reinforced the worst gender stereotypes, attributing all power to a male hero and all frailty to a damsel in distress. The surgeon was alert, erect, and skilled, and the patient, asleep, supine, and helpless—that is, without animating or humanizing virtues of any kind. Life-saving surgery, in other words, seemed to require the total degradation of a woman's spirit as well as of her flesh. This abasement, so integral to the surgical ordeal, was to color every aspect of treatment for most of a century.

"A paragon of surgical precision": the rise of the Halsted mastectomy

A good part of the surgeon's interest in breast cancer arose from the easy accessibility of the breast. Considered an appendage rather than a vital organ, one lying outside the body, gave it advantages as a site for both clinical investigation and surgical intervention, well before the arrival of modern anesthesia. This did not make the surgery safe, but the postoperative survival rates of patients undergoing breast surgery were higher than those associated with many other amputations.[31] And compared to the risks associated with surgery performed on the lungs or liver, for instance, breast surgery had the virtue of allowing quick and relatively direct access to diseased tissue. In other words, it made surgery look good. Mastectomies, in fact, remained the most popular and the safest cancer surgery well into the twentieth century.[32]

In the nineteenth century, a great many well-known surgeons, both European and American, introduced changes to the basic procedure. But ultimately, in the United States, breast cancer became indissolubly linked with the operative technique introduced by Halsted. This association between man and method signified a coming of age for American surgery. Halsted had gone to Austria and Germany as a young man to complete his training. But by the end of the century, the emergence of first-rate modern medical institutions like Johns Hopkins had helped to tilt the balance of power (and the direction of professional traffic) toward the United States rather than away from it, conferring legitimacy and status on its own surgeons.

The proprietary aspect of the claim did not pass unnoticed or uncontested. Counterclaims were made on behalf of European pioneers in breast surgery, notably for the British Mitchell Banks and the German-born Willy Meyer.[33] All had advocated some version of an extended operation that, like Halsted's, would include the removal of lymph nodes and pectoral muscles in addition to the breast. These battles to settle the question of who got there first may not, 100 years ago, have had the practical consequences they do now in terms of determining access to research grants and commercial patent rights. But they foreshadow these latter-day consequences in highlighting the competitive process of technical innovation at the expense of a more inclusive perspective on the disease.

Of course, the attribution of a surgical procedure to a single practitioner follows in the well-established tradition of marking territorial claims for tissues and organs inside the body, to honor the first scientific "explorers" who isolated and defined them. The exploration of the terra incognita of a woman's body has left a landscape so cluttered with "discoveries" (such as Fallopian tubes, named after Gabriele Falloppio) that they fill a book designed explicitly to memorialize them.[34]

What distinguished Halsted's version of mastectomy from that of his colleagues was his insistence on the *routine* performance of the procedure for the removal of the breast exactly as he had defined it. The emphasis here is on the word "routine." The glands and tissues specified by Halsted were no longer to be removed (or not) at the discretion of the individual surgeon determining his approach on a case-by-case basis. They were to be removed by him on a regular basis. The Halsted approach, in other words, signaled the standardization of surgical treatment for breast cancer. Radical mastectomy became the unvarying response to every set of symptoms and every medical history.

At the end of the nineteenth century, medical interest in cancer surgery far outstripped any parallel interest in tumor biology. Practical treatments for the disease (whether legitimate or illegitimate) ran well ahead of any scientific capacity to test theories of causation. In the 1880s, there were no special labs for medical research in the United States, no governmental support for biological scientists.[35] Cell biology remained in its infancy. The histories of cancer surgery and cancer research ran along separate grooves. By the end of the nineteenth century, surgery had its own laboratory and guinea pigs—the operating theater and charity patients—and its own source of funding—the private patient. Scientific research had to wait considerably longer for either.

An operation was deemed to be successful if it appeared to "work"; doctors did not have to understand why it worked.[36] The answer to the latter question required scientific inquiry at a level of financial and organizational complexity that would not be coordinated until the second half of the twentieth century. Until then, apparent success was all that was required; the radical mastectomy could survive as a proximate solution if not a final one. As a stand-in for a true cure, it had an astonishingly long run.

The operation was backed up by a scientific theory of disease that was easy to grasp and plausible. Cancer, Halsted believed, behaved in an orderly fashion, appearing first in the breast and spreading outward along known pathways. As a surgeon, he was less concerned with the origins of the disease than with its behavior once it showed itself symptomatically. For the most part, surgeons kept well away from the loaded speculations broadcast by gynecologists to explain the origins of a malignancy (which often involved blaming women for bringing the disease on themselves). They understood from early on that female hormones played a distinctive role in promoting many breast cancers, but their response to this finding remained narrowly surgical. From the end of the nineteenth century, they knew that removing a woman's ovaries could reduce the risk of a cancer recurrence but they did not really understand the endocrinology behind this practice (estrogen was not isolated and identified until 1923).

Medical (as opposed to surgical) doctors had much more reason to seek explanations for the onset of breast cancer. None of the vast array of caustic pastes and poultices they had prescribed, some of which were quite toxic, had proved to be effective. Knowing they had no cure for the disease, their only hope was to find a way to prevent it. Passing the blame onto women themselves was a reflection of their desperation. Surgeons, on the other hand, reversed these priorities. They wanted the opportunity to demonstrate that they did have something to offer. They were, accordingly, far less motivated to prevent the disease than to treat it. With nothing standing in their way, no competing therapies to oust or outperform, they moved easily into what was essentially a treatment vacuum. There they exploited to the full the advantages of early arrival and, like any founding fathers, left their indelible mark on the culture of all subsequent generations.

The impact of surgery

The repercussions of the surgical dominance of breast cancer are hard to overestimate. They have been felt in every corner of breast cancer's modern history—in patient attitudes, in the pace and direction of research, patterns of treatment and pastoral care, in the transformation of medical hierarchies, education campaigns, even the definition of the disease itself. How much of this is attributable to its own dynamics and how much to the lack of any countervailing treatment alternatives (until after the Second World War) is impossible to say. But from the moment the radical mastectomy was installed as the universal standard of treatment, its influence was enormous.

First, the surgery had a dramatic effect on the lives of many women who agreed to have it. It is easy today to forget that many of these women had tumors that were crippling as well as painful. Erupting through the skin, they could spread across the chest in a profusion of suppurating lesions that made it impossible for a woman to leave her bed. Although surgery for advanced disease could not have saved a woman's life, it might at least have provided some real palliative relief, releasing her from constant pain and enabling her to participate once more in domestic routines—to sit at the table, for instance, or to receive visitors. Surgery offered a reprieve, and more of a chance of dying with dignity. Without it, disease was allowed to run rampant, to consume the body of its victim.

The experience of Sarah Sim, a wife and mother living the pioneer farm life in Nebraska in 1880, reveals the kind of suffering and death from untreated disease that may have been common before the twentieth century. Her husband Francis had not been afraid to name his fear: "I think it is a cancer," he wrote to her sister. Her brother John, in another letter to this sister, describes Sarah's condition to her:

Sarah has been confined to bed constantly since Thanksgiving. Her right breast is enlarged to nearly the size of a lady's head and is as hard. A tumor or outgrowth from the lower right side as large as my fist and 3 smaller ones, 2 of which have opened on the upper part. Occasionally she is taken with bleeding from the larger tumors which weakens her greatly and great care is exercised in dressing the breast to prevent bleeding. She is able to lay only in one position and is only out of bed once in 24 hours . . . long enough to have the bed arranged. . . . I have little in fact no hope of her recovery. Sim thinks unless she improves, she can not last to exceed 3 months. . . . What more to say, what more to report I know not.[37]

Her husband's prediction proved to be accurate; Sarah Sim survived this twilight life for another ten weeks. The day before she died, her brother wrote to their mother that she was "so weak, so feeble that we shall greet Death as her rescuer from suffering and as a Friend."[38] She died at home, treated by a doctor who made occasional visits and nursed by her sister and her sister's daughter who had come from Connecticut to care for her.

The grotesque proportions of Sarah Sim's breast tumors and the pain they produced made her disease and her suffering impossible to disguise. Surgery, when it arrived on the scene, made it possible for breast cancer to be hidden from view. A woman who recovered from a radical mastectomy could now hide her illness from the world. She could reenter society or play a more active role in domestic life without drawing attention to her physical loss. While this may have preserved her sense of privacy and restored some sense of normalcy, it implicitly placed a higher value on the social denial of the disease than on the private need to unburden oneself. A woman with breast cancer, in other words, soon discovered that surgery itself created some disturbing conflicts.

It is doubtful that any woman facing surgery would have been unduly concerned about the long-term consequences of treatment itself. It is much more probable that she feared the surgery itself rather than its aftereffects. The procedure had to be performed in a hospital, an institution not far removed from the poorhouse in the minds of many middle-class patients, and known to be unhygienic. But there was more to fear than the risk of infection. The mortality rate from the radical mastectomies itself was high. It is not known whether a woman agreeing to surgery understood that postoperative death was precipitated by the procedure itself rather than by accelerated disease. It would certainly be understandable if she failed to distinguish one cause of death from another. She may also not have known how extensive the surgery would be, that it would permanently disable as well as disfigure her, depriving her of the full use of her arm on the operated side. She might have imagined the removal of a breast but not the more invasive "clearance" of her chest and underarm tissue and muscles.

The longer-term repercussions would have crept up on her unawares as she regained strength and reawakened the hope to stay alive. Her recovery would be mediated by her own particular circumstances, whether she expected to remain an invalid or to return to a more active social life. She would probably not have understood this process as a conflict between the demands of her private and public selves; the explicit recognition of competing demands, particularly those based on gender, is of relatively recent origin.

Before the 1970s, there were few alternative narratives a woman could construct that recognized the primacy of her own experience, or that encouraged her to separate it out from the more powerful sense of obligations that defined her. A woman ill with a fatal disease had little or no sense of entitlement. If she thought at all about the contradictions between the physical limitations set by her body and the worldly expectations of society, she would not have understood it as a confrontation or a form of oppression. More likely, she would have attempted to accommodate the demands of domestic or social propriety wherever possible. The pain or discomfort this caused her would be interpreted as a necessary part of the recovery process, just one more in a series of adjustments that society now required of her, and that she was willing if not very well able to make.

A woman's not knowing what to expect was another clear expression of the absence of breast cancer from the culture. Knowledge of the disease was not part of any oral or written tradition handed down from one generation of women to the next, like advice about childbirth or sex, advice designed to help a woman cope with natural apprehension about the unknown or ambivalence about the known. It was not an occasion that generated any comforting sense of continuity based on the sharing of experience between mother and daughter. Breast cancer was a rare event, and one in any case more likely to strike women of the older generation. These were women whose mothers were probably already dead, who had no natural comforters to advise them, and no common language with which to overcome their terrible isolation. For most of these women, the submissive role they were scripted to play barred them from expressing any curiosity about their own bodies, at any stage of their lives. Given their earlier habits of compliance, they were hardly likely to take a stand against the damaging side effects of surgery when they knew that any expression of concern would be understood as a challenge to their doctor's authority.

If Pygmalion represented the male desire to create a woman from scratch, in order to fall in love with (and control) her, the heroic surgeon perpetuated the same myth of heroic rescue through creative re-modeling. (Traces of this myth still cling to the plastic surgeon reconstructing the breast of a mastectomy patient today, as Chapter 8 describes.) An onlooker in Halsted's operating room likened his performance to the work of an artist, "akin to the patient and minute labor of a Venetian or Florentine intaglio cutter or a master worker in mosaic."[39] The surgeon was master of his craft, the female patient, his handiwork. With unfettered access to a woman's body, he could achieve miraculous transformations, re-shaping it to restore her health. Although few surgeons would have openly espoused such an extreme view, most would have been comforted by it in the operating theater. Given the pain and disfigurement inflicted by the surgery they performed, how else would it be possible to believe without hesitation that the benefits associated with a radical mastectomy always outweighed the risks?

The notion that women believed only what they were told by men suggests that their curiosity could be easily satisfied. It would be highly unlikely, therefore, for a patient to be properly informed in advance of the true extent of the surgery she faced. Her preoperative ignorance would then leave her vulnerable to a postoperative anguish she would be forbidden to express. The surgeon who had saved a woman's life could hardly be chastised for depriving it of quality. After all, a woman, once recovered, would be restored "good as new" for all the world to see, confirming her surgeon's expectations of success. Private pain would once again be the price women were asked to pay to uphold society's reverence for male accomplishment.

However a woman interpreted this scenario, it must have been disturbing. Whatever her level of comprehension, the overriding response to the prospect of a radical mastectomy would be one of justifiable dread. Anything she knew about it would be overlaid by an association with death. There was, in fact, no outcome that was satisfactory—the rejection of medical treatment could lead to a death every bit as painful as one following surgery. Neither action nor inaction offered an escape from pain or mutilation.

The double dilemma of radical surgery has left a permanent scar on the idea of treatment itself. It carried risks of death and deformity as great as those associated with untreated disease, and it also required the collusion of women in a drama that seemed to communicate, often in a public arena, all of the late nineteenth century's ambivalence and hypocrisy about the role of women in society.

The 1889 painting of a mastectomy by Thomas Eakins ("The Agnew Clinic") deftly captures these contradictions. A popular illustration today for the jackets of medical histories,[40] it was painted in the same year that Halsted was appointed professor of surgery at Hopkins. It portrays another famous surgeon, David Agnew (1818–92), presiding over an amphitheater of attentive male medical students. As Bridget Goodbody has pointed out, the painter has eliminated almost all signs of disease or surgical injury from the canvas. The patient's body shows little trace of having been violated but still appears to be whole. Her face and body are those of a younger woman, not those of the typical middle-aged breast cancer patient. The side of her body where the breast has been removed has been artfully draped, leading the viewer's attention to the young, healthy, and eroticized breast that remains. This exposure contradicts common surgical practice; normally, all of a woman's body would be covered except the surgical site. But it allows the painter to portray the surgeon as someone who appears to have conquered disease without sacrificing the virtues of idealized womanhood by destroying her sexuality—affirming "the viewer's sense of the doctor's all-powerful authority."[41]

Ironically, although Agnew has now become almost an icon of the nineteenth-century surgical hero, he had serious doubts about the value of radical mastectomies. "I do not despair of carcinoma being cured in the future," he wrote, years before the painting was commissioned, "but this blessed achievement will, I believe, never be wrought by the knife of a surgeon."[42] Any such doubts he might have expressed while modeling for Eakins have clearly been airbrushed out of the painting. Painted as he approached the end of an eminent career, Agnew exudes the confidence of someone passing on the torch to the next generation. In many respects, the painting presents a visual equivalent of the heroic medical history (of the type mentioned in the last chapter), written by a young acolyte tracing his own surgical lineage back through the accomplishments of distinguished mentors. In the painting, Agnew appears to have retired from the fray, with his scalpel at rest, watching from a distance as his residents finish the job he started, demonstrating their own grasp of the skills he has passed on to them which they, in turn, are now passing on to the next generation. Those eager students on the bleachers, if they took up where their predecessors left off and kept the faith, would collectively have gone on to perform thousands of mastectomies themselves, until they reached retirement age just before the outbreak of the Second World War.

During the interval between the careers of men like Halsted and Agnew and the training period of surgeons who have retired in the 1980s, the grip of radical surgery on breast cancer treatment remained undiminished. It has been described by Bernard Fisher as an era "which must be viewed as incredible both in terms of its longevity and in its freedom from criticism."[43] Those changes that did occur in the understanding of the disease were not inconsiderable, but they nonetheless show traces of having evolved under the shadow of radical surgery. This is not to disparage the improvements that emerged over the first half of the twentieth century but to make it clear how much they were shaped by the overriding imperatives of surgery. The complacency that surrounded the automatic use of the radical mastectomy must surely have played a role in suppressing interest in breast cancer research. The sense of its shadowy existence as a medical backwater is conveyed by Michael Shimkin, formerly associate director for field studies at the National Cancer Institute, who recalled being surprised, when he began his medical career in the 1930s, "by the low status accorded to breast cancer in the hierarchy of medical concerns."[44]

The misrepresentation of "success"

Once the radical mastectomy was enthroned as the "gold standard" of treatment, the clinical interpretation of symptoms lost its primacy. Where clinical skills had formerly determined the appropriateness or extent of surgery on a case-by-case basis, they were now preempted by the automatic choice of radical mastectomy. All suspicious symptoms led to one recommended treatment. Inevitably, the adoption and dissemination of the procedure had the effect of devaluing the diagnostic capacity of clinical skills.

The standardized use of one procedure as *the* primary treatment for all breast cancers logically suggested the underlying existence of a standardized pathology as well. How else could the practice be justified? It was not that clinicians renounced their investigative skills. But once the prescribed treatment was foreordained, there was certainly some loss of urgency and incentive to sharpen them. If the recommendation for treatment was always going to be the same, the benefits of a more detailed clinical investigation would be gratuitous. The effect of this demotion of clinical findings was to flatten the profile of breast cancer as a disease. The diagnostician had only to determine whether the presenting symptoms were likely to be malignant or not, that is, breast cancer or not. If radical mastectomy followed in every instance of a suspected malignancy, there was little point in monitoring the different behaviors and outcomes of different kinds of breast cancer. Inevitably, the simplified diagnostic response contributed to the delay in recognizing the wide diversity of breast cancer as not one but a collection of diseases, each with its own biology and pattern of behavior and each responsive to treatment in its own individual way.

Ironically, the recognition of diversity in the pattern of disease and the need for an individualized response on the part of the doctor were fundamental to another, radically different approach to medical treatment that was fast disappearing. The practice of homeopathy, on the wane just as surgery first rose to prominence, depended upon a doctor's capacity to listen creatively and patiently to a patient's entire medical history and to respond with a treatment that was individually tailored to her unique set of symptoms.

Surgical treatment for breast cancer lacked this subtlety, in both its theory and practice. Its one-size-fits-all approach proved to be no match for the slippery cunning of a disease that took so many shapes and forms. The inexplicable behavior of many of these cancers showed up in postoperative survival data. Early follow-up studies revealed that many women continued to die within a few years of surgery while others lived for decades. Even women with apparently small tumors could sometimes die surprisingly fast. Operating on the belief that breast cancer was a local disease rather than a systemic one left surgeons without any rational explanation for these wide variations in outcome. But rather than adjusting the theory, in the light of evidence that contradicted it, they chose instead to adjust the practice. A more careful selection of patients, they hoped, might help them raise the survival rates and so provide a better track record for the procedure.

Early classification systems that defined tumors by their stage of development were a first step in the process of differentiation. They were designed to enable the surgeon to distinguish between "operable" and "inoperable" tumors. This was clearly a proxy for the distinction between "curable" and "incurable," though it was not the same thing. Drawing up informal guidelines that set limits on "operability" allowed surgeons to exclude tumors that were already too far advanced to offer the patient any hope of recovery. Eliminating those cases with the worst prognoses would raise the average postoperative survival rates. Since these were the only statistics ever publicized, rates of survival quickly became synonymous with rates of "cure." Any apparent increase in survival might therefore raise a woman's expectation of a cure from surgical intervention.

In the first half of this century, a great deal of evidence in the medical literature demonstrated just such an upward trend in survival rates.[45] The table below summarizes the changes over the period 1894 to 1941 in the percentage of women surviving five years after a radical mastectomy. All the women (approximately 2,000 of them) were patients at the Massachusetts General Hospital in Boston.

CHANGES IN THE PERCENTAGE OF
WOMEN SURVIVING AFTER 5 YEARS

TREATMENT PERIOD	5-YEAR SURVIVAL, PERCENTAGE
1894–1904	19
1911–1914	27
1918–1920	30
1921–1923	35
1924–1926	41
1927–1929	43
1930–1932	45
1933–1935	50
1936–1941	51

SOURCE: Taylor and Wallace 1950.[46]

The series shows a steady improvement in results; over an almost fifty-year period, each group of patients did better than the last. No one disputes the overall trend that these figures suggest, but their significance for the treatment of breast cancer is open to interpretation. Many of these incremental improvements are attributable not to radical mastectomies themselves but to the benefits of earlier detection, a more careful selection of surgical candidates, improvements in anesthesia and in pre- and postoperative care. In other words, they reflect *the accommodation of the disease to the treatment*, rather than the more expected accommodation of treatment to the disease. The surgical procedure (and the scientific theory that endorsed it) remained more or less undisturbed throughout this period—and in command. All the adjustments that collectively enhanced the reputation of radical surgery took place outside the operating theater. The improved survival rates, therefore, were less a demonstration of the increasing curative powers of radical mastectomy than a demonstration of the prevailing power of surgery. Lacking any check on its authority (from either competing therapies or internal criticism among colleagues), it was able to dictate the adaptations it needed in order to improve its performance record.

A closer look at the results from the Boston hospital illustrate the sacrifices involved in producing more optimistic results. These are not at all disguised by the authors of the study, but they involve a level of detail that would fail to attract much interest beyond the readership of medical journals. They certainly did not form part of the public relations message about the effectiveness of treatment for breast cancer.

First of all, the statistics include only those women who were actually treated. As the authors themselves attest, "a more careful selection of cases" contributed to the improved results. Not surprisingly, over the fifty-year period, surgeons narrowed the definition of operability, particularly after the introduction of therapies such as radiation that offered palliative rather than "curative" treatment. "Throughout the half century," wrote Taylor and Wallace, "radical operability has remained at about the same level, ranging from 72 per cent to 80 per cent of all primary cases admitted to the hospital. A progressive sharpening of operability has tended to lower this percentage."[47] In other words, at least one of every five women who appeared at the hospital with breast cancer was turned away from surgery and hence excluded from the survival rates. Whether given some form of palliative care or not, these women were expected to die. But their deaths from breast cancer were not incorporated into the history of the disease because that history has been expressed primarily as the history of treatment.

In setting the criteria for admission, physicians were acting as gatekeepers to history as much as to treatment. Only those women whose disease conformed to the standards doctors had set would be included in the records. The others would be lost to history altogether. And it was not just their lives that were set aside. In rejecting advanced or anomalous expressions of disease from the operating theater, surgeons were essentially banishing them from the realm of scientific inquiry. Their proper investigation was put on hold, as was any attempt to provide curative rather than palliative treatment for them.

Not everyone was blinded by this approach. Americans, however, were much less likely to voice their objections than their European colleagues. R. McWhirter, for example, a Scottish proponent of conservative surgery and radiation therapy in the United Kingdom, admitted in 1947 that "cases considered to be beyond a method of treatment are just as much failures of the method as cases actually treated and failing to be cured."[48] This was much too open an evaluation of radical surgery for any American clinician to make publicly at the time, tantamount to professional heresy.

Beyond the realm of medical controversy altogether was an even larger group of women who, as far as the historical record is concerned, were statistical nonstarters. These were women who never took their symptoms to a doctor at all, but allowed their disease to run its course without any medical intervention. Well into the twentieth century, the number of women who remained beyond the reach of treatment is significant, if impossible to pin down. Although hospitals (and departments of surgery) began to multiply from the end of the nineteenth century on, they may nonetheless have failed, even decades later, to keep pace with the ever-growing population of women with symptoms of disease. In individual hospitals, surgical case-loads were limited. At Johns Hopkins Hospital in Baltimore, the average number of radical mastectomies carried out each year in the decade ending in 1930 was just 24, exactly the same as it had been twenty years earlier, in the years between 1900 and 1910. In the fifty-year period 1889 to 1939, the number of breast surgeries performed annually at the Presbyterian Hospital in New York rose from 6 to 60 but the number of newly diagnosed cases of breast cancer in New York City had risen by 1939 to an estimated 3,000, more than double the figure ten years earlier.[49]

How many of these women ever received any medical advice, let alone treatment, is impossible to say. Although we know that, in the first half of the twentieth century, the number of women dying of breast cancer exceeded the number treated for the disease in a hospital setting, there are many explanations for this shortfall.[50] We don't know where to draw the line between inadequate supply (a shortage in skilled manpower or in available surgical beds) and inadequate demand (a shortage in the number of women who could afford to pay for treatment or who were convinced that the benefits of surgery outweighed its risks). The ranks of the untreated also included those who presented themselves for treatment but were rejected, and those who rejected the treatment they were offered.[51] Last but not least are the women (and men) who were too ashamed or terrified ever to consult with a doctor at all. All we can say for sure is that none of the experience or suffering of any of those who did not make it into a hospital, even for palliative care, has been factored into the published survival statistics.

There was, in fact, no pressing need to keep track of these women at all, to pin down the size and shape of the disease population. Breast cancer was not an infectious disease and so it did not arouse the concern of public health agencies on the alert for the warning signs of epidemics. Physicians were under no obligation either to collect or to pass on information about new diagnoses of breast cancer, as they were for diseases such as measles, tuberculosis, and smallpox. As with so many other aspects of this disease, information about it remained largely in the hands of surgeons. Their single-minded focus on survival following treatment reflected their own interests. Preoccupied with the drive to reduce mortality, surgeons tended to overlook the alarming growth over the course of the century in the numbers of women newly diagnosed with the disease.

The primary emphasis on dying from rather than living with the disease was already well established. Breast cancer had first appeared in the U.S. Census in 1900 as a "cause of death" rather than a "reportable disease," suggesting that, unlike smallpox or measles, there was little that society could do to restrain it. It entered the national consciousness as it entered the record books: as a disease that kills. And as census after census amply illustrated, its power to kill remained undiminished, rising from a rate of 9 deaths (for every 100,000 Americans) in 1900 to a rate of 17 deaths 20 years later.

The high mortality rates were a constant reminder of the uphill battle that surgeons faced. Surgery would mount a challenge to these figures, and would gradually force the statistics of death to give way to the statistics of survival. As more women survived—and survived for longer—the formal follow-up period steadily lengthened, extending from one to three years and then to five and even ten years after surgery. The follow-up evidence was neatly framed to demonstrate, over time, signs of improving odds against the disease. Survival rates set the standard for competition between surgical departments across the country, each vying to push the prevailing limits higher and higher. Although comparisons were often meaningless, institutional reputations were often built upon and sustained by the cumulative follow-up "success" rates for surgical procedures. Keeping the rates elevated was essential.

This uniformity in approach to the disease clearly made it harder to generate much enthusiasm for alternative perspectives that were more concerned with possible causes than with apparent cures. The historic lack of data on the incidence of breast cancer, for example, reflects the relative lack of concern with the social, demographic, and environmental aspects of the disease.[52] These are all factors that have turned out to be quite significant. But it is only over the last few decades that we have really begun to grapple with them, to begin to measure their impact on the numbers and distribution of breast cancer diagnoses. Before that, the profile of those living with the disease had to be reconstructed retrospectively from the data of those dying from it. In a reversal of expected practice, statisticians relied on rules of thumb (like the formula of "three cases per recorded death")[53] to breathe life into the population of those diagnosed but not *yet* dead. This was the administration of science from the grave, with the dead presiding as independent variables. Death from breast cancer, such a practice implied, was a foregone conclusion, dragging down its victims at a rate that was apparently fixed in stone.

Such a view cast a pall over scientific efforts to uncouple the relationship between incidence and mortality. The former had to be liberated from the latter before inquiries into the causes, distribution, and control of the disease could even be conceived of, let alone carried out. Any approach to prevention, whether theoretical or experimental, required a radical shift in outlook. Rather than accepting the notion of unvarying disease that standardized treatment implied, it highlighted the importance of *the individual patient*—suggesting that her own genetic makeup and environmental history (taken in the broadest sense) might play a role in determining her risk for the disease and her response to it. A diagnosis of breast cancer, in other words, might be the result of a complex interaction between biology and the patient "host" rather than just the crude assault of disease on an inert body that the surgical model implied. If biology and epidemiology could isolate those factors that, in combination, seemed to predispose a woman to breast cancer, then, at least theoretically, the odds might be altered in her favor.

The presumption that science could intervene at a much earlier stage, not to treat but to eliminate the need for treatment altogether, would not be likely to emerge from the world of clinical practice. Surgery, after all, was focused on reducing the number of deaths, not on reducing the number of diagnoses (the same may be said of chemotherapy today). Equally important, it was an approach to the disease that could be effectively implemented within the private practice of medicine. The pursuit of prevention, by contrast, involves the coordination and primarily public financing of large-scale and complex research projects that draw upon a wide array of skills from many disciplines. Paradoxically, the identification of risk factors that might benefit women on an individual basis can only be derived from the study of very large populations.

The newer perspective on prevention, which bypasses the skills and outlook of surgery altogether, did not have much hope of thriving as long as information on the incidence of breast cancer remained tethered to treatment. Once again, the persistence of this dependency is clearly demonstrated in the statistical history of the disease. Until 1974, national estimates of new cancer cases in the United States had to be derived from data from just two cancer registries (in Connecticut and New York). Although epidemiological studies of breast cancer have grown enormously over the past few decades, there is still, in 1999, no national cancer registry mandated to collect and monitor information on new cases of disease in every state.[54] Current cancer registries still cover only about 14 percent of the U.S. population. This is as much a symptom of the historic precedence of treatment over prevention, as it is an expression of the surgical stranglehold on the direction of scientific enquiry.

୨●

The strategies adopted to promote better surgical results went beyond restricting access to surgery. Although the screening process appeared to be filtering out the undesirable, there was an equally powerful (if more covert) dynamic at work in the opposite direction as well. Just as important as the careful exclusion of "unfavorable" cases was the inclusion of women with cancers that were thought to be more "favorable": those with very small or equivocal tumors whose surgeries were more likely to boost the results.

The history of all twentieth-century campaigns promoting early detection starts here. The logic of surgical case selection was driven by the need to pin down exactly that range of breast tumors that allowed surgery to operate at optimal levels of efficiency. Surgeons were as eager to screen in those cancers that were considered likely to raise the survival rate after surgery as to screen out those that were likely to lower it. Whether or not small tumors needed radical mastectomies, radical mastectomies needed small tumors.

To the extent that surgery did catch breast cancer before it had spread to other organs in the body—and it often did—the survival benefits it conferred were distributed statistically among *all* surgically treated breast cancers, at whatever stage of advancement. Average survival rates rose accordingly. These encouraging results may have inadvertently helped to delay or at least to slow down the pace of research into early-stage breast cancers or any other forms of the disease that deviated from the so-called norm. Standard treatment had, after all, implicitly hypothesized a disease prototype. The drive toward early detection sought to bring all tumors within the scope of that prototype, which was essentially defined by operability. The increasing trend toward the discovery and presentation of smaller and smaller tumors (through the promotion of early detection, breast self-examination, and, finally, screening (mammography) certainly did save lives. But it also, by improving surgical results, helped to prop up the use of and rationale for a therapy that could never provide a true cure for the disease.

Part
Two

3 ?

"A Really Hideous Mutilation":

THE RADICAL MASTECTOMY IN THE CORRESPONDENCE OF A BREAST CANCER PATIENT AND HER SURGEON, WILLIAM STEWART HALSTED (1917–22)

Introduction

The two chapters that follow reproduce two correspondences, each between a breast cancer patient and her surgeon, each running from diagnosis to death. The first set of letters was exchanged between Barbara Mueller and William Stewart Halsted, over the years 1917 to 1922; the second set between Rachel Carson and George Crile, Jr., from 1960 to 1964. Although separated by more than forty years, both women's experience of disease was dominated by the culture of the Halsted mastectomy. For Rachel Carson, as it had been for Barbara Mueller before her, the surgeon was still male, still the gatekeeper to breast cancer treatment, and still reluctant to disclose the truth to his patient. Surgery still held center stage. Even hormonal therapies, aimed at reducing the level of circulating estrogens, were achieved by surgical means (by removing a woman's ovaries) rather than by drugs.

From an end-of-century perspective, the fifty years spanned by these two correspondences seem to represent a plateau in the history of breast cancer treatment. In the United States at least, there was little serious challenge throughout this period to what became known as the "gold standard" of treatment. Surgeons may have genuinely believed that the clear superiority of the modern procedure (in its earlier intervention, its relative safety, and its improved survival rates) entitled them to sit back and rest on their laurels. But what looked like the onset

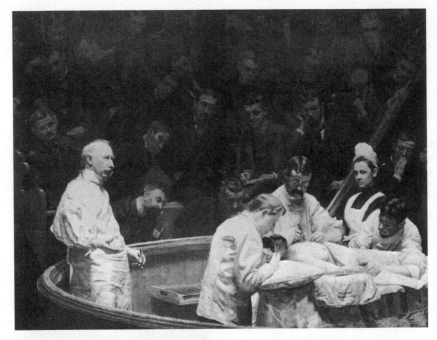

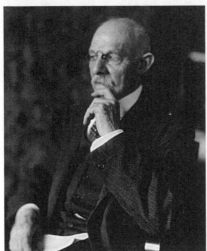

(Above): Agnew Clinic by Thomas Eakins. *Permission of The University of Pennsylvania Archives.*

(Left): William S. Halsted, M.D. *Permission of The Alan Mason Chesney Medical Archives of the Johns Hopkins Medical Institutions.*

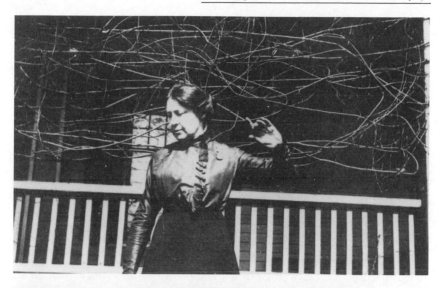

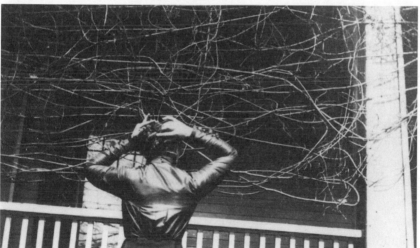

Unidentified post-mastectomy patient of William S. Halsted, M.D. *Permission of The Alan Mason Chesney Medical Archives of the Johns Hopkins Medical Institutions.*

of a golden age was really more the creation of a medical backwater. In the absence of any challenge from competing therapies, which would have kept it under active scrutiny, surgery grew complacent. It had no natural predators. Rarely put on the defensive, it was never forced to demonstrate its legitimacy or reexamine its theoretical underpinnings.

If many more women were undergoing surgery, it did not necessarily follow that mortality rates fell. On the contrary, they rose. Breast cancer claimed 8,500 lives in the year that Barbara Mueller died. By 1964, the year of Carson's death, the number of deaths had tripled, to almost 26,000. Some of this increase was attributable to a population that was aging, but the death rate, which adjusts for this, also rose dramatically, almost doubling over the 42 year period (from 7.8 deaths for every 100,000 people in 1922 to 13.7 in 1964).[1]

Campaigns for early detection brought more and more women to the operating theater and got them there earlier and earlier, allowing postoperative results to appear ever more promising, as seen in the last chapter. But among clinicians, there was no sense of a race for the cure, no urgent quest for the origins or causes of breast cancer. Surgery was not, after all, designed to prevent disease but to treat it. With no protest from any other quarter and nothing to stand in its way, the practice of radical surgery soon fossilized into dogma.

By the mid-1930s, some dissenters did begin to raise their voices, suggesting, in the first instance, that a combination of less radical surgery and radiation might yield survival rates comparable to those associated with radical mastectomies. But since their recommendations failed to disturb the fundamental scientific paradigm, they were easy enough to dismiss.[2] The first real threat to the hegemony of the radical mastectomy came from biology, not from surgery, and not until the late 1950s, that is, close to the end of the period spanned by these letters.[3] The correspondences, then, occur during a period that, for breast cancer, was an age of inertia.

The letters that follow provide a better understanding of the human cost of this failure, offering a more intimate view of the consequences of the Halsted era for individual women caught up in it. They spell out, in considerable detail, the nature of the suffering it imposed and the quality of courage it demanded of those who chose to be active participants in their struggle for survival. In a sense, the letters share the same perspective as all the other chapters in this book. That is, they were all written midstream, when the final outcome of the story was still unknown. In the letters, there remained—always—a hope if not a certainty of cure. For the history of the disease itself, that hope has been attenuated over time to an intolerable thinness as the certainty of cure continues to recede before us.

This first correspondence is between a woman diagnosed with breast cancer 80 years ago and her surgeon, William Stewart Halsted, whose radical mastectomy remained the standard form of treatment for breast cancer for almost 100 years. In the absence of any alternative, close to two million American women submitted themselves to this procedure before the 1970s, and yet hardly a trace of the extraordinary pain and disfigurement they suffered survives. So complete was the collective denial of breast cancer that few women ever overcame the conspiracy of silence to document their own experience of the disease. Most women never discussed it with anyone outside their own families; many tried to keep it a secret even from their children.

The most frequently cited, extremely rare, exception to this self-censorship is the early nineteenth-century account by the English novelist Fanny Burney. Best known for her novel *Evelina*, published in 1788, Burney was an inveterate letter-writer and diarist, married to a Frenchman and living in France. Nine months after the event, she wrote an extremely intimate yet carefully observed account of her experience with breast surgery in a long letter to her sister. Anesthetized only with a "wine cordial," and with a handkerchief spread over her face, she endured the removal of her breast in her own home by a team of seven surgeons and a nurse. Surviving the operation by 30 years, Burney died in 1840 at age 88.

Critics have been interested in the graphic and novelistic rendering of Burney's operation as a precursor to the new genre of "pathography," a kind of memoir that allows the marginalized female patient to reconstruct her own encounter with the medical establishment as part of the process of recovery. It has been described as "a performance of recuperation," allowing the patient to put her experiences into order and shape, and enabling her to "reassert ('re-inscribe')" herself "as a complete whole being." With the assertion of narrative control over past experience, "the once dependent, puzzled and anxious observer, now proclaims—erects—herself as the bearer of a knowledge of equivalent stature to the doctor's."[4]

The authors of breast cancer diaries that almost two centuries later have become part of mainstream literature are the direct descendents of Fanny Burney. Though varying widely in quality, these accounts all view the act of writing as part of the healing process, a therapeutic reordering of their own ordeal.

The letters of the patient in this correspondence (whom we will call Barbara Mueller)[5] are not really part of this tradition. First, they were not written self-consciously with a view to publication, but were prompted instead by the patient's immediate need to understand her situation and to obtain the treatment most likely to save her life (she may also have felt that the act of keeping in touch with her doctor would enhance her chances of survival). Rather than unfolding a story told in retrospect, from the safe haven of recovery, the Mueller/Halsted correspondence tells its tale prospectively, moving forward, sometimes at irregular intervals, through the messy uncertainty that accurately reflects the patient experience. The contrast in outcomes is striking. Fanny Burney survived her mastectomy by almost thirty years; Barbara Mueller survived only five. Her letters, therefore, express an urgency that is missing from the more reflective chronicles of illness reassembled by longterm survivors.

A second crucial distinction arises from the differences between personal narrative and a professional correspondence. While the former gives us a private and often intimate view of experience controlled wholly by its author, the latter is a partnership of sorts, one that reflects the social restraints and inhibitions governing the roles of doctor and patient at the time and also obeys the prevailing rules of epistolary etiquette. Until the mid-nineteenth century, it was common for doctors to evaluate their patients' complaints without actually touching them; the patient's own narrative, sometimes conveyed by letter, often served as the only basis for diagnosis.[6] The Mueller/Halsted correspondence certainly refers back to this tradition with its archaic forms of courtesy.

The entrenched social mores embedded in these letters impart to the material a rich and unusual historical sense of the tone of the relationship between the two correspondents. (That the letters do not tell the whole story is evident from other accounts of Halsted's life and work cited in the previous chapter.)

The language of the exchanges between Mueller and Halsted (their literary conventions and formalities) gives us some idea of the quality and scope of their interactions in person, whether in the doctor's office or at the bedside. The forebearance and courtesy communicated by Mueller in the face of terrible pain demonstrate the impregnability of medical authority at the time her letters were written, the inadmissibility of doubt about the competence or wisdom of the male medical establishment. The permitted range of patient response was narrow, limited to dutiful submission, gratitude, and silence.

Barbara Mueller pushed against these boundaries in her letters, seeking to play a more active role in determining the course of her treatment. But, as her correspondence makes clear, she was trapped, as much a prisoner of early twentieth-century literary proprieties as of its rigidly prescribed sexist codes of behavior. She was not a revolutionary thinker or a professional writer but an intelligent if otherwise unexceptional middle-class woman. Her letters are direct and artless, totally lacking in pretension. Nonetheless, they position her on the cusp of modern consciousness, making her unspoken thoughts sometimes almost audible.

It is, in fact, the implicit conflict between her possibly half-realized suspicions and the permitted forms of expression open to her that make this correspondence so compelling and such a valuable contribution to the silent and largely undocumented history of women's suffering.

The Mueller/Halsted correspondence

Barbara Mueller came to Halsted in 1917, late in his career. Halsted had been recommended to her by her brother, an eye, ear, nose, and throat specialist who had been trained in Maryland and had worked for a time at the Baltimore Medical College. Because her family was medically well-connected, Mueller had access to the best advice and treatment then available. By anyone's standards, she was a remarkable patient. She was well educated and took an active interest in every aspect of her case. At a time when only about half of cancer patients ever saw a surgeon and the average lag between the discovery of a lump and the first consultation with a doctor was over a year,[7] Mueller took herself to be examined just seven weeks after first noticing a lump in her left breast. She took an intelligent interest in monitoring her health (weight, temperature, minor illnesses) and the progress of what she believed was her full recovery. When worrying symptoms appeared, such as the swelling of her arm and hand, she carefully charted their course, taking note of their changing size and tenderness, and she took the initiative in bringing these concerns to the attention of her surgeon.

Until her death, she remained unfailingly devoted to the doctor she believed had cured her. She never once questioned the wisdom of the surgery she had undergone and was, in fact, willing to put herself under his knife a second time. She never learned—from her doctor or anyone else—that her cancer had metastasized. The letters she exchanged with Halsted illustrate her enduring faith in the wisdom of decisions he made on her behalf. They also reveal a great deal about the unspoken protocols and proprieties that defined a woman's experience of the disease eighty years ago, providing a useful look at the nature of the doctor-patient relationship in the days before the psychological consequences of breast cancer had been acknowledged or played any part in disease management. Finally, they make us much more aware of the things that have changed since then, and of those that have not.

Barbara Mueller was diagnosed with cancer on March 14, 1917, and admitted to a private ward at Johns Hopkins Hospital for a radical mastectomy on March 27. She was fifty years old, a single woman working as a private secretary with no family history of cancer. The lab tests carried out by the pathologist, Dr. Joseph Bloodgood, showed no evidence of cancer in the axillary lymph nodes.[8] Her clinical exam, however, had revealed that the nipples of *both* breasts, not just the one with tumor, were drawn back (retracted). The pathologist thought the presence of this sign, together with evidence of chronic cystic mastitis, might warrant the removal of the second breast "for protection" (that is, prophylactically). Halsted did not agree. While acknowledging that "the disease in the operated breast was evidently of long duration so that she [Barbara Mueller] probably has unremoved glandular metastases," he adopted a wait-and-see approach rather than choosing to carry out any further surgery at the time.

Like today's patients, Barbara Mueller was immediately concerned with the financial implications of her illness. As a working woman, she would have lost income during the period of her hospitalization and convalescence. (In fact, we don't know whether she ever returned to work.) But unlike almost all of her contemporaries, she had health and accident insurance. In fact, in 1905, when she first purchased a policy from the Fidelity and Casualty Company in New York, coverage for women was virtually unknown. Many companies expressly forbade it.[9] The policies that became open to women at just about the time Barbara Mueller bought hers were an early recognition of the rapid rise of women in the workforce.[10] Mueller would have purchased her policy through her employment; originally, coverage was designed to protect against the loss of income (arising from illness or accident) rather than to pay medical bills or hospital costs.

Fidelity and Casualty had been a pioneer in offering coverage to women.[11] At the turn of the century it introduced a policy offering health and accident coverage to schoolteachers (mostly women). In 1905, for a premium of $15 per annum, the policy paid $7 a week indemnity in the event of sickness up to a maximum of $3,000.[12] It also paid $700 for death from "sunstroke, freezing, suffocation by gas or hydrophobia." Extraordinarily, Barbara Mueller's policy actually included the word "cancer" in its register of covered diseases although, at the time, it was far down the list of recognized causes of death, well behind tuberculosis and pneumonia.[13] But its presence on the list meant that Halsted was forced to reveal to Mueller her true diagnosis so that she could submit a proper insurance claim. So in a way, Halsted's unprecedented candor, which would not become routine practice for another fifty or sixty years, can be described as a consequence of Mueller's entry into paid employment. But, as these letters demonstrate, this still left a wide gap between "naming" and "knowing."

Correspondence 1917–22

MAY 13, 1917
My dear Dr. Halsted,[14]

When referring to my Health & Accident Policy which has been in force about twelve years, I find that the Health clause contains a very limited number of ailments for which the Insurance Company would pay weekly indemnity. However among the ailments, cancer is specially provided for, but no provision is made for tumors, unless the latter be under some technical name which I do not recognize. I have not heretofore had the courage to ask you nor any of the J.H.H. [Johns Hopkins Hospital] staff with whom I came in contact, whether the trouble in my breast was of a malignant type or not. Under existing conditions therefore, it is necessary for me to know if I can claim indemnity by reason of cancer. Will you please therefore advise me at your earliest convenience. The Insurance Company advise me that if I can prove that the growth is a result of accident I can also make claim under this part of the policy but it would be impossible for me to state whether the trouble arose from accident or not. However, any expression of opinion you can give me in this respect would be appreciated.

I am glad to be able to tell you that I am feeling in pretty good shape and each day find that I am gaining in strength and assurance. My leg has healed very nicely [where skin had been taken to graft onto the surgical wound] and beyond itching is giving me no trouble. The breast likewise seems in good shape though one very small spot towards the chest shows a disposition once in a while to discharge slightly. It will doubtless please you to learn that I practically have full use of my left arm which is a comfort indeed.

I would greatly appreciate [it] if you will let me have your bill promptly as I am endeavoring to get my affairs in shape.

With best wishes, Yours very cordially,
Barbara Mueller

MAY 15, 1917
My dear Miss Mueller,

The tumor in your breast was a cancer. I hope it will be a comfort to you to know that we believe it has been entirely excised and that you will see no signs of its recurrence.

I am glad to know that you are steadily improving in health and that the wounds are nicely healed. It is also gratifying to me to know that you are rapidly regaining the use of your arm. If you are still in town at the end of June, I shall hope to have the pleasure of seeing you.

Very sincerely yours

W. S. Halsted

MAY 22, 1917

My dear Dr. Halsted,

I was indeed very glad to receive your reassuring letter and on that am building hopes of never having a recurrence of my recent trouble.

Am enclosing herewith Health Indemnity Claim of the Fidelity & Casualty Co and would greatly appreciate if you will do the needful and fill out the Physician or Surgeon's Certificate. I was at the J.H.H. for five weeks—March 22 to April 26 inclusive but on account of the condition of my leg was unable to go out until ten days after leaving the hospital. I think the date on which I first consulted you was March 14th.

It does seem strange, does it not, that the Health Policy provides for cancer but this policy has been in force for about twelve years. Unfortunately, however, the Company allows no surgeon's fee for this sort of operation. It is considered a very limited policy and I believe the new forms are much more liberal with regard to operations.

. . . I failed to find your bill enclosed with letter and shall be glad to send you the check promptly upon its receipt.

Inasmuch as I expect to be in town during the summer, I shall surely make it a point to see you about the end of June.

Very sincerely,

Barbara Mueller

[It seems, from the next letter, that Halsted waived or reduced his surgical fee for Barbara Mueller's mastectomy. His fees were known to be high but it is impossible to determine the relationship between his fee and her generous voluntary payment.][15]

JUNE 14, 1917

My dear Dr. Halsted,

Referring to my visit to you yesterday and our conversation relative to compensation for my recent operation—While highly appreciating your generous attitude towards me yet in reviewing the situation I feel that out of gratitude for my restoration to health which I owe to your great skill that I should do something in a material way towards helping others. To this end therefore I am enclosing you my check for $500 [about $7,000 in 1999 prices] which I will ask you to accept and use according to your best judgement.

Again I wish to thank you for your wonderful attention and interest and to assure you that the recollection of these favors will never be effaced from my memory.

With kind regards and hoping you will have a pleasant summer.

Yours very gratefully

Barbara Mueller

[Dr. James B. Murphy, 1884–1950, mentioned in the next letter, studied medicine at Johns Hopkins and in 1910 was appointed as assistant in pathology and bacteriology at the Rockefeller Institute (now University) in New York City. At his death, he was the head of its Laboratory of Cancer Research. At the time of his correspondence with Halsted, he was conducting experiments with x-rays; these can legitimately be described as one of the earliest attempts to provide "adjuvant" therapy to breast cancer patients. Murphy believed that low doses of x-rays would increase the number of lymphocytes in the blood and that this in turn would increase the body's resistance to tumors, preventing their further growth. He began clinical tests of his theory in 1916, enlisting breast cancer patients who had just had their breasts removed.[16] Unfortunately, Murphy was never able to establish any correlation between the number of lymphocytes in the body and the progress of the disease and his experiments were discontinued in 1922.

It's not clear whether Barbara Mueller learned about Murphy's work from her brother or from Halsted; Halsted knew Murphy from his days at Johns Hopkins but either man could have known about it either from the newspaper or from contemporary medical literature.[17] In any event, Barbara Mueller was eager to participate in Murphy's experiments, and probably knew that Halsted was drafting the following letter to Murphy.]

JUNE 21, 1917 [Halsted to Dr. Murphy]

Dear Murphy,

Do you care for any more of our cases of breast cancer? Probably you do not care to burden yourself with further work this summer.

A case I had in mind for you is a nice woman, in quite moderate circumstances, upon whom I operated about three months ago. The prognosis is not absolutely bad, but there is a little retraction of the nipple of the opposite breast which the patient is quite sure has come on within the past few years. If you care for such a case I will question her more carefully and write you again.

Very sincerely yours

W. S. Halsted

[Dr. Murphy writes back a few days later to say he has lost two of his assistants and can't take on any new cases. Halsted writes to tell Miss Mueller on June 26 that "it will be impossible for (Dr. Murphy) to treat any cases at present."]

OCTOBER 9, 1917

My dear Dr. Halsted,

Doubtless by this time you have returned from your summer vacation and I trust have been benefited by the rest.

Am sorry not to have seen you before leaving Balto to take up my residence in New York but on Sept 26th I went to the Johns Hopkins Hospital for Dr Reid to make an examination and he seems to have found conditions satisfactory, and perhaps he has made a similar report to you.[18] Under these circumstances therefore will it be necessary for me to come down to Balto for an examination by you in the near future or when do you think it advisable for me to come down?

Are there any further developments in Dr Murphy's experiments that would be applicable to my case and which you would consider an advantage for me to follow up?

Yours very truly

Barbara Mueller

[In his reply, Halsted appears to misunderstand Barbara Mueller's renewed interest in Murphy's experiments with radiation, forgetting that he wrote to her on the subject just four months earlier.]

OCTOBER 15, 1917

Dear Miss Mueller,

Thank you for your kind note of October 9th. I hope that you may have occasion in the near future to come to Baltimore and that I may have the privilege of examining you.

During the summer I wrote to Dr. Murphy of the Rockefeller Institute, having particularly your case in mind. He replied that his experimental work at present is so heavy that he cannot at this time undertake the treatment of human subjects.

With kindest regards, I am,

Very sincerely yours

W. S. Halsted

DECEMBER 9, 1917

My dear Dr. Halsted,

It is my purpose to come to Balto on Saturday 15th for about a three day visit and this is to inquire if it would be possible for you to see me say on Monday 17th and if so at what hour and place. . . . While a very recent examination by my nephew Dr. H. L. Mueller did not reveal any indication of a recurrence of my trouble yet I should be gratified if it were possible for you to pass an opinion as to my present condition.

Should my visit not fit in with your plans will you kindly advise me promptly and I can then defer it to a more opportune time.

Yours very truly

Barbara Mueller

DECEMBER 11, 1917

Dear Miss Mueller,

I shall surely be able to see you sometime on Monday. Unfortunately, I cannot at this moment name the hour because my time is so filled.

Please phone my secretary, Miss Stokes a little after noon on Monday.

Sincerely yours

W. S. Halsted

OCTOBER 8, 1918
My dear Dr. Halsted,

When I saw you last December, you requested that I come to Balto for examination during October 1918.

During the past two weeks I have noticed a very decided swelling in my left forearm (side of operation) and while there is no great discom fort arising from it, yet there is quite some soreness manifested on the inner side of the arm below the bend when touched. Otherwise, I am happy to say I am feeling very well and retaining my normal weight.

Today I learned of the meeting of the College of American Surgeons scheduled to begin Oct 23rd in New York City. It occurred to me that if you contemplated attending this convention that I might be so bold as to ask if you could make it possible to examine me while you are in New York at such time and place as you may select. If however this plan is not practicable then I will endeavor to come to Balto especially to see you whenever is convenient for you. Will be glad to know your wishes in the matter.

Hoping this finds you well and with all good wishes
Yours ever gratefully
Barbara Mueller

OCTOBER 18, 1918
My dear Miss Mueller,

It will give me great pleasure to see you. Unfortunately, I shall not be able to attend the meeting of the American College of Surgeons.

It will, I think, be well to postpone your visit to Baltimore until the epidemic of influenza has somewhat subsided. The Johns Hopkins Hospital is admitting only cases of influenza, emergencies excepted.

With kindest regards, I am,
Sincerely yours
W. S. Halsted

NOVEMBER 12, 1918
Dear Miss Mueller,

I fear you think that I have forgotten you, but it is only within the last few days that we have been admitting surgical patients to the hospital.

It will give me pleasure to see you whenever it may suit your convenience to come. Please advise me at least ten days in advance in order that a room may be reserved.

Sincerely yours

W. S. Halsted

NOVEMBER 29, 1918

My dear Dr. Halsted,

Up until now I have not been able to state definitively when I could come to Balto as I had a slight attack of grippe. Inasmuch as I am now feeling quite well again, [I] would like to know if you could arrange to see me on Monday Dec 9th and if so at what time and where. While I am hoping there will be no occasion for hospital treatment or operation, yet if you deem it advisable for me to secure a room at the Johns Hopkins Hospital even tentatively I shall be very grateful if you will make such provision for me. I would state however that the forearm swelling previously referred to seems to be gradually subsiding.

Awaiting to hear from you as early as practicable, and with kind regards,

Yours very sincerely

Barbara Mueller

DECEMBER 2, 1918

Dear Miss Mueller,

It will give me great pleasure to see [you] on Monday, the ninth of December. Unfortunately I cannot at this moment arrange the hour. Will you kindly telephone Miss Stokes, my secretary, on your arrival.

I am so pleased to know that the swelling of the arm is subsiding, and I hope that it may not be necessary for you to enter the Hospital. In any event, I am quite sure that it would not be possible to secure a room for December 9th.

Sincerely yours

W. S. Halsted

[Sometime over the year that passed between these December 1918 and 1919 letters, Halsted must have seen Barabara Mueller and decided to admit her for further surgery, most likely to remove lymph glands in her neck.[19] We do not know which of her symptoms prompted this decision; we do know that it came less than two years after her original mastectomy. But, as the following letter from Dr. Edward Mueller, Barbara Mueller's brother, to Dr. Halsted shows, the decision was made for her that her family duties took precedence over the medical plan.]

DECEMBER 11, 1919 [Dr. Mueller to Halsted]

My dear Dr. Halsted,

No doubt you are awaiting an explanation as to the reason for the change of plans regarding the operation on my sister, Miss Mueller. My sister called me up on the phone and reported that you had advised an operation on her in the left supra-clavicular region and I suggested that she have it done at once. However, after my talk with her, I felt that owing to my mother's condition, besides various other attending difficulties, it would be inadvisable for my sister to have the operation performed away from New York. I therefore advised her later to come home.

I wish she could have remained in your skillful hands, as it was by my advice that she first consulted you, but there would be so many demoralizing features surrounding my sister's absence, that I felt compelled to take this course. Miss Mueller was very much annoyed that I had changed my mind, but I feel that I am doing what is best under the circumstances. I am going to ask Dr. John Erdman to see my sister tomorrow and should his opinion coincide with yours, I will ask him to operate.

There seems to be a unanimous lack of opinion [consensus] regarding the cause of the tense swelling of the forearm and oedema of the hand. Is it possible that it is a malignant process in the arm and is not due to pressure on the lymphatics and blood vessels? I would greatly appreciate an expression of your opinion on the case.

Trusting you will understand how keenly I feel the necessity for advising my sister as I have done, and hoping you will not feel annoyed, but realize that I did it with great reluctance.

Most sincerely yours

Edward L. Mueller

DECEMBER 12, 1918 [Halsted to Dr. Mueller]

I think you are quite right in desiring another opinion, and I should have entire confidence in Dr. Erdman's judgment.

My feeling is that in the absence of symptoms of nerve pressure it is unlikely that the swelling of the arm is due to glandular involvement. It was my intention to try to determine the matter through as small an incision as possible, for an extensive exploration might lead to further impairment of the lymphatic circulation.

With kind regards, I am,

Sincerely yours

W. S. Halsted

JANUARY 18, 1920 [Barbara Mueller to Halsted]

My dear Dr. Halsted,

Your kind letter should have had a prompt reply but for the fact that I have been sorely pressed for time due to mother's illness during the past ten days.

You are mistaken about the swollen arm being the cause of your remaining in my thoughts—am happy to say I have only the pleasantest recollections of you and a deep feeling of gratitude. That left arm did give me some worry when the swelling manifested itself, but now I no longer am disquieted, as the swelling has to some extent diminished though the arm still remains considerably larger than the right, and I am suffering no discomfort. As a matter of fact I am feeling generally well and Dr. Mueller Jr. [her nephew] has examined me at intervals of three or four months since I saw you last and can find no indication of a return of my old trouble. I had hoped to have gotten down to Balto. to see you but mother is rather dependent upon me and it is not very easy for me to get away even for a day. However, as soon as I see my way clear to come to Balto will let you know in advance and arrange to be there when it suits your convenience, again assuring you of my undying gratitude and with all good wishes.

Yours very sincerely

Barbara Mueller

NOVEMBER 2, 1920

My dear Miss Mueller,

You are so constantly on my mind that I must write to ask about the swelling of the arm.

I am more than ever interested in those swellings because I now believe that many of them are determined by a very mild grade of infection, occurring sometimes at long periods after the operation. These infections do not necessarily give any outward signs or constitutional symptoms but not infrequently there is slight redness at some period or other—the redness usually accompanied by a little rise in temperature, slight malaise, and perhaps nausea.

Can you recall in connection with the first appearance of the swelling in your arm (which, if I remember rightly, occurred about one year after the operation) whether there were any local or constitutional disturbances?

Had you perhaps had the influenza, or a cold, or pharyngitis [sore throat], or anything of an infectious nature at sometime not long before the unexpected appearance of the swelling?

Has the arm since you saw me diminished or increased in size? and have there been periods when it seemed definitely larger than at others?

I trust that you are well, and shall greatly appreciate a rather detailed reply.

With sincere regard, I am,

Very truly yours

W. S. Halsted

[What Halsted took as an infection in his patient's arm is today understood as the result of the surgical disturbance with lymphatic or vascular drainage as a result of the lymph node dissection under the arm.]

NOVEMBER ? 1920

My dear Dr. Halsted

Please pardon delay in replying (to) your very solicitous letter of 2nd but I purposely postponed answering so that I could thoroughly refresh my memory concerning my health and general condition since my operation in March 1917.

It is now twenty six months since the swelling first manifested itself or rather when it became annoying—which was therefore about eighteen months after the operation. Between the time of operation and Sept. 1918, I had had no ailments of any kind that required medical attention—particularly no cold nor pharyngitis, and I went through the influenza epidemic without being disturbed by it. I can recall no rise in temperature nor any nausea. About the middle of November 1918 I was indisposed for a few days—my symptoms were a general achiness throughout my system, though no rise in temperature, but to the contrary, for a short period was sub-normal. This you will note was about two months after the swelling became so pronounced.

In February 1919 I had a little grippy attack of a few days duration, with but a slight rise in temperature and at the same time had some slight intercostal neuralgia.

About fourteen months ago or in September 1919—had an attack of bronchitis which was not a very stubborn case.

In March 1920 had an attack of head neuralgia and in October 1920 another attack of intercostal neuralgia.

This is as complete a history of my condition since March 1917 as I can furnish and I think you will agree with me that outside of the discomfort which I suffered by reason of the arm swelling, my health has been generally good.

I do not think that the arm has diminished in size since I saw you in Balto in December 1918, but I am suffering practically no discomfort. The only time when there is any disturbance is when I am wearing a sleeve or glove which contracts the arm or hand, then there is a perceptible swelling and discomfort, but I try to prevent this as far as possible by wearing sleeve or glove that allows for expansion.

Am happy to be able to tell you that I am feeling very well at present and while I should like to be able to get down to Balto in order to have you examine me again, yet I do not see how it will be possible in the immediate future. In accordance with your instructions I had been having my nephew Dr. Henry L. Mueller examine me from time to time and he always found my condition satisfactory. For the past three months though I have not given the matter any thought or attention as death claimed this fine young man on August 5th—he was stricken with cerebral hemorrhage while on duty at Mt. Sinai Hospital where he had been intern and house surgeon.

I want to thank you for your deep interest in my welfare as it is indeed flattering to know that I am still in your mind. However I want to assure you that I shall always feel the deepest gratitude to you for the wonderful success you achieved in my operation.

Yours very sincerely

Barbara Mueller

NOVEMBER 13, 1920

Dear Miss Mueller,

I thank you very much for replying so fully and satisfactorily to my questions. I am happy to know that the swelling of the arm has not increased and to be able to assure you that it surely is not caused by a return of the growth.

The death of your nephew is indeed most sad. I am mourning the loss of Dr. Leltzer who was a true and precious friend.

With kind regards, I am,

Very sincerely yours,

W. S. Halsted

[The correspondence ends here and resumes abruptly eighteen months later with the announcement of Barbara Mueller's death. The following letter suggests that Halsted had been unaware of—and uninvolved with—his patient's final illness.]

APRIL 19, 1922 [Dr. Mueller to Halsted]

My dear Dr. Halstead [*sic*]:

My dear sister Barbara passed away last Sunday evening after fifteen months of great suffering, especially so in the last few months. She was kept in ignorance in spite of her suspicion of her disease. There was no recurrence in the operated area. The first manifestations showed about October 1919 by some lameness on the left side. Several radiographs showed changes in the pelvic bones. She received x-ray treatment from Dr. M. J. Sittenfield without any apparent benefit, but an indurated gland behind the ramus of the jaw on right side seemed very much improved from x-ray and radium.

I want to thank you most fervently for your skill and most generous interest that you manifested in my dear sister. She was a wonderful character and to praise her would be like painting the lily. This may be thought to be a brother's pride. No, I say this because I knew her so well. My mother & sister came to cold? [*sic*] New York, but in a short time my sister made a host of loyal friends who showered her with the most lavish hospitality—showing what a magnetic nature she possessed.

My dear Doctor Halstead trusting you are enjoying good health and mental peace.

Yours very sincerely

Edward L. Mueller

APRIL 22, 1922 [Halsted to Dr. Mueller]

Dear Dr. Mueller,

It grieves me to receive the sad tidings of the death of Miss Mueller and I beg to tender you my deep sympathy. I can well understand your distress at the loss of such a sister. She made a great impression upon all those who were privileged to take care of her. The sweetness of her disposition and the nobility of her character endeared her to us all. Her gratitude and generosity I shall never forget. I wonder if you know that she presented the Hospital with five hundred dollars.

Naturally it is a satisfaction to me to know that there was no local return of the growth, but how sad it is that she should have suffered so dreadfully. I have been particularly interested in the story of the swelling of her arm and should greatly like to know if this increased after her visit to me about three and a half years ago. I am sending you a reprint of a recent publication of mine which will explain to you the nature of my interest. The swelling of the arm attracted her attention about one year after the operation and she came to Baltimore to consult me about it. I could find no evidence of any glandular involvement above or below the clavicle and assumed that the swelling must have been due to an infection so slight as to cause no constitutional symptoms and no blush of the arm. She may however have had slight symptoms such as malaise or unobserved rise of temperature prior to or coincident with the swelling. Can you recall any mention on her part of indisposition for a day or two about the time that the arm began to swell? Was a post mortem examination made of the axilla, supraclavicular region and mediasternum? I shall greatly appreciate your kindness in replying to these questions.

Very sincerely yours

W. S. Halsted

JUNE 22, 1922 [Dr. Mueller to Halsted]

Dear Doctor Halstead,

Your very kind letter to me has not been answered earlier because it has been hard for me to dwell upon my poor sister's fate. There was no autopsy and none proposed, although Dr. Eli Moschowitz, a pathologist, was my sister's attendant. I received your reprints on the oedematous arm. My sister did not seem to put much stress upon her swollen arm. She had temperature of one or two degrees above the normal in her last days with a pulse of 90. I wish I could give you more information about my sister's case as I know how intensely you are interested in your work and I know how important the knowledge of end results is to all of us.

With my kindest regards and best wishes for your continued and uplifting efforts on behalf of suffering humanity.

Yours very sincerely

Edward L. Mueller

≈

One of the most striking features of this correspondence is the absence from it of any women other than the patient. There were, of course, few women doctors (and fewer women surgeons) at the time of Mueller's illness, so her dealings as a patient with a predominantly male medical establishment were not unusual. But having both an older brother and a nephew who were physicians may have intensified her role as a patient even within her own family. The gender disparity in access to medical information and decision-making illustrates, within this one family, the more widespread contrast between educational and professional opportunities available to men and women at the time.

Mueller's experience does, however, suggest that she made good use of the privileges of her class; her confidence and capacity for articulate self-expression reveal the relative advantages of a middle-class upbringing. But these were often outweighed by the disadvantages of her gender. Although she clearly benefited from her brother's professional standing, it proved to be a double-edged sword. While his connections gained her access to Halsted in the first place, they also made it possible for him to prevent her returning to Halsted for further surgery, by being in a position to recommend a local substitute. Barbara Mueller clearly wanted to go back to Halsted and her brother knew it ("Miss Mueller was very much annoyed") but he summoned the classic paternalist justification—"I feel that I am doing what is best under the circumstances"—to keep her in New York where their mother was ill.

Edward Mueller did not, apparently, think it inappropriate to expect his sister to help look after his mother as well as herself, to be a caretaker as well as a patient. It's hard to imagine who, if anyone, looked after her when she was dying, or to know whether she had any emotional support at all. There was neither husband nor children in the wings nor does there seem to have been any other female relative capable or willing to lobby on her behalf. Her letters offer few clues about her private life. While her brother mentions "a host of loyal friends," it would have been exceptionally unusual for Barbara Mueller to share her illness with them. Did her mother or sister-in-law ever step in on her behalf? With her mother ill herself and her sister-in-law grieving for the loss of her own son, it may be that Mueller was as truly alone as the letters suggest. Their stripped-down quality, with their sights set narrowly on survival, suggests the absence of any emotional allies and makes Mueller's courage and determination even more poignant.

A modern feminist sensibility might be forgiven for noticing how, in the final exchanges between her brother and Halsted, Barbara Mueller's individual story is transmuted into medical case history. In his last letter, Edward Mueller responds to Halsted's request for postmortem information, supplying the particulars of his sister's terminal illness. He then moves on, whether from a sense of delicacy or obligation we shall never know, to a more formal acknowledgment of Halsted's "uplifting efforts on behalf of suffering humanity."

Beyond the formalities of this final exchange lay Halsted's more disturbing reaction to treatment failure. Halsted can admit that he could find no signs of cancer anywhere near the original tumor site but he cannot admit that it could have spread elsewhere, beyond his surgical reach. Having earlier in his career disparaged the idea that breast cancer cells could early on travel undetected through the bloodstream to develop tumors at other sites in the body, he found himself without a satisfactory explanation for Mueller's death. The idea that disease could spread discontinuously rather than in a connected fashion required too much of an imaginative leap. Boxed into his own paradigm, Halsted is forced to fall back on the idea that an infection arising from the swelling in Barbara Mueller's arm must be the culprit. "The most common cause of the last postoperative swelling," he wrote in a paper published in 1921, while Barbara Mueller was still alive, "is, of course, the recurrence of the disease, a recurrence which blocks new channels ... lymphatic obstruction predisposes to streptococcal inflammation."[20] So determined was he that Barbara Mueller's death should validate his theory that he solicits corroborating evidence from her brother. In desperation, Halsted insinuates that the early warnings of a fatal infection were, in fact, present (in "slight symptoms") but that they were overlooked *by the patient.*

Less than three months later, these posthumous interrogations came to an end. Halsted himself was dead, of pneumonia following surgery for gallstones. The surgery that bears his name, however, lived on as the treatment of choice for another 60 years. But if the Halsted procedure did not change much during that period, everything surrounding it did. Every passing decade witnessed important changes in society (influencing expectations and interactions between physicians and patients). It also extended the reach of scientific knowledge, in, for example, physiology, pathology, and cell biology, while at the same time introducing improved anesthetic techniques that increased the safety of surgery. Equally significant were changes over the course of the century in the appearance of the disease at the moment it first came to the attention of a physician. The success of campaigns promoting early detection combined with improved diagnostic techniques changed the disease from one that was identified through its symptoms to one that could be identified subclinically, that is, before the appearance of any symptoms.

In other words, the relationship between the radical mastectomy and the social and medical environment in which it was performed continued to change even if the basic procedure remained more or less constant. What Halsted and his contemporaries saw and what they knew of the disease formed part of a surgical outlook that died with them, reemerging in a new form (with new pre-occupations and priorities) in every subsequent generation of surgeons. This means that the strategies employed to keep the radical mastectomy viable (acceptable to both surgeons and patients) had to be continuously adjusted as well. Inevitably, the theoretical justification for the procedure and the medical infrastructure supporting its use carried meanings in the late 1970s very different from those they had called up 60 years earlier, during Halsted's lifetime.

In 1979, the Consensus Development Conference of the National Institutes of Health finally gave its approval for the first time to less radical surgery for primary breast cancer.[21] This confirmed a trend toward treatment that allows most newly diagnosed women with early stage cancer to keep their breasts, if that is their choice.

Keeping their lives is another story. The survival rate for the kind of metastatic cancer that Barbara Mueller suffered from has not changed for over a century. As one former president of the American Cancer Society has written, "over a period of 100 years, breast cancer treatment has evolved from no treatment to radical treatment and back again to more conservative management, without having affected mortality."[22]

4 ✒

"A Private Little Hell":

THE LETTERS OF RACHEL CARSON AND
DR. GEORGE CRILE, JR., 1960–64

Introduction

In 1960, almost forty years after the death of Barbara Mueller, Rachel Carson was also diagnosed with breast cancer. Already an acclaimed ecologist and nature writer, she had embarked on the writing of what would become her best-known book, *Silent Spring*. Mueller had been 50 at the time of her diagnosis and survived 5 years. Carson was 53 and survived 4 years. Both had radical mastectomies. Single women, with no known family histories of cancer, both had access to what was thought to be the best medical care of their day. They took an educated interest in every aspect of their own treatment, even expressing an enthusiasm for unproven experimental therapies that were not available to most patients.

Rachel Carson's 1960 diagnosis of breast cancer falls on a timeline about halfway between Barbara Mueller's encounter with the disease and that of a woman today. It would be tempting, therefore, to locate her experience of treatment in a parallel position midway between the standard practices prevailing in 1920 and those in place around the year 2000. But from our contemporary vantage point, Carson's experience seems to have had much more in common with Mueller's than with any breast cancer patient's today.

The medical advances between 1920 and 1960 were modest. Radical mastectomy remained the cornerstone of treatment, although by 1960 radiation had developed into a widely used and powerful adjuvant

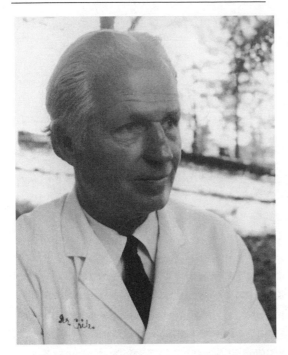

George Crile, Jr., M.D.
Permission of Helga Sand-
burg Crile. Photograph by
Dwight Boyer.

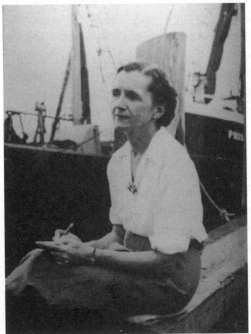

Rachel Carson, 1950.
Courtesy of Rachel Carson
History Project, Rachel
Carson Council, Inc. Photo-
graph by Edwin Gray.

therapy. In 1955, the National Cancer Institute received authorization and funding for research into the possible uses of chemotherapy. By 1959, about 3,000 cancer patients were enrolled nationally in NCI-sponsored clinical trials that were testing new drugs.[1] Carson's doctor, in fact, tried but failed to get her into what was probably the first clinical trial of a treatment for breast cancer, evaluating the postoperative use of thiotepa.[2] But the anticancer drugs that have become a standard component of treatment today were not even on the horizon then. Nor, significantly, was the use of mammography, which meant that women could not be treated at all until their tumors had grown large enough to be manually detected. The American Cancer Society had, however, begun to encourage earlier detection through the promotion of breast self-examination; by 1953, films demonstrating the technique had been shown to more than three million American women.[3] It's impossible to say whether Carson knew of this campaign or whether she had ever been to a demonstration screening; it is certain that by the time she learned the true nature of her own disease, it was too late.

In effect, then, although Carson's handling of her own breast cancer might appear to be very different from Mueller's, the treatment she endured was not radically different. But what separates both of these women's experiences from the late twentieth-century version is not so much changes in the nature of treatment but more a radical shift in the nature of consciousness. For Carson, and even more starkly for Mueller before her, breast cancer was a disease with no separate identity and no history. Until after the Second World War, cancer was considered more a monolithic disease than a vast collection of different diseases with widely different biologies and behaviors. Breast cancer was not listed as a separate disease in the annual reports of the National Cancer Institute until 1965, the year after Carson's death. Many cancer treatments reflected this lack of differentiation. They were more generic than specific, aimed at large groups of cancers rather than targeting particular sites. The physicians providing these treatments also tended to be more generalists than specialists.

But if the conditions of "supply," that is, the medical responses to cancer, seem outmoded to us today, the conditions of "demand"—the socially sanctioned attitudes that the patient brought with her into the doctor's office—seem almost unimaginable. Although Carson's *Silent Spring* played a crucial role in arousing a national awareness of environmental concerns, Carson herself fell ill and died before the advent of feminism; Betty Friedan's *The Feminine Mystique* was first published just before her death. Without an awareness of any of the issues brought into the public arena by the early women's movement, it would have been very hard even to conceptualize such a thing as a woman's disease. Although it may seem like quibbling, a disease to which women are vulnerable is not quite the same as a "woman's disease," just as the eventual shift over time from "cancer of the breast" to "breast cancer" denotes more than a semantic distinction. However subtle the changes in usage, they nonetheless convey the now enhanced status of the disease. Breast cancer is no longer one among many but a disease in its own right, one women have publicly identified with.

Breast cancer remained practically as invisible in Carson's time as it had been in Mueller's. It belonged to no tradition of shared experience among women. Given this absence, it is extremely unlikely that either Mueller or Carson ever thought to compare her own experience of breast cancer with that of women who suffered from the same disease before them. Nor would they necessarily have been aware of friends or even other family members afflicted with it. Although Carson and Alice Roosevelt Longworth, for example, had met each other at social gatherings, it is almost certain they neither knew nor exchanged notes about their respective mastectomies—Roosevelt had her first mastectomy in 1956 and would live to undergo another one twenty years later. Women of this generation simply had no sense of breast cancer as something to be shared with other women, no consciousness of undergoing a common ordeal. And without an identity of its own, the disease could not attract or cultivate the concerted attention of its victims. Lacking a public presence, it generated no media interest, expressed in either stories or statistics, to bolster its visibility.

How powerful this connection between women could be is glimpsed in Carson's correspondence with George Crile, Jr., the physician she turned to after she had undergone a radical mastectomy. In

January 1963, while she was still his patient, Crile's wife Jane died of the disease. Jane Crile had been a friend of Carson's and unusually open about her disease. Her ordeal, and her willingness to share it with Carson, had clearly provided some comfort. "When she wrote me after my visit with you two years ago, that she shared my problem, it was as though a great tide of courage flowed into me. If she, so vibrant, so gay, so full of the love of life, could live with the problem so fearlessly, I could at least try to do the same."[4]

This kind of mutual support is now so common that it is easy to take it for granted. But feminism has irrevocably altered our view of our own bodies and our sense of responsibility for them. The need to "bear up," to be courageous like Carson, now competes with the need to be angry, that is, to turn our response outward rather than inward. So much more confident have we become of our right to question everything that affects the experience of disease (our relations with professional caregivers, with research funding agencies, with insurance companies, and so on) that it becomes harder to remain sympathetic with the more self-denying behavior of earlier generations of women. We have a mistaken sense, in retrospect, that we have seen these changes coming all along, that their arrival was always a foregone conclusion and that women living before us might have done a better job of anticipating them as well.[5]

The sense of enjoying what we consider a superior perspective sometimes makes us impatient with those who came before us. We can be frustrated, for instance, by the apparent prostration of earlier generations of women before all forms of male authority, whether embodied in teachers, husbands, employers, or doctors. We lack imaginative sympathy with the limitations of their culture. It is sometimes hard, for instance, to understand a woman's enthusiasm for immediate and radical breast surgery when we now know that it is only rarely justified on medical grounds. But until very recently, almost all women facing this prospect really did believe that the so-called heroic procedure offered the only chance for survival. Unless and until the culture supports alternatives, there can be no choice and no doubt.

Just as we overestimate the resources available to earlier generations of women with breast cancer, so we also tend to underestimate the courage of those who did try to push against prevailing prejudices. Because they were fighting battles that have now been won, we lose sight of the difficulties they faced at the time. The wild success and importance of *Silent Spring* makes us overlook the considerable prejudice Carson faced throughout her life as a female scientist seeking employment. Even with impressive academic credentials including long work experience in government service, and after the publication of a critically acclaimed book (*Under the Sea Wind*), she was still turned down for jobs at both the Audubon Society and the New York Zoological Society.[6]

It is equally easy to underestimate the paternalism that Carson encountered in her role as patient. But she did, in fact, express remarkable determination in the handling of her situation. She negotiated directly with her caregivers rather than designating a husband or other male relative to serve as an intermediary; she asked for full disclosure of her condition so that she could participate directly in the choice of appropriate treatments; she expressed her lack of confidence in some of those treating her, refusing to be intimidated by any of them; she sought a second opinion from an unorthodox consultant; and, finally, she researched and pursued alternative therapies despite her doctors' lack of support for them. These aspects of her approach to treatment may seem uncontroversial today, but in the early 1960s such behavior was not just unusual; it was unheard of.

George Crile, Jr.

George Crile, Jr. ("Barney" to his friends) was almost as exceptional a correspondent as Carson herself. Born in 1907, the son of a famous surgeon and founder of the Cleveland Clinic, he played an active role in bringing the subject of cancer into the public realm. In 1955 he published a book, *Cancer and Common Sense*, that was aimed at the general public. In it, he tried to dispel some of the misconceptions surrounding the disease, and some of the terror they caused. Many of the ideas he raised in this little book, besides the very idea of a doctor appealing directly to the public, were considered highly unorthodox by the medical profession, who did not welcome them. Among these ideas was the heretical suggestion that the radical mastectomy may be no more effective in improving the chances for survival than more modest surgery. The evidence he presented in support of this idea came from a clinical trial conducted by a British surgeon. Given the universality of the Halsted mastectomy among American surgeons at the time, it would have been impossible to get support for such an experiment in the United States.

Crile also took issue with the secrecy surrounding the issue of disclosure. "Do not be afraid to ask your surgeon to tell you the truth," he urged his readers. "If you do not ask him he may evade the issue." Rachel Carson read this book; perhaps she remembered these very words. She had met Crile three years prior to its publication. Crile's wife was a member of the family that owned Halle's Department Store in Cleveland. Carson had met her there at a book-signing session for *The Sea Around Us* in November 1952 and became friends with her and her husband. Jane died of breast cancer just a year before Carson. In 1973 Crile's second wife, Helga Sandburg Crile (daughter of the poet Carl Sandburg), was also diagnosed with breast cancer. She survives her husband, who died in 1992.

A decade after Carson's death, Crile entered the fray yet again with a book called *What Women Should Know About the Breast Cancer Controversy*. Here, in a carefully worded, clear, and readable format, he presented the history of the debate surrounding radical mastectomy and marshaled evidence from clinical trials supporting the use of more conservative surgery for early stage breast cancer. For the time, it was a radical manifesto, and it earned him the outspoken contempt of some of his peers. "The trouble with Crile," one of them ranted, "is that he advocates so many goddamn different things. . . . He has introduced a sense of chaos into breast treatment. Now any surgeon can do anything he pleases for breast cancer and call upon Crile as his authority. I'm afraid that much of the progress we've made . . . will recede if you do all this crappy small stuff."[7] Small was clearly not beautiful to proponents of super-radical surgery.

Crile's position can be described as occupying the very opposite end of the surgical spectrum represented in the late nineteenth century by Halsted. Born about a half-century apart, these two men had working lives and philosophies that span the century of the radical mastectomy, from its hopeful inception through its rise to dominance to its final, much delayed exposure as a scientifically discredited and usually medically unnecessary procedure. Halsted practiced medicine at a time when surgery constituted the only treatment for breast cancer. By the end of Crile's working life, radiation and chemotherapy (including hormone therapies) had reduced surgery to only one among many alternatives.

Rachel Carson as a patient

Rachel Carson clearly would have been forgiven if she had remained the well-behaved ladylike patient she was expected to be. But she was no more orthodox in her response to this terminal illness than she had been to the manmade assaults on the natural environment that had fired her scientific imagination. But as with her battles against the giant chemical corporations, she had to be selective; she couldn't challenge the established treatment of breast cancer on all fronts. It is remarkable that she managed to confront it at all. But, without ever losing her poise, she chose to reject the role of compliant patient and to become instead an advocate for herself, to be her own "case manager" in the days before such a phrase had even been coined.

It was one thing for doctors to confer or correspond with each other behind their patient's back. It was quite another for a patient to play this game herself. Carson violated the implicit confidentiality of the doctor/patient relationship (traditionally binding on the patient but not on the doctor) by reconstructing her own narrative of illness. Relying upon the clinical detachment she understood as a scientist, she pieced together a summary of her experience which she took to Dr. Crile, a man who had been her friend before he became her consultant. She wanted a second opinion and independent advice well before such things were common practice. Her direct appeal to Crile was an end run around her own doctor. Although she hadn't objected to a radical mastectomy, she *did* object to not being told the truth, or the whole truth, about the results of this surgery. More than two years later, when looking back on her ordeal with a more experienced eye, she regretted having chosen Dr. Sanderson in the first place: "How differently I would handle it now—how carefully I would select the surgeon. It's hard to see how I could have given so little thought to the possibilities."[8] But even if her uneasiness about her doctor's response was, in the immediate aftermath of her surgery, more an apprehension than an articulated grievance, it was nonetheless sufficient to prompt her to contact Crile, generating the correspondence reproduced below.

Just how atypical Carson's response was in 1960 can be glimpsed from a breast cancer diary published in the same year. Written by a woman who described herself as a "gray-haired professor of Bible in a church-related college," it was one of the very earliest attempts by a breast cancer patient to provide a source of emotional comfort to fellow sufferers. With a foreword written by her doctor after her death, the memoir recounts anecdotes and offers advice that highlight the virtues of Christian resignation. As the author puts it, "When I first learned of the possibility of cancer, I stood on a street corner and cried inwardly, "This is too big for me to handle, Father! Please take over!"[9] Rather than actively participating in the decision-making process, she preferred to put herself in the hands of her physicians, relieved that "God has led me to efficient doctors." Carson's response could hardly be more different. She approached her own ordeal without the comfort or conviction of religious faith, relying instead on her own clear-eyed intelligence to shepherd herself over the rocky terrain of her illness.

It's hard to imagine anyone diagnosed with breast cancer in 1960 who was more aware than Rachel Carson of the controversies surrounding both the causes of cancer and many of its treatments. Her files for the cancer chapters in *Silent Spring* show an interest in the evidence of cell damage caused by manmade chemicals used in industry and agriculture; she also kept track of the possibly harmful effects of chemicals and other substances used in cancer treatments. Just months before undergoing radiotherapy herself, Carson was clipping newspaper articles suggesting that "even small amounts of radiation may entail some risk of biological damage,"[10] that there was "no threshold dose, or dose rate, below which medical x-rays fail to cause genetic mutation."[11] Her awareness of the risks of conventional treatment added to her well-documented suspicion of chemical companies as manufacturers of pesticides made her much more open to experimenting with alternative treatments that lay beyond the reach of the medical-industrial complex.

Carson insisted on running her public and personal lives on separate if parallel tracks, each one sealed off from the other. This old-fashioned code of conduct strikes a 1990s sensibility as extraordinary. We have grown so accustomed to first-person rather than third-person narratives of illness that the reticence of someone of Carson's generation and class now seems positively self-denying. By its absence in much of Carson's writing, we see that the first-person narrator in others' accounts serves in some way as the reader's protector and companion. When a story of illness is recounted in a contemporary memoir, the narrator takes the reader by the hand and leads her through every stage of the labyrinth of treatment, pausing along the way to share her reflections and interpretations of events. Most important, at the end of the story, she often puts the treatment behind her, living proof that there is a way out of the medical maze, back to "normal" life. Of course for Carson, as for Mueller before her, there wasn't a way out. The bleaker, less modulated narrative of her experience was a reflection of her writing in active battle mode rather than in peaceful retirement.

Carson's apparent professional detachment toward her illness may suggest an impoverished emotional life to the modern reader. But though even her friends could remark on her "incapacity for chit-chat," she had many close friendships. During the years of her illness, she was perhaps closest to Dorothy Freeman, a near neighbor of hers in Maine. Their letters to each other, recently published,[12] were often warm and intimate. But their correspondence also respected a code of conduct of its own, distinguishing between letters that could be shared with other family members and letters that could not (the latter were referred to as "apples" and were sometimes folded inside the former).

This unyielding sense of privacy, which valued a clear and unbridgeable separation between the public and the personal, can be hard for more modern sensibilities to grasp. Its clarity is perhaps emblematic of an earlier culture where social behavior was neatly compartmentalized, each chamber clearly defined and subject to its own set of rules.

In fact, the rigid separation of public and private experience that is built into Carson's perspective on her illness is really an accurate reflection, at the individual level, of a much more pervasive pretense that operated across society at large. The broader public refusal to acknowledge the existence or the extent of the disease or to reveal the extraordinary physical and emotional suffering it caused operated as a powerful taboo. Public denial of private anguish added the ingredient of shame to the mix of terror and pain that the disease itself inflicted. Something so terrible that it had to be hidden away—both literally and figuratively—brought disgrace rather than compassion in its wake.

In rejecting the reality of breast cancer, society dismissed as insignificant the suffering and death of all those women who experienced it. Lying beyond the limits of the public imagination, breast cancer was virtually outlawed. Any reference to it, therefore, was a dangerous and unwelcome reminder of one's outsider status.

In this context, Carson's handling of her own situation was entirely consonant with the social mores of her time. She never chafed against the prevailing conventions. For her, breast cancer simply occupied a place in two spheres of her life. As an illness that had to be treated, it became the subject of medical attention and experiment; as a personal catastrophe, it remained strictly private, hers to consider and to control. The two were not to be confounded. Even when she was visibly suffering, she worked hard to keep her pain private. "There is no reason even to say I have not been well," she urged her friend Dorothy Freeman. "If you want or think you need give any negative report, say I had a bad time with iritis that delayed my work, but it has cleared up nicely. And that you never saw me look better. . . . I know what happens when even an inkling of the other situation gets out. As last night, scraps of dinner table conversation about poor Senator Neuberger: 'You know she had a cancer operation' . . . 'They say she's down to 85 pounds' . . . That's the sort of thing I couldn't bear and the reason I have told so few people. Whispers about a private individual might not go far; about an author-in-the-news they go like wildfire."[13]

Illness was, of course, not the only aspect of one's private life to keep beyond the reach of the public, particularly in the early 1960s. The possible disclosure of sexual infidelity was a far greater threat to public reputation than the revelation of illness. Just how important it was to seal off any hint of private impropriety from public view is revealed in the media's handling of the private life of Jack Kennedy, newly elected to the presidency. The willing collusion of the press in the conceal-ment of Kennedy's promiscuity reveals the extent to which the secrecy of private life was still considered to be culturally acceptable. It also reflects the clear understanding that the "truth" was a plastic con-cept that could be easily molded to honor the terms of a "gentle-man's agreement" between the White House and the Washington press corps. It was, after all, still possible in the early 1960s for male-dominated interest groups to manage the release, exchange, and reten-tion of information as they liked, without having to answer to any higher authority. This was just as evident and unobjectionable in the corridors of Washington hospitals (where Carson was treated) as it was in any Washington press room.

To tell or not to tell?

In 1960, the unquestioned authority of the surgeon remained intact. Still almost always male, his judgment alone determined the "best in-terests" of his patient. He chose the "appropriate" treatments for her and recommended doctors to carry them out. But he also had to decide whether or not to tell her what it was she was being treated for, that is, whether or not to disclose to his patient her diagnosis of cancer. Almost universally, he chose not to tell.

A survey carried out about the time of Rachel Carson's diagnosis asked cancer surgeons "What is your usual policy about telling pa-tients? Tell? Don't tell?"[14] Ninety percent of those who responded said they would regularly withhold the truth. Only when patients refused to undergo treatment would doctors raise the stakes and introduce words and phrases calculated to signal to the patient the seriousness of her condition, in the hopes of securing her cooperation. But even then, physicians evaded the real issues, resorting to euphemisms rather than meeting the challenge head-on. Words like "lesion" or "mass" were substituted for "malignancy" and tumors were described as "precancerous" or "in the early curable stage."

The doctor's rationalization for misleading the patient was that it protected her from the despondency and loss of hope that often accompanied a cancer diagnosis. In the words of one participating physician, "I would be afraid to tell and have the patient in a room with a window."[15] But an article published at virtually the same time in the *Ladies' Home Journal* ("Should Doctors Tell the Truth to a Cancer Patient?")[16] gave a very different view of patient preferences. Reporting on a nationwide survey carried out by the Canadian Cancer Society, the story revealed that two-thirds of the women interviewed gave a "yes" answer to the question. They wanted to know the truth.

Despite physicians' insistence that their silence was motivated by a concern for the "best interests" of their patients, it was clear to some medical researchers that the issue was more complex than it appeared. There was a growing awareness beginning in the 1960s that the evasion tactics used by doctors to sidestep the word "cancer" might have as much to do with protecting the physician as with protecting the patient. Doctors too looked at a cancer diagnosis as "a death warrant" and brought their own pessimism and despair into the cancer wards. Their prevarication with patients may have had more to do with a sense of failure or with their own unexamined fear of death than with any reasoned approach to patient care.

Delay in physicians' diagnosis of their own cancers has been "well documented" since the 1930s: "Not only do physicians postpone seeking medical care, but their doctors delay further, perhaps because the diagnostician must especially avoid recognition of cancer in a patient so like himself." There was, in fact, no sound evidence that doctors could cite to link a disclosure of cancer to suicide or even to depression. There was no evidence of any kind because doctors spurned potential research into medical attitudes, preferring instead to project their "strongly held rationalizations into the vacuum of knowledge."[17]

From the 1940s on, however, a small group of medical researchers had taken up the problem of cancer disclosure,[18] so it is fair to locate the origin of the debate on truth-telling within the medical profession itself. It soon, however, attracted the interest of medical sociologists, feminists, and bioethicists, whose appearance on the scene reflected broader changes in the culture at large. But despite the burgeoning academic interest in the complexity of the doctor-patient relationship, progress in the cancer wards remained slow. As late as the mid-1970s, a decade after Carson's death, researchers could still point to an array of subterfuges that were in common use.

Medical sociologists began to classify this behavior. One identified the typical evasion of breast surgeons as a type of "functional uncertainty."[19] This was defined as the pretence of uncertainty used by doctors to disguise the underlying clinical certainty of cancer. It was a concept that allowed surgeons to pass smoothly from a positive biopsy of breast tissue to a radical mastectomy, without consulting the patient.

The following verbatim account of a breast surgeon's report to his postoperative patient illustrates the practice:

> Well . . . Miss . . . that mass in your breast contained some suspicious cells so we thought it was best to remove it. It's just as well that you had it done because in a year or so it would probably have been serious. We also took away some glands from your armpit. Although there didn't seem to be anything in them, it's always best to be on the safe side.[20]

The language used here avoids any words likely to raise alarm. Neither "malignancy" nor "mastectomy" appears. The words that are spoken suggest that the patient's breast was potentially but not actually malignant. This was clearly untrue. But it had been true until the moment the surgeon was informed that the results of the frozen tissue section taken from the patient's breast did show the presence of cancer. Up until that moment, the surgeon's clinical experience may have told him that the tumor was likely to be malignant but he could not be certain until the pathology report confirmed it. After that moment, of course, he had no further doubt. His patient, however, still remained in a state of innocence, asleep on the operating table. Although present at the time the diagnosis was revealed, she remained ignorant of it.

The fact that her surgeon was unable to communicate the results to her directly did not deter him from acting on them unilaterally, that is, without her agreement. Afterward, he simply recalled his own retrospective uncertainty about the diagnosis and stretched it to cover the mastectomy as well. More a sign of magical thinking than of scientific logic, this sleight-of-hand offered a way for the surgeon to circumvent the difficult interpersonal aspects of surgery and allowed him to focus exclusively on the technical requirements of the job.

There was no compelling medical justification for this pervasive practice of moving immediately from diagnosis to mastectomy other than the argument that it spared a woman the risks of a second round of general anesthesia.[21] But that left unexplained the necessity for performing the biopsy under a general rather than a local anesthetic in the first place. The practice of fusing diagnosis with primary surgical treatment, universal at the time of Rachel Carson's surgery, survived well into the 1980s. A study carried out years after Carson's death reported that "half of the physicians surveyed [still] thought it medically proper and thirty percent ethically proper for a physician to perform a mastectomy with no authorization from the patient other than her signature on the blanket consent form required for hospital admission."[22]

Carson never raised this as an issue. What we now routinely accept as distinctly separate stages of care (biopsy, diagnosis, decision-making, and treatments) she still regarded as one event. The progressive disaggregating of primary treatment into its constituent parts alerts us to the scale of the changes that have occurred—social as well as medical—over the past forty years. Advances in the quality of local anesthesia have been matched by the rise of "informed consent," which extended the legal doctrine of self-determination into the medical arena, requiring that patients be informed in advance of the risks and possible benefits of any procedure recommended to them.[23]

A second important strand in the complex weave of change has been the marked increase in our tolerance for cancer and in our shared beliefs about its behavior. Now that breast cancer is no longer perceived as a medical emergency, it's sometimes hard to remember that women facing surgery often believed that every moment counted and wanted their surgeons to remove the offending mass as quickly as possible, believing that days or even hours might make all the difference in "catching" the disease before it was too late. Though it's hard to picture Rachel Carson in a state of panic, she was certainly subject to the same prevailing convictions about the "dread disease." What we know of cancer biology today takes some of the urgency out of decision-making, although even now the desire to "get rid of it as quickly as possible" still colors our judgment in the doctor's office. Patients, after all, are no more immune to magic thinking than are their doctors.

The Carson/Crile correspondence, 1960–63

Although Rachel Carson was not diagnosed with breast cancer until 1960, she had had prior experience of breast disease.[24] Fourteen years earlier, in 1946, when she was 39 years old, she had had a breast cyst removed. Four years after that, a physical checkup revealed a lump in her left breast. She knew it might turn out to be serious but approached the possibility circuitously. "There is a small cyst or tumor in one breast," she wrote to her agent Marie Rodell, "which the doctor thinks I should get rid of, and I suppose it's a good idea. . . . The operation will probably turn out to be so trivial that any dope could do it; but of course there is in such cases, always the possibility that a much more drastic procedure will prove necessary." The tumor, "about walnut-size and very deep," was removed on September 21, 1950. According to her biographer, when Carson specifically asked her surgeon whether the tissue biopsy showed any evidence of malignancy, she was told it did not. Her doctors recommended no further treatment.[25]

While it is possible that this tumor was benign—benign forms of breast disease do often precede malignant disease—given Carson's subsequent medical history it seems most unlikely. If it was a cancer, how did the pathologist miss it? A negative finding on a biopsy is always inconclusive; it does not rule out the possibility of cancer cells in other parts of the tissue not sampled. But with no other reason to suspect a malignancy in a 43-year-old woman, perhaps the biopsy was less rigorous than it might have been. Or perhaps the whole tumor was not removed, despite what Carson had been told. With surgeons all too ready to perform radical mastectomies, it seems unlikely that the misdiagnosis, if that's what it was, was deliberate. And though it might be tempting to imagine that the earlier detection of Carson's cancer might have saved her life, the virulence that her disease displayed later on suggests otherwise. Earlier treatment might have prolonged her life but metastatic cancer would still have killed her.

In March 1960, ten years later, Carson discovered what she thought were more breast cysts. Surgery at Doctor's Hospital in Washington on April 4 revealed two tumors in her left breast, one "apparently benign" and the other "suspicious enough to require a radical mastectomy."[26] Carson, unlike most cancer patients at the time, had actually asked her surgeon, Dr. Sanderson, whether the tumor was malignant. Whether he was prepared for such candor is not known. He certainly did not respond in the same spirit of openness but told her instead that she had a "condition bordering on malignancy." The fact that he prescribed no follow-up treatment must have reinforced Carson's understanding that there was really nothing to worry about. But less than nine months later, she came to realize that she had been deceived.

Carson must have found Dr. Sanderson's prevarication doubly galling. As a woman who had achieved remarkable success both as a scientist and a writer at a time when women were still largely excluded from public and professional life, she would have been stunned by the paternalism of her surgeon's remarks. But as a scientist, and one who paid a high price for her own integrity (in the face of opposition from the chemical industry), she might also have seen Dr. Sanderson's lie as a kind of data falsification that violated the ethics of clinical medicine as of science. She certainly tried to preserve an impartial view of her own "case"; how could her doctor fail to do so? Whatever her reaction, it was strong enough to galvanize her to get in touch with her friend Barney Crile (Dr. George Crile, Jr.) at the Cleveland Clinic.

It was a fortuitous decision. In a sense, it lifted Carson's experience of disease out of the doctor's office and created a parallel universe for it on the page, where she felt most at home. To approach Crile, she had to draw on those very skills that had already brought her so much success—a capacity for meticulous observation coupled with considerable interpretive skills. If writing gave order to her life and engendered a sense of competence, then the very act of reconstructing her own experience, however grim the details, must nevertheless have had therapeutic value for her. The clinical detachment she displays in documenting the increasing signs of terminal illness may appear to the reader as strangely dissociated, but it might have been just what Carson needed to continue her life on a business-as-usual basis, comforted by the familiarity of the process if not by its implications. That she also relied upon writing to express more intimate reactions to her ordeal is evidenced by the letters she wrote during the same period to her friend Dorothy Freeman, excerpts from which, included below, amplify the story that enfolds in her correspondence with Crile.

DECEMBER 7, 1960
Dear Dr. Crile,
My apologies for a hand-written letter, but I've had flu and am still abed. Yesterday I tried to reach you at the clinic and learned you would return Friday, so I thought it might be as well to write you a few details, after which I shall telephone.

I hope I'm not imposing by asking your opinion on a personal medical problem but after rereading your fine book on Cancer I'm sure you can give me the advice I need on how to proceed.

Briefly, this is the story. During the past 12 years or so, I'd had two operations for breast tumors, both benign. Then last March it was discovered I had two more in the same breast. An operation was advised. The preliminary sections in the operating room aroused enough suspicion that a radical mastectomy was performed. However, the permanent sections did not reveal definite malignancy, although something was said about "changes." No follow-up with radiation was considered necessary.

All was presumably well until early November when a curious, hard swelling appeared on the 3rd or 4th rib on the operated side, at or near the junction with the sternum. At first I wasn't sure I was seeing anything, but within a week or 10 days it became obvious enough to send me to my internist and at his suggestion to my surgeon. X-ray pictures were taken and are said to show that the swelling is not the rib itself, but something lying between rib and skin. (It is, however, very hard, and not moveable.) Although both doctors acknowledge it "may" have some connection with the former trouble, they profess to be puzzled. With no further diagnostic work, they recommended x-ray therapy. The man I was referred to may be quite competent, but he does not specialize in therapy.

I had treatments last week—Nov. 28 and 29—and promptly became ill with what was first said to be either an unexpected reaction or flu. Presumably it was the latter, for I've been in bed a week with fever, aching and nausea. No more treatments, of course.

At least this has given me time to think and I now feel the whole procedure has been rather slap-dash in an area where that is hardly desirable! I have told the doctor (whom I've known for many years so it was easy to talk it over) that I don't want to resume these treatments at least until we have had a new evaluation of the whole thing by someone else.

Now this is where my problem lies—where my questions to you come in. What *kind* of person do you think I should see? And what kind of investigation should I wish to have made in order to determine first, whether this is anything significant, and assuming it is, which of a variety of treatments would make sense? I don't want to get into the hands of an over-zealous surgeon. And I know too well that both radiation and chemo-therapy are two-edged swords.

Perhaps you can make recommendations of actual names here in Washington. If not, knowing the kind of person you would go to would help.

Several medically well informed people have suggested Dr. Louis Alpert, who is Medical Director of the Warwick Cancer Clinic here at George Washington Hospital. Dr. Alpert himself specializes in chemotherapy. However, all types of therapy are used at the clinic and I suppose an attempt would be made to fit the treatment to the situation. However, I know the Clinic is working in chemotherapy under a grant from NIH [National Institutes of Health]—which, of course is eager to have more and more chemicals tested, and all this makes me feel just a little like a guinea pig!

I'm sure this has given you the picture and that you will understand my need of understanding advice. I want to do what must be done, but no more. After all, I still have several books to write, and can't spend the rest of my life in hospitals!!

Since I do want to see someone next week, I shall try to reach you at the Clinic Friday afternoon. Of course I shall be very grateful for your help.

Sincerely,
Rachel Carson

This letter provides a baseline narrative for the treatment scenario that follows. It also inadvertently betrays more evidence of the doctors' prevarication. Carson writes that her doctors "profess to be puzzled" by the hard swellings that appeared between her ribs on the side of her operation. But having eliminated (through x-ray) the possibility that the swelling was caused by the rib itself, and knowing that tumors do not show up on film, they knew almost for a certainty that the hard mass was malignant.

In responding to Carson's appeal, Crile asked for her medical records to be forwarded to him. Dr. Michel Healy, Carson's internist, replied that "Dr. Sanderson did not tell Miss Carson that she had a malignancy, but said that she had a condition bordering on a malignancy. Because of [this] . . . her present management is quite difficult."

Carson had by now figured it all out herself. "I know now that I was not told the truth last spring at the time of my operation," she wrote to her editor Paul Brooks at Houghton Mifflin. "The tumor was malignant, and there was even at that time evidence that it had metastasized, for some of the lymph nodes also were found to be involved. But I was told none of this, even though I asked directly. . . . My doctors still tried to keep me in the dark by pretending to be puzzled, but did recommend radiation. I had actually started treatment just before I got flu. But by that time I was beginning to realize the deception, and while laid up with flu did a lot of thinking, the result of which was a decision that I wanted a more skilled judgement brought to bear on the problem than any then concerned with it."[27]

Crile was an exceptionally good choice for Carson. He was interested in her work, not intimidated by her formidable intelligence or reputation, and he was a writer himself. He was also quite knowledgeable about the disease and, for a surgeon, remarkably open-minded about what constituted appropriate treatment. He assured Carson's radiologist that he had been "much interested in radiotherapy for breast cancer for a number of years . . . so perhaps I do know a little bit more about what to expect . . . than some surgeons who have employed it only under quite hopeless circumstances."[28] He was something of a maverick in his own profession. His early and visible stand against radical mastectomy was underlined by his refusing to perform one after 1955. In this, he had exposed himself to the same kind of criticism and scorn that Carson herself regularly experienced at the hands of the chemical-industrial complex. Most reassuring to Carson, perhaps, he met her request for candor head on. Just as he had advocated in his 1955 book on cancer, he told Carson the truth about her situation, that is, that she had cancer and that it had spread to her lymph nodes.

In considering a treatment plan for his patient, Crile had access to all the therapies available today, with one important exception—chemotherapy. This is the primary systemic treatment now prescribed for patients with breast cancers at all stages. At the time of Carson's illness, the NIH had just started its first clinical trial of a drug (thiotepa) designed specifically to control breast cancer, but Carson did not enroll in it. The absence of any of these drugs from Crile's armamentarium left him with hormone therapies as the only available treatments that could address Carson's cancer as a systemic disease rather than a local one.

But to start her off, he recommended only local radiation to the area where she had had surgery. Before undergoing that treatment, however, he wanted her to have her ovaries removed (oophorectomy).[29] Carson, at 53, was still menstruating and therefore still producing estrogen. Crile reasoned that removing estrogenic stimulation from her body would tell him whether the tumor was hormone-sensitive or not. If it shrank as a result of estrogen deprivation, then the association was positive. This was intelligent and appropriate treatment and the suggested sequencing was a part of it. If the radiation had been done first and been followed by sterilization, it would have been impossible to identify any estrogenic effects that might have been present.

Carson must have been relieved by this initial response and comforted by the kind of relationship it promised. Whatever her feelings, they prompted a more reflective and poignant follow-up letter. In it, Carson reveals attitudes and behavior that may be common today but that were unprecedented in 1960.

DECEMBER 17, 1960
Dear Barney,
Ever since early November when my problem became apparent I had been trying to clarify my own initially obscure ideas of the kind of person I wanted to ask for a solution. Now it seems to me strange that in the very beginning I did not think in large enough terms to think of going to Cleveland and to you. Your kind of mind combines everything I wanted, and it would be hard to express fully the feeling of relief I have now that the direction of the treatment is in your hands.

You smiled when I suggested that medicine could ever be scientific, but one of the things I appreciate in you, and one of the things I mean by "scientific," is your awareness of what is *not* known and your unwillingness to rush in with procedures that may disrupt that unknown but all-important ecology of the body cells.

I appreciate, too, your having enough respect for my mentality and emotional stability to discuss all this frankly with me. I have a great deal more peace of mind when I feel I know the facts, even though I might wish they were different.

There is much more I might say, but I want to report a couple of developments. In conversation with Dr. Healy yesterday I learned that

Dr. Andrews will be out of town until Monday. Dr. Healy will call him then, but is quite doubtful that he will undertake my case. This apparently is based on his own experience in trying to refer cases to NIH, and meeting with no success unless they fitted into some project underway.

Dr. Healy mentioned several other radiologists (including the Washington Clinic's Dr. Cole, who started this work, who is not a specialist on therapy, and for various reasons is not one I want to return to.) At that point I said that if he encountered difficulty with Dr. Andrews I would ask that he not contact anyone else, but return the problem to you, for I felt that on the basis of your own associations with Dr. Andrews you might be able to get him to make an exception and undertake it.

If, because of some NIH red tape, even that does not work, I am going to ask, Barney, that you make the alternative suggestions, and that you be the one to discuss the problem directly with whatever radiologist is going to undertake it, and work out the procedure with him and not through a third party.

I know I am speaking very bluntly and undiplomatically (and that is why I have marked this letter "personal") but in a matter of such importance I am just not willing to let what I achieved by going to you be destroyed by any little professional associations here. Dr. Healy is a fine internist and usually a very open-minded man, but if I had felt him fully competent to advise on this problem I would not have gone to Cleveland! He is associated with Dr. Cole at the Clinic, and perhaps it is natural that he should be trying to keep Dr. Cole in the picture, but I cannot go along with this. There was enough mention of Dr. Cole's opinions and procedures yesterday that I had a feeling that it will take a little diplomacy to ensure that he does not have a voice in the way this is handled. That is one reason for repeating my request that arrangements be made directly by you with the radiologist.

What I should like, of course, would be to be able to come to Cleveland and let you and your staff handle it, but because of my little household that would present some pretty large difficulties.[30] But I want to come as close to that as possible, and I think it can be done if you, in whatever way you think proper, will let it be understood that I am your patient and you are directing the procedures.

I shall promise not to burden you with a spate of letters like this, but it does seem most important to get this started on the right foot.

It was such a delight to visit all of you, and I did thoroughly enjoy all of our conversation. Don't be too surprised if I ask you to read a little chunk of manuscript some time.

Again my deepest gratitude.

Sincerely,

Rachel

Crile responded immediately.

DECEMBER 22, 1960

Dear Rachel,

First let me thank you for your lovely letter. I am glad that you feel as you do. I have always believed that intelligent people in responsible positions not only wish to know as much as possible about any ailment they have, but also that such people are entitled to know everything that is known about such ailments.

The lovely blonde poinsettia arrived at our house last night, and all of us have been admiring it. . . . Of course, I would be greatly flattered and delighted to read any manuscript that you send on.

With best wishes in your work and for the Holiday Season, I remain,

Yours very sincerely,

Barney

Crile arranged for Carson to see Dr. Ralph Caulk, chief radiologist at the Washington Hospital Center. In January 1961, she underwent sterilization and subsequently began a course of daily radiation treatments, which ended in mid-March. Soon after the sterilization, Carson was optimistic about its effects. She wrote to Dorothy Freeman: "Dr Caulk is inclined to agree with me that there is already a suggestion of shrinkage. He confirms my thought that once we are sure it is going down, he can go ahead with local radiation." The next day she wrote again, "As I understood Dr. Crile's estimate, the chances that the swelling would go down on withdrawal of hormone stimulation were 50–50."[31]

In addition to cancer, Carson had long been suffering from arthritis. Her efforts to locate the best treatment for this condition provide a wonderful example of Carson the irrepressible scientific sleuth. Like today's newly diagnosed and educated patient, she turned to the medical journals, confident that they would provide her with the information she needed to make an informed decision. She also tracked down a well-known specialist in the field but was not prepared to accept either his diagnosis or his recommendations for treatment without subjecting them to her own critical assessment—and to that of Crile.

Later on, her longstanding arthritic condition would make it harder to recognize the first signs of metastases to the bone.

MARCH 18, 1961
Dear Barney,

I have been waiting for my various problems to settle down a bit before bringing you up to date. Now, besides reporting, I want to ask you a question or two, so will go ahead.

I am to see Dr. Caulk next Tuesday for a check-up, following completion of radiation about two weeks ago. He will report all details to you after he examines me, so I'll just give the general facts. In order to get the radiation of the tumor started, I spent a week in the hospital beginning February 12. By the following week, I was able to make daily trips to the hospital via car, wheel chair, and assorted bearers and pushers, so it was quite a safari each day, but we managed it. I was supposed to be having 10 treatments, but no real change in size or appearance of the tumor was evident until the 8th or 9th treatment, so the course was extended to 14. By that time (two weeks ago) it was definitely shrinking. This it has continued to do, although I can still clearly see a slight circular bulge. Whether this is satisfactory progress of course I don't know until you and Dr. Caulk have spoken.

My joint problem has held the center of the stage since January 18th. After we last talked Dr. Darrell Crain, a specialist in arthritic disease, came to the house and I have been under his care ever since. He felt my difficulty had all the earmarks of acute infectious arthritis . . . and has continued to give me weekly injections of hydrocortisone in both knees and the ankle. It was a month before I could even stand, and at that time putting any weight on my feet was agony. . . .

Now this is where my major question to you comes in. Dr. Crain suggested that in order to speed things along, he might want to use intramuscular injections of gold. As you know, I'm not an especially tractable patient, and don't just go along with such things without doing some inquiring and thinking on my own. I know just enough about the use of gold to be reluctant. I know, for example, that one of its toxic effects can be exerted on the bone marrow. My feeling about this is that I've already had to subject my bone marrow to a certain abuse via radiation. There, I had no alternative, but in this case I wonder whether it might be preferable to put up with a certain amount of arthritis rather than do something that might tip the scales and bring on really serious trouble.

Does my hesitation make sense? I would really like very much to have your opinion.

I have every reason to feel that Dr. Crain is excellent in his field. . . . But I feel that, like most specialists, he is looking chiefly at his own problem without much regard for the whole picture, which by this time is rather complicated. . . .

Aren't you, or you and Jane, coming to Washington this spring? Do let me know if you are, and have a little time to spare. Perhaps I could meet you down town if you haven't time to come out here.

My warmest greetings to you both.

Sincerely,

Rachel

Crile spoke with an arthritis specialist he knew, a Dr. Scherbel, who confirmed for Carson that Dr. Crain was "an excellent authority in the field." Scherbel did not feel that any harm would be done by the gold treatment suggested by Crain but thought there were simpler ways of doing the same thing. He had had good results with nitrogen mustard mixed with cortisone and injected directly into the joints.

MARCH 23, 1961

Dear Barney,

. . . Re the proposed gold treatment, I find Goodman and Gilman's *Pharmacological Basis of Therapeutics* specifically says this treatment must not be used for patients who have recently had radiation! So I guess my hunch was not far off. They characterize the treatment of arthritis with gold as treating a "disease of unknown etiology with a drug of unknown action." And really I'm not in such desperate condition that the various risks that attend the use of gold seem justified.

From comments given me anonymously by an authority at N.I.H. I judge that this diagnosis of rheumatoid arthritis may be rather shaky, and I felt yesterday that perhaps you had the same feeling.

We shall coast along and venture nothing new until after I have seen you.

Sincerely,

Rachel

That same day she confided to a friend that she was "now itching to get to the N.I.H. library for some reading on arthritis."

Two days later she wrote to Dorothy Freeman, "from my work at the N.I.H. library, I was familiar with the standard reference work on the pharmacology of various drugs, and knew that details were always included on any adverse effects, precautions to be taken, etc. I asked [a friend] to read the section on gold for me. The whole picture of its hazards is pretty appalling, but for me the high point in the account is the specific and urgent statement that gold should not be administered to any person who has recently undergone a course of radiation! So there I had the answer to my own hunch. Yet this man, knowing perfectly well I'd just had radiation, was quite ready to give it to me. What this does to my already great cynicism about doctors you can perhaps imagine."[32]

When Carson next returned to Caulk in March 1962, she reported her discovery of hard, painful lumps in the lymph glands of her right side. This was the first evidence of her cancer showing up outside the radiated area. The lymph nodes of the left internal mammary chain run close to those on the right and Carson's cancer appears to have crossed over from one to the other; this is called contralateral spread. It indicated that she was no longer benefiting from the hormone response following her sterilization. The protective effect of the removal of her ovaries had lasted for a year and a half. (From this result, an oncologist today would estimate that she would be likely to benefit from a second line of hormone therapy, but for a period only half as long.)

Carson flew to Cleveland to seek Crile's advice. His biopsy revealed gross involvement of the whole mammary chain on her right side. He recommended to Dr. Caulk that he proceed with field radiation of the axilla and supraclavicular region (that is, under her arm and at the base of her neck). Carson began these treatments mid-March, 1962, and suffered from their side effects: "There is now considerable skin reaction, especially under the arm. Rather like a sunburn, and very sore. Nivea cream helps some. Dr. Biskind told me heavy doses of CVP would help on the radiation sickness, and in other ways reduce the ill effects, especially by reducing destruction of capillaries. I wish I'd called him, for ideally I should have started a week before radiation. He feels, also, that faithful use of the liver compound will help in the control of the malignancy. This agrees with much experimental work I've read. I must try to stay with it. But such an array of medicines! Marie once said her answer to the question of what to take to a desert island would have to be 'a pharmacist'. Mine too."[33] Another enlarged and painful node was soon discovered deep in her armpit, indicating that the radiation had not been successful in stopping the cancer's spread.

Carson had corresponded with Dr. Biskind as part of her research into effects of pesticides on human health. Biskind, a world-renowned nutritionist and retired toxicologist, had made himself unpopular with the chemical industry by presenting damaging evidence at hearings to amend the Pure Food and Drug Act. Carson trusted his judgment.[34] Now she was consulting him again, this time regarding nutritional approaches to her cancer, a remarkably original involvement at the time for either patient or physician. "He has great confidence in the anticancer factor present somewhere in the B-complex—it isn't known exactly where so that is why he urges a whole-liver preparation. This is borne out by research I'm familiar with—animal studies, I mean. Dr.

B. has had patients on such a program who have simply had no recurrences, even though the cancer had metastasized at surgery. Of course one should also make a strong effort to eliminate the chlorinated hydrocarbons from one's food, because they cause loss of the B vitamins and also damage the liver. But civilization has made it so very difficult to do that!"[35]

Caulk told Carson that she would soon have to undergo yet more radiation, of about two weeks' duration. She confessed to Dorothy Freeman "that there had been pain and soreness recently quite far up in the armpit, and that I thought I felt 'something.' And I did—there is another enlarged node. It is just about on the border line of the former treatment area—would have received some radiation but not enough to prevent its going bad. Dr. C[aulk] does not want to resume immediately, and will try to wait until after my Easter trip—if I go. I'm to see him a week from Thursday and he will see how it's developing and decide.

"I was quite prepared for this, as I intimated, because the pain one night was quite definite, and something new. It has not continued, but soreness has. There has also been soreness in the neck, and of course I was afraid of new trouble there, but Dr. C. says it is just the effect of treatment. So that was good news. Also, a report on the spinal X-rays showed nothing but some arthritis quite consistent with my age. I may not have told you there was some concern because my back hurt while lying on the treatment table, so Dr. C. wanted pictures. The trouble with this business is that every perfectly ordinary little ailment looks like a hobgoblin, and one lives in a little private hell until the thing is examined and found to be nothing much."[36]

If Carson's breast cancer took her to a private hell, the publication of her book *Silent Spring* in June 1962 brought her undreamed-of public acclaim. Given the increasing pace of her symptoms, her treatments, and their side effects, it seems astonishing that she had another life at all, let alone one that required the prolonged concentration, imagination, intellectual rigor, and passionate commitment to its subject that a book like *Silent Spring* would have done. Would such an achievement have been possible if its author had not maintained such a rigid separation between her lives? As a professional woman of her generation, Carson was already quite familiar with the need to keep up a firewall between her working life and her private life; she would not have been tempted to display photographs of her loved ones on her desk at work. But her determination, like her intelligence, seems also to have been exceptional. As she put it, "It was something I believed in so deeply that there was no other course; nothing that ever happened made me even consider turning back."[37]

Her doctors may, in some small way, have felt themselves to have been midwives to this book. They were clearly pleased to see it in print. Caulk acknowledged its publication to Crile and he responded: "It has been very satisfactory to me to know that she has been able to complete her book, and it is with great pleasure that I have been reading the installments of it currently running in the *New Yorker*."

The pain in her back did not abate. X-rays of her spine taken in December by Dr. Caulk revealed no change in her condition. When the pain failed to subside, Caulk, fearing metastases, advised five radiation sessions to her back. Crile concurred, saying that it might take two or three weeks to get the pain under control. "If it really is a metastasis, then we have gotten it quite early, before any real damage has been done. So there is much reason for optimism."

Jane Crile died at the end of January, 1963, of breast cancer that had metastasized to the brain. In February, Carson's visit to Dr. Caulk revealed new lymph tumors above the collarbone, midway to the shoulder and another higher in the neck.[38] Although Crile was reassuring, it was clear that Carson's cancer had metastasized to her bones.

FEBRUARY 17, 1963

Dear Barney,

You have been much in my mind. . . . I am glad you have the book to work on, and above all, glad you and Jane had those months to work on it together, giving it form and substance. It may be emotionally hard in some ways for you to carry it through to completion, and yet I think it will be a satisfaction.

Jane meant many things to me—a friend I loved and greatly admired, and a tower of strength in my medical problems. When she wrote me, after my visit with you two years ago, that she shared my problem, it was as though a great tide of courage flowed into me. If she, so vibrant, so gay, so full of the love of life, could live with the problem so fearlessly, I could at least try to do the same. Over the months since then the feeling I've had could best be explained by an analogy. Once, years ago, my mother and I were driving at night in uninhabited, unfamiliar country near the North Carolina coast. For the 50 or more miles through those wooded lowlands we were able to follow the lights of a car ahead. As long as it progressed smoothly I knew our way was clear. Jane was that kind of reassuring light to me. Now, without that light to follow, I admit my courage is somewhat shaken.

But you, Barney, for different reasons, are also a great source of strength. So now I'm writing you of my current problems. I didn't want to bother you while Jane was ill, and for that matter the more important ones have just happened, or at least have just been noticed.

First: I finally saw a cardiologist, Dr. Bernard Walsh, about three weeks ago. I definitely have angina[39] (even the cardiogram is now abnormal, but he said the diagnosis was perfectly clear from symptoms alone) of the less common type in which the pains come on without physical provocation, the worst ones during sleep. Dr. Walsh said frankly the implications are serious and it is most important to get the situation under control. So—I'm virtually under house arrest, not allowed to go anywhere (except as you will see later) no stairs, no exertion of any kind. I had to rent a hospital bed for sleeping in a raised position. . . .

The second problem is in your department. About two weeks ago I noticed a tender area above the collar bone on the left (operated) side, and on exploring found several hard bodies I took to be lymph nodes. Dr. Caulk was just going out of town for several days and said he would come to the house on his return. By that time I was so sure I was going to need treatment that I just had myself taken down to see him. . . . They are definitely lymph nodes "gone bad," some lying fairly well up in the neck. This is the side opposite last year's trouble spots and is an area never previously treated. So we have begun—5-minute treatment 3 days a week to keep my hospital trips to a minimum.

Now there is a further complication. At the time I went in about my back in December I kept making remarks about having "arthritis" in my left shoulder, but no one paid much attention. It has been increasingly painful, and now there is some difficulty about certain arm movements. I had begun to have suspicions, so now I've tackled Dr. Caulk about it again. They took a picture Friday and there does seem to be trouble. He let me see the x-rays. It is the coracoid process of the scapula—the edge of it looks irregular and sort of eroded. For some reason Dr. Caulk seems rather puzzled—says he wants some of his associates to look at it and may want a picture from another angle, but on the whole he does feel it is a metastasis.

Well, all this brings questions in my own mind, which leaps to conclusions that may or may not be justified. Oh—the back trouble cleared up, but so slowly that Dr. Caulk had about decided it wasn't a metastasis. Treatment was begun just before Christmas and completed December 31. I was still in considerable pain in mid-January. Then rather rapid improvement set in and now it's ok. But now this bone deterioration in the shoulder makes me think all the more I had a metastasis in the spine. Dr. C. says not necessarily, but I think he's just trying to reassure me.

Barney, doesn't this all mean the disease has moved into a new phase and will now move more rapidly to its conclusion? You told me last year that it might stay in the lymph nodes for years, but that if it began going into bone, etc., that would be a different story. If this is the correct interpretation I feel I need to know. I seem to have so many matters I need to arrange and tidy up, and it is easy to feel that in such matters there is plenty of time. I still believe in the old Churchillian determination to fight each battle as it comes, ("We will fight on the beaches—" etc.) and I think a determination to win may well postpone the final battle. But still a certain amount of realism is indicated, too. So I need your honest appraisal of where I stand.

Jane continues to give me courage. Kay told me of her question to the doctors: "Which of you is in charge of not giving up?" How like her! Well, I nominate you to that post. I would like so much to discuss some of this with you, and wonder if you'd call me some day soon. . . .

My love to the children. As ever,
Rachel

Caulk wrote to Crile on March 6 to report on the completion of Carson's radiation therapy. This had been directed to the lower left cervical, supraclavicular, and subclavicular areas of the neck. Caulk informed Crile that "the areas treated have undergone excellent involution [shrinkage]." Carson received further radiation to her left shoulder, which provided some benefit in terms of pain relief, and to a left rib, which showed little improvement. "As agreed upon, we will observe the effect of the current dose of x-ray therapy upon her pain, and at such time that the pain in these areas recur or new areas of bone pain occur, we will then consider institution of androgen therapy for a one-month trial to determine if the current tumor will prove to be endocrine sensitive." (Androgen was thought to antagonize estrogens by competing with them but some of its possible side effects—beard growth, acne, and the deepening of the voice—were clearly undesirable.)

In mid-March Carson decided to try Krebiozen, an unproven anticancer substance circulating in the 1950s and 1960s whose story was a bit like that of laetrile in the 1970s.[40] Krebiozen was a substance advertised as a serum extract from horses injected with a deadly fungus. Later tests revealed that it contained mineral oil and a form of creatine, a substance normally excreted by the body. Neither of these components has any proven anticancer activity.

In July of 1962, the government blocked interstate trade of the drug. Krebiozen users protested soon after and picketed the White House, with placards that announced their demonstration as a "Death Watch. We want to live. Krebiozen is our life-line."[41] The next year, the federal government carried out a comprehensive evaluation of the records of 500 patients who had allegedly benefited from this treatment but found no evidence of any therapeutic effects. Despite this, Carson was still willing to give it a try but had to find a physician in Washington willing to give her the injections. Caulk did not want her to have it but not because he knew it was ineffective. "I hope we can avoid having her receive the Krebiozen," he wrote to Crile, "because if any coincidental improvement should accrue, such benefit by a well-known person as she, would give the sponsors of this product unwarranted support."[42]

APRIL 3, 1963

Dear Barney:

Dr. Caulk tells me he has heard from you and that you approved his decision to resume radiation of the spine when the new x-rays showed damage of the vertebra. I was sure you would agree that there was no time to be lost. I've just completed the new series. Heaven knows (and I suppose Dr. Caulk does) with how much radiation that poor vertebra has been bombarded; I've certainly lost count and I must say I'm somewhat discouraged for I still go about stiffly and painfully. But it was slow to yield in December, so perhaps time will bring some improvement.

I am about 99 percent sure you will not approve of what I'm about to tell you, but at least I hope you will not feel actually opposed to it. Perhaps I should preface this by saying that I am unable to feel any enthusiasm about the hormone approach for the present. If I understand you correctly, the use of testosterone would be only a means of determining hormone dependence of the tumor, and would not, in itself constitute a continuing or final treatment. This, it is my understanding, would be adrenalectomy and/or removal or destruction of the pituitary[43]—either of which I would at present be most reluctant to submit to. And according to reports I've seen recently from the *J.A.M.A.* [*Journal of the American Medical Association*], neither promises a great deal, really, in terms of prolongation of life.

With this preamble, I shall then tell you that I have recently looked over all the available information on Krebiozen and have decided I want to give it a trial. I'm not expecting miracles. I'm well aware there is no claim it is a cure, and also aware it is a 50–50 chance as to whether I'd be helped at all. But if I'm in the lucky 50 percent bracket, I feel I might live more comfortably and perhaps somewhat longer than otherwise and avoid the side effects of hormones. There is, of course, no reason why I could not also have further radiation if it should be indicated.

I have discussed this with Dr. Healy and he is willing to give me the injections. I've also brought up the subject with Dr. Caulk and, as I really expected, he is not in favor—simply for the negative reason that he doubts it will do any good. My answer was that as far as I've been able to learn it will do no harm, so what do I have to lose?

I am well aware of the controversy over Krebiozen and of the AMA's longstanding war against the Foundation and Dr. Ivy[44]—but then I have seldom if ever found myself in agreement with the AMA! Their attacks on Krebiozen resemble so closely some of the methods used against those critical of pesticides that the parallel is quite suggestive. . . .

I hope you will at least view this venture of mine indulgently, Barney. If it gets me nowhere we can then think about other things later. If the past few months are typical there will be no dearth of symptoms to work on.

My best to you and the children.

As ever,

Rachel

APRIL 5, 1963

Dear Rachel,

I know how discouraging it is to have the tumor popping up unexpectedly here and there, and I do not blame you at all for wishing to employ some agent, which has the possibility of effecting systemic control. In so far as the use of Krebiozen is concerned, I have nothing at all against it. It becomes rather expensive, but that is a minor consideration and the one good thing about it is that I have never known it to do any harm. The difficulty with Krebiozen is, of course, that no one knows exactly how it is prepared and what it is, nor have there ever been any clinical trials made of it with objective controls.

I have known at least fifteen patients who have been treated with Krebiozen and have followed their course. I have never seen any indication that the drug was effective in the cases that I watched, although one of our orthopedic surgeons did note what he considered to be a regression of an embryonal type of sarcoma following its use. I think the main thing in the treatment of this disease is to keep busy doing something, and certainly Krebiozen would be as good as anything else except hormones.

I think you are underestimating a little the potential benefit of hormones, because there are well-documented cases in which patients with extensive systemic metastasis have obtained remissions of from four to six years. One of these I had occasion to document followed prolonged use of large doses of stilbestrol, and I have observed a number of remissions following hypophysectomy [removal of the pituitary gland] that have lasted from two to four years. We are at present in the course of developing a very simple method of ablating the hypophysis by radioactive yttrium. We have now done about twenty patients, to date there has been no morbidity or mortality, and the ablation appears to be just as complete as following the formidable operation of hypophysectomy. The radioactive material is inserted through the nose under stereoscopic image amplifier control so that it can be positioned exactly in the center of the sella turcica. Doctor Dohn in our Neurosurgical Department has had a great deal of experience with this type of implantation, because he does all of the steretactic destructions of brain tissue for Parkinson's disease and so forth. I think that this is going to replace all other forms of major endocrine ablation and that it will give just as high (40 percent) incidence of objective remissions as did hypophysectomy.

What I would do if I were you would be to go right ahead with Krebiozen for the present, and I hope that you will be fortunate enough to obtain a remission from its use. If not, however, I would certainly go directly to yttrium implantation which involves none of the side effects of the use of male hormones and gives the maximum chance for prolonged remission.

. . . . Keep up the good work, Rachel, and remember that the endocrine approach to the problem of breast cancer employs alterations in the specific chemicals that control the growth of specific tumors. This is the type of biologic specificity that you are looking for in your ecological problems and that to date have shown the greatest promise in the control of malignant tumors.

With best wishes. . . .

Yours very sincerely,

Barney

Carson began Krebiozen injections in April and stopped in July. The drug had no effect on her symptoms or pain whatsoever. In September she was back at the Washington Hospital Center for more tests. She wrote to Dorothy Freeman, "I've been x-rayed practically from chin to ankles . . . there is new trouble. All of the pelvic bones on the left side are involved, and there is ample explanation for the pain and lameness I've experienced most of the summer."[45] Caulk conferred with Crile and, with Carson's consent, decided to begin a course of testosterone phosphorus to ease her pain. On each of three days in the beginning of October, she was given an injection of phosphorus for the control of pain. By October 23, the phosphorus still had not had any positive effect.

She then began to experience numbness in her right arm which gave her difficulty writing. There was new involvement in her upper back and numbness in her right hand. Dr. Caulk and Dr. Healy, disappointed with the results of the phosphorus, decided to try a regimen of steroids which Crile recommended to suppress Carson's adrenal function and so—he hoped—to slow down the metastatic spread.

Carson confessed to Dorothy Freeman that she minded "the difficulty in my arms most. When I drop something it is almost impossible to pick it up. . . . I believe . . . that for the most part I do manage to be 'matter of fact' in my own thinking about the situation. Oh, I don't deny there are periods of depression and of dark thoughts. There is still so much I want to *do*, and it is hard to accept that in all probability, I must leave most of it undone. And just when I have attained the power to achieve so much I feel is important! Strange, isn't it? And there are times when I get so tired of the pain and especially the crippling that if it were not for those I love most, I'd want it to end soon. But I seldom feel that way."[46]

In November Crile sent Carson to see a neurologist, Dr. Hunstead, about the pain in her hand and arms. He told her he wasn't sure that the trouble was metastasis to the bone—"says it could perhaps be arthritic. And the upper vertebra that has been giving some trouble is definitely not the cause, for it would not affect the right nerves. This proves the wisdom of consulting someone who really knows the anatomy, etc. I'm sure Dr. Caulk would just have gone ahead and treated that vertebra. So once again I'm indebted to Barney for sensible advice."[47]

By the end of November, her hand still showed no improvement. Caulk arranged for her to have some x-rays of her neck vertebra which revealed trouble at the base of her skull. A large area of her back was irradiated. Caulk took in "a rather long area, beginning about the base of my skull, all the cervical vertebrae, and I guess a few of the dorsal. On further study he found one of them has undergone compression, so my troubles are easily understood. Applying hindsight, it would seem all this might have been deduced from the symptoms in my hands and the treatment started weeks ago. But I guess that there was still faith in the phosphorus; no doubt it is hard to know. Anyway he thinks that in time my hands will improve."[48]

Carson knew that her disease was by now "widely disseminated." Dr. Caulk, she wrote, "a very kind-hearted man, said yesterday, 'I do hate to be the purveyor of so much bad news to you.' Then he added, 'But you know, it is three years since you first came to me, and you had very serious problems then.' I felt that he left unsaid, 'Don't expect too much more time.' "[49]

From this point until her death three months later, the symptoms became an onslaught. She lost her sense of smell and taste. A few weeks later she was put on prednisone and antibiotics and then hospitalized with staphococcal meningitis and shingles, a common side effect of radiation. From mid-February on, she suffered from uncontrollable nausea. Blood tests revealed severe anemia, another consequence of radiation to her vertebrae, and a condition that could well have put her heart under greater stress. When she failed to respond to other measures, she received four or five blood transfusions at home. These relieved her nausea and made her feel stronger. Crile and Caulk both agreed that it might be a good time to try the hypophysectomy. Some of her friends disagreed. She took her doctors' advice and flew for the last time to Cleveland. On March 18, doctors implanted radioactive yttrium-90 to kill functioning pituitary tissue. For nearly a week, Carson lay near death, severely jaundiced and suffering from serious heart irregularities. Gradually, her clinical condition stabilized but on April 14 she suffered a heart attack and died.

Engaging the enemy

After reading this correspondence, it becomes much easier to understand why the experience of cancer relies so heavily on military metaphors. The relentless succession of symptoms and side effects that Carson experienced really was a bombardment. Over the last two years of her life, the pace seemed hardly to let up. And yet we know that, however time-consuming, debilitating, and demoralizing the treatments, they did not succeed in destroying the other lives (both private and professional) that Carson worked so hard to seal off from her illness. She kept up a furious pace of lectures and professional engagements held to honor her work. She stayed in touch with a wide circle of friends and colleagues. It is almost as though she believed that she could safeguard these other lives by cordoning them off from her breast cancer. And the weapon she used to encircle her disease was, of course, her writing. If the charms of language could pacify illness, Rachel Carson would surely have recovered. Her very attentiveness to her disease, her flattering chronicle of all its manifestations, were an implicit recognition of its awful power. She fought back with the only artillery she had. Her writing had, after all, proved remarkably effective in the battle against the chemical giants, where the odds against her were surely no less. Perhaps that same defiance could prove itself once again.

Carson's writing never failed her. Wherever she found herself in possession of a few free moments—in airplanes, under hair dryers, in hospital cafeterias, even while undergoing treatment—she reached for a pen and paper. So perhaps it is not surprising that her writing kept up with the accelerating pace of her illness despite the extraordinary obstacles that illness put in her path. Perhaps most cruelly for a writer, the metastatic spread to her spinal column sent pain and numbness down her right arm to her right hand, her writing hand. Yet even this difficulty did not stop her putting her thoughts into words. It was as though she believed that as long as she could muster the imaginative capacity to observe and interpret, she would remain a contender. In other words, as long as she was writing, she was not dying.

Something of this same impulse infects the writing of contemporary memoirs as well. Keeping up with one's disease demonstrates a willingness to engage with the enemy on its own terms. Finding out how it behaves—what treatments inhibit its growth, what treatments it ignores, who it kills, who it spares—is one tactic that may contribute to the design of a larger defensive strategy. Gathering evidence from whatever source (medical journals, media, friends, doctors) may have a protective value in itself, perhaps simply by enhancing the illusion of preparedness.

But the written chronicle of illness from diagnosis to death, exemplified by these letters, is also clearly an exercise of mind, one that allowed Carson to apply the skills she was most familiar with, in a process of observation and analysis with which she was entirely at home. It is the consistency of her approach, the identifying marks of her own intellectual rigor, that, revealing itself wherever she turned, created a sense of congruity—and a bridge—between her public and her private selves. She did not experience these lives as separate or discontinuous. Her writing engaged with both equally and forged all the connections she needed.

Part
Three

5 ?◦

The Battle for the Breast

AT THE TIME of Rachel Carson's death in 1964, an individual's experience of breast cancer was still a private affair. The disease was still an iceberg, a killer in the dark, without even a visible tip to draw attention to itself. And yet the number of American women dying from it every year had already surpassed 25,000 and seemed to be rising. By the mid-1960s, most women with symptoms were being treated. None of them had any idea of just how large a sorority they belonged to. Some may even have thought their experience was unique, that they were the unfortunate victims of a freak disease. Society offered them very few clues to their real situation.

How had they come to be such unwitting partners to this apparent conspiracy of silence? And why did it survive as long as it did? To begin to make sense of this, it helps to return to the beginning of the century and to reconstruct, from there, the history of women's participation in the experience of disease. The history of breast cancer, after all, depends as much on the assimilation of women into the medical establishment as it does on the pace of medical progress.

The average life expectancy of an American woman at the turn of the century was just under 49 years. Infectious diseases were still the primary killers. In 1900, a woman was much more likely to die from tuberculosis, the flu, or pneumonia than from any kind of cancer. Infectious diseases together accounted for roughly 1 of every 3 deaths; cancers accounted for 1 in 25. The situation changed rapidly as the century progressed. By 1940, the positions of cancer and tuberculosis were virtually reversed; cancer had become the second leading cause of death (after heart disease), TB was now the eighth. The dramatic inversion of the death rates was attributable to two primary changes: improvements in public health (in sanitation, nutrition, basic health care) and the aging of the American population. The average life expectancy of women born in 1940 had risen to just under 67 years, a gain of almost 18 years in just four decades.[1] Paradoxically, it was the elimination, or at least the decline, of other diseases that had killed women prematurely that now opened up the vista of old age, the breeding ground of cancer. By 1930, there were more than twice as many women over 65 as there had been in 1900. As their odds for overall survival increased, so too did their exposure to breast cancer.

Alas, the triumphs of twentieth-century medicine over diseases such as smallpox and polio were not to be repeated with breast cancer. What American medical science did achieve was not the eradication of the disease but its representation. The continuing failure of clinical medicine to make any headway against a rising tide of deaths forced medical science to take a much closer look, to employ ever more sophisticated criteria in its effort to pin down the characteristics of this intractable disease. Over the century, the concept of breast cancer has expanded continuously. The single textbook standard has been replaced by a complex taxonomy of diseases, incorporating a broad collection of malignancies, each with widely divergent characteristics and behaviors.[2] But an understanding of this more heterogeneous reality did not pass into public knowledge until very near the end of the century. For most of the past 100 years, women reacted to breast cancer as one invariant malignancy that was, invariably, fatal. Their limited knowledge was a direct consequence of the engineered response to symptoms and to treatment that has been the hallmark of almost a century of public health campaigns.

The campaign for early detection in the context of consumer culture

Today we know that the incidence of breast cancer is more than ten times higher in women over 50 than it is among younger women. We also know that there has been a steady increase in the overall incidence of the disease that still defies explanation. But before the early twentieth century, cancer statistics in the United States could not really be relied upon to tell us very much at all about its behavior. In the absence of any national standards governing the collection of information, it was impossible to discover underlying trends in cancer mortality, or to know anything much about women who died from the disease (or indeed, about those who suffered with the disease but lived to die from another cause). There was little consistency from one state to the next in the approach to death certificates; many were not even signed by doctors.

The arrival of the twentieth century marked the beginning of significant improvements. In 1900, the U.S. Bureau of the Census, for the first time, introduced annual mortality reports in ten states. After the census of 1910, therefore, it became possible to construct the first time-series tables showing the changes that had occurred over the previous decade.

Frederick Hoffman, a statistician for the Prudential Life Insurance Company and a pioneer in the development of cancer statistics, understood the potential influence of statistics on health policy. In 1913, he delivered an address to a meeting of the American Gynecological Society on "The Menace of Cancer."[3] It laid out, in painstaking detail, incontrovertible evidence demonstrating the rise in cancer deaths, for both men and women, for all types of cancer and for almost all age groups. The trend established by these figures pointed to the desperate need "for a nation-wide effort to bring about a better public understanding of the accepted facts of cancer." Accordingly, Hoffman offered a plan for the establishment of a new organization "for the study and prevention of cancer, primarily for the purpose of educating the public at large in the absolute necessity of operative treatment at the earliest indications of cancerous growths."

This first mission statement of the American Society for the Control of Cancer (the ASCC, the organization that would in 1945 would become the American Cancer Society) was a bold move into unknown terrain. But with the benefit of hindsight, it also reveals the essential dilemma facing the new organization, one that would only catch up with it later on. This was the contradiction between a commitment to the *prevention* of cancer and a commitment to cancer *control*. In 1913, many of those active in the cancer community might well have believed that the two could be folded into each other. Medical science at the time still understood breast cancer as a local disease. If, therefore, early detection was pursued vigorously enough and women came to their doctors at the very first sign of disease, then theoretically the disease could be run down virtually to its source, preempting the manifestation of symptoms, if not eradicating the disease entirely. The long-term goal of prevention, then, however poorly defined, would depend on the effectiveness of early detection.

This attitude to cancer control may help to explain why the new organization made no commitment to research and why its focus on educating the public seemed at the time a reasonable approach to prevention. In the case of breast cancer, all of the Society's efforts were devoted to the promotion of early detection. In reality, this may have been as much a pragmatic response to the limited means available to the fledgling operation as it was the outcome of a carefully worked out strategy. The organization had no expectations of large-scale financial support and operated on a shoestring for decades. Even if members of the Society understood that cancer prevention would require long-term investment in biomedical research, the Society would never have been able to afford such a commitment. It did not, in fact, undertake to support scientific research until after the Second World War, when its financial position was much more secure.[4]

But if it had little financial leverage in its early days (with no endowment or philanthropic support behind it), the ASCC did nonetheless wield exceptional influence over the direction and development of national policy. The special relationship that has come into prominence over the past fifty years between the cancer charity and the federal government has, in fact, been there from the very beginning. One of the first acts undertaken by the new organization was to petition the Bureau of the Census, urging it to prepare "a more detailed statement of the deaths from cancer and other malignant tumors."[5] From this request came a special Census Report published in 1914 that acknowledged the suggestion of the ASCC and provided perhaps the first comprehensive set of time-series data on cancer mortality in the United States. The report demonstrated an almost threefold rise in the number of cancer deaths between 1900 and 1914 and an almost fourfold rise in the number of breast cancer deaths over the same period.

Ten years later, another government report confirmed the persistence of this trend, documenting an unprecedented rise in breast cancer deaths between 1910 and 1920. Worse, it revealed that the increase in the mortality rate was, in some age groups, almost double the increase for all cancers taken together. So, for example, while deaths from all cancers had risen by 36 percent among women aged 50 to 59, deaths from breast cancer had risen by 71 percent in the same age group.[6] Even for women over 70, the rise in breast cancer deaths exceeded those from all cancers combined.

The detailed findings of these early reports make it quite clear that the trend that would characterize the behavior of breast cancer for the rest of the century was already well documented, if still poorly understood, by 1925. Over the first half of the century, while the population of the United States doubled, the rate of death from breast cancer almost tripled and the actual number of deaths rose fivefold.[7] But these figures, carefully recorded and published year by year, did not set off any alarms in the general public. What was finally picked up and broadcast in the 1990s was not the remarkable climb of the death rate but the alarming rise in the *incidence* of breast cancer. The overall lifetime risk for the disease was found to have grown from about 1 in 20 in the 1960s to about 1 in 8 today.[8] The fact that breast cancer activists adopted the incidence rather than the death rates as their rallying cry in the nineties may suggest a subtle change in the perceived odds for survival and the emergent confidence of a well-organized demand for it.

The campaign for early detection

In 1925, the statistical guideposts were still those of deaths, unmitigated by any countervailing trends. For breast cancer, these showed no signs of abating. The bleak findings recorded in the 1925 government cancer report were finally enough to goad the ASCC into action. The primary inference that the cancer charity drew from these discouraging statistics was that not enough women were reaching their surgeons *in time.* What was needed, therefore, was a drive to raise public awareness.

By the late 1920s and 1930s, public health campaigns were in a position to draw on the techniques and psychology of modern advertising. Wartime propaganda generated by advertising gurus to sell war bonds and to recruit men into the armed forces had demonstrated that "it is possible to sway the minds of whole populations, change their habits of life, create belief, practically universal, in any policy or idea."[9] In the decades following the First World War, advertising had come into its own, riding the coattails of the boom in mass-produced consumer goods (cars, radios, and electrical appliances in particular).

The ASCC, seeking to alter the American woman's perception of breast cancer, knew that advertising had the capacity to change consumer consciousness. It had witnessed, in 1920, the transformation by advertising of Listerine from a product that had been in use as a general disinfectant since the nineteenth century into a mouthwash to ward off "halitosis." The change in packaging alone, without any corresponding change in product, raised the profits of its owners, Lambert Pharmaceuticals, from $100,000 in 1920 to $4 million in 1927.

The success of the Listerine campaign revealed the vulnerability of the American public to what advertising historian Roland Marchand has called the culture's "social shame." Trading on this sense of fear, advertising moved quickly to fill a perceived vacuum in personal advice, adopting a tone of intimacy through person-to-person copy that addressed delicate failings of personal hygiene that "even your best friend won't tell you." Advertisers created fictional female personae to serve as personal confidantes to women in distress. Deodorants, douches, and mouthwashes provided the remedy; they were the antidotes to social disgrace. Even disposable sanitary pads could now be advertised. A hugely successful campaign for Kotex in the early 1920s demonstrated that advertising could be applied effectively to subjects that had once been considered taboo.[10]

Women, of course, were the primary targets of most advertising. In the 1930s, trade journals estimated that they accounted for about 85 percent of all consumer spending. Advertisers were merciless in exploiting what they considered to be a woman's "natural inferiority complex," raising doubts wherever possible about her sexual allure. Aimed particularly at wives with disposable income, advertising emphasized a woman's responsibility to remain as youthful and as physically attractive as possible: "so often a woman has only herself to blame if she fails to stay young with her husband" ran the copy for a typical ad. The message was clear: only the regular use of marketed beauty products could keep her husband's interest alive—and without it, she would perish. So negative were the messages conveyed by advertising copy in the twenties and thirties—"she evades all close-ups . . . dingy teeth and tender gums destroy her charm," "once pursued, now shunned"—that women often emerge as pitiable creatures who have been banished from society, skulking furtively along dark alleys away from the glare of streetlights.

Almost any body part or bodily fluid could put a woman at risk. Nothing was safe from the predations of consumer marketing that ranged freely over a woman's body like a lunar probe, stirring up a cloud of fear in its wake, as it searched for ever-new sources of profit. Certainly breasts were not spared. "The great majority of women, probably nine-tenths or more," wrote the author of a breast self-help book in the late 1930s, "have a bust problem to a greater or lesser degree. . . . [Contemporary fashions] have made womankind more bust conscious than before, with the result that much time, attention, and money is being devoted to bust culture."[11]

The consumer marketing culture aimed at the breast created one standard of perfection against which nine-tenths of American women were doomed to fail. This failure, like so many others, could be laid at their feet. Although some of the many deviations from the so-called norm could be ascribed to "natural" causes (to pregnancy, nursing, wasting illnesses), many others were "unnatural," that is, brought on by women themselves. These included "tight binding of the breasts to achieve the boyish form; reducing and fasting fads . . . [which] often leave the breasts limp, loose and hanging; poor diet, faulty hygiene, lack of suitable exercise, incorrect posture, weak abdominal muscles . . . all may contribute to soft, flat, or drooping breasts."[12] Each of these deficiencies could spin off its own mini-industry of correctives. Some, like those caused by reducing and fasting aids, were themselves the legacy of earlier rounds of product marketing, demonstrating the usefulness of women as a renewable source of profits.

Bringing breasts within the scope of consumer culture heightened a woman's sense of her body as inherently defective. The culture provoked a clear association between beautiful breasts and healthy breasts; anything less than perfect was intrinsically unhealthy. So well before any hint of real disease entered the picture, women were already expecting it. After all, the Victorian belief in women's physical inferiority still stalked the culture, even if it was now more a shadowy presence than a central tenet of social life. It was still there, and the psychology employed by the new consumerism had little difficulty in reviving it.

Women, in other words, were conditioned to accept responsibility for whatever calamities befell them. A woman's role as household manager put her in charge of everything within her domain, herself included. A well-maintained household required a well-maintained wife. Anything that threatened to disturb the integrity of either would be her failure, and would put her at risk. This was as true of a burned casserole as it was of disease. But a disease that not only compromised her role as household manager but also threatened to destroy her sexual charm left her totally vulnerable to the husband she depended upon. If bad breath and body odors could justify a husband's desertion, what would follow from his discovery of a breast lump, the first sign of a potentially "dis-figuring" disease?

Unlike bad skin or bad hair, cancer of the breast was neither a temporary embarrassment nor a manufactured problem. There were no products on the market that could restore an afflicted woman to "picture perfect" health and so guarantee her place of safety in the home. But if consumer capitalism could not solve the problem of breast cancer, it could, and did, influence its reception in the culture. The fear of rejection that it whipped up to manufacture and sustain its product markets might have been designed with minor physical imperfections in mind, but it inevitably spread to encompass all the ills that women's flesh was heir to. The relentless undermining of women's self-esteem left them ever more vulnerable to the belief that breast cancer was just another flaw in their makeup, a flaw that, like all the others, they alone were responsible for repairing.

The discovery of a lump, then, forced a woman to make an impossible choice between her social survival, on the one hand, which demanded the preservation of an intact body at whatever cost, and her physical survival on the other, which demanded the mutilation of that same body. Both sides of this dilemma had been created by the culture she inhabited.

From the 1920s on, all the public education campaigns targeting breast cancer incorporated this inescapable contradiction. They made good use of the permissive and persuasive powers released by these "missionaries of modernity," the advertising copywriters, to change women's attitudes toward their own health. (This included, of course, the power to mislead as well as the power to inform.) But the public education campaigns were also conducted within a culture that traded increasingly in women's physical insecurities, bringing more and more of their bodies within the reach of consumer marketing.

The conflict this set up in women was really the expression of a deeper conflict between opposing male views of what constituted the "best interests" of women. The medical profession wanted to sell the idea of surgery as a cure for breast cancer. To succeed, they had to convince women that their survival mattered, that the loss of life was more terrible than the loss of a breast. The only obstacle was fear. "There is one thing so often encountered in women with cancer of the breast," wrote the surgeon William Rodman, "that it might be looked on as a symptom of the disease, to-wit, a tendency to suppress all knowledge of its existence, not even confiding in those to whom one would ordinarily go for advice, but on the contrary, deliberately and artfully concealing its presence from them."[13] On the other side, consumer product manufacturers and other beauty consultants worked hard, as we've seen, to keep this fear alive, promoting, wherever possible, the dread of physical impairment: "Badly shaped breasts may prove a definite vocational hindrance . . . or it may result in a woman's failing to gain the man of her choice and thereby affecting her entire future life and happiness."[14]

This struggle between medicine and commerce for the hearts and minds—and bodies—of women shows just how contested a territory it was. Whatever the underlying dynamics of this clash of interests, it did not go away. Although sometimes more accommodating and at other times more adversarial, the relationship between corporate capital and (now) corporate medicine remains as focused on this battle today as it ever was in the past (see Chapter 8).

Perhaps understanding something of what was at stake, the ASCC, in pursuing its mandate to educate women about the perils of cancer, chose to bring them inside their public relations campaigns from the very beginning. Drawing upon the demonstrated success of person-to-person advertising in the Kotex campaigns, the Society elected to ask women themselves to carry their message directly to other women. In 1929, the ASCC produced a small pamphlet, "What Every Woman Should Know about Cancer." The recommendations set out for a woman in this pamphlet clearly convey the full range of responsibilities enjoined upon her by society at large. A woman is asked to have a medical examination once a year, but she is also asked to:

1. make sure that a copy of the pamphlet is distributed to every woman in her club;

2. see to it that a qualified speaker is invited to "give a lecture on some aspect of the cancer question at least once a year";

3. make sure "that the members of her family are protected as far as possible against cancer and, if attacked, that they are promptly provided with the best medical attention."[15]

What appears to be an early acknowledgment of a woman's special vulnerability to cancer becomes an opportunity to remind her of her obligations to others—to her family, to other women, even to the objectives of the ASCC. Even though the pamphlet purports to be concerned with potential fatal illnesses that may strike *her*, the message it conveys confirms her continuing responsibilities for the welfare of others. She cannot be disencumbered, isolated from her roles as social secretary and family manager, even as she's being addressed as an individual in need of information, care, and consolation herself. She cannot, in other words, become a patient in a world that has cast her as primary caretaker.

The references to women's clubs and the need to seek the "best medical attention" are clear indications of the limited audience targeted by the new campaign. This concentration on the social elite had been there from the Society's very beginnings. One of its most successful early fundraising efforts had been a letter-writing campaign to 2,000 people listed in New York's *Social Register*. Following in that tradition, the leaflet "What Every Woman Should Know about Cancer" was drafted with an affluent middle-class audience in mind. But although its text made no concessions to the circumstances of less privileged women, the pamphlet was nonetheless translated into seven other languages (including Slovak, Russian, and Polish). Some elements of its message, therefore, must have reached lower-income and ethnic minority women. For the most part, they might have been expected to learn about cancer through a "trickle-down" of information, from employer to employee, mistress to servant, much as last year's ball gown might have been passed along. In fact, Mary Lasker, engineer of the postwar transformation of the American Cancer Society, first became interested in the disease when her housekeeper was diagnosed with uterine cancer, so one might call this as much a "trickle-up" effect as "trickle-down."

In the days before the development of mass communications (including television and direct mail), a mass distribution of this kind required extremely labor-intensive support. Pamphlets had to be handed out one at a time to passersby at subway stations, schools, supermarkets, cinemas, and so on. The success of this early campaign—an estimated 668,000 copies were distributed—rested almost entirely on the willing participation of an army of volunteer labor, almost all of them women, from the General Federation of Women's Clubs (GFWC), the YWCA, and the Metropolitan Life Insurance Company as well as from the ASCC itself.

The lives of women caught up in these campaigns had changed in important ways since the turn of the century. First, they were healthier. The use of antiseptic methods in delivery had greatly reduced maternal deaths from puerperal fever. Improvements in gynecological surgery had made it possible to correct debilitating conditions associated with multiple childbirths (such as fistulas, prolapsed wombs, incontinence) that had turned women into chronic invalids in the classic Victorian tradition. Women also began to have fewer children, regulating their own fertility through the use of a variety of birth control methods, not all of them legal. All of these trends demonstrated the power of improved medical intervention to alter women's lives. Together, they helped to undermine the nineteenth-century belief that women were creatures completely at the mercy of their uterine disorders.

A second important change for women early in the century was dress reform. They were finally liberated from the corsets that had emphasized their sexual functions at the expense of their freedom of movement. Looser clothing enabled them to participate in exercise and competitive sports. More important, liberating clothing brought into closer alignment the public and private expressions of the female body, minimizing the extraordinary contradictions between a woman's natural shape and the upholstered version she presented to the world at large. This loosening of restrictions of course made itself felt in women's social and professional lives too. Having won the vote in 1920, many women saw, or at least hoped for, broader opportunities outside the home.

Volunteer work for many women provided the perfect halfway house. It offered a way out of their homes but did not expose them to the harsher realities of paid employment. Nor did it threaten the underlying domestic dynamic. Women volunteers did not relinquish their responsibilities as wives, sisters, and mothers; they simply extended their reach to encompass public libraries, hospitals, and gardens as well. Since the nonworking wife was more commonly middle-class than working-class, it is not surprising to find a conservative bias among many voluntary associations. The General Federation of Women's Clubs, for example, withheld its endorsement of women's suffrage until late in the day. Their members, for the most part, would not have described themselves as feminist. But they certainly saw themselves as willing and very able.

The Women's Field Army

The American Society for the Control of Cancer recognized the potential resource that the GFWC represented and incorporated it in one of the most powerful campaigns it ever mounted on behalf of early detection. It was prompted by the belief that more women than men die of cancer, and especially of cancers that are still curable in their early stages. If women consulted a doctor earlier, more lives could be saved. The average period of delay had, in fact, already been halved, falling from about seventeen months in 1911 to about eight months in 1933.[16] But this was still much too long. The ASCC wanted to eliminate it altogether. The agency set up expressly to accomplish this mission was the Women's Field Army (WFA).

To garner support for their program, the ASCC approached the GFWC to seek their cooperation in what they hoped would become a national crusade. Based entirely on the voluntary participation of women, the Army's work was conceived as a military operation, in line with the Society's general approach to cancer. The early posters of the ASCC portrayed a battle between St. George and the dragon, and almost all its promotional materials made generous use of war legends and battle imagery.

But the promotional material added a softening touch to the imagery as well, one that conjured up women's role as nurses rather than soldiers. "When the dead and dying from cancer are regarded in a similar light to the slain and wounded on the field of battle," wrote one doctor involved in the establishment of the Women's Field Army, "the same compulsion that leads to victory against an invading army will operate in the struggle to vanquish this disease."[17]

To "man" this new Army, women were "enlisted" by appointed "Commanders" in every participating state. Their primary task was to encourage women in their local area to report, like military recruits, for

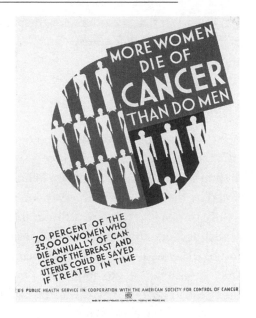

A poster from the 1930s promoting early detection. *Library of Congress, LC-USZC2-1009.*

periodic "physicals" that might detect early signs of cancer. They were expected to "invade" homes and family life across the country with a mission to save lives, drawing women's attention to the early warning signs of disease, softening their fears of treatment, brightening their prospects of survival. But, in a distinct departure from military tradition, women recruited into the Army were asked to pay an enlistment fee of one dollar, in effect paying for the privilege of volunteering. In performance of this duty, Field Army workers, who recruited over 100,000 members in the first year, acted as the primary fundraisers for the parent organization (in some years supplying it with the majority of its operating income).

In addition to their delivery of pastoral care, the volunteers also organized far-reaching media campaigns and helped to finance and administer the very first cancer prevention clinics.[18] They organized public lectures and exhibitions. They staffed Society booths at every kind of conference and fair and distributed millions of brochures and cancer labels. (At the 1939 World's Fair, they exhibited a life-size trans-lucent plastic model of "Cancer Woman" that demonstrated electroni-cally, beginning with a single spot of light in the breast, the progressive growth and spread of a tumor through the lymph nodes of the armpit and neck to the lungs and bones.) They also spent time soliciting free advertising and editorial space in hundreds of newspapers and maga-zines, and on subway cars and billboards.

From the start, there were many physicians and state medical socie-ties that were suspicious of the Army's objectives and refused to partici-pate. Paradoxically, their fears may have been aroused by the vehe-mence of the martial tone adopted in the WFA's public relations material. The WFA's planned campaign was considered by many to be an act of trespass that could interfere with medicine's own campaigns against the disease. According to one historian of the movement, "some nervous physicians needed reassurance that the women in their enthusiasm would not break over into realms reserved for the medical profession."[19] However successful martial metaphors might be in incit-ing women to join the battle against breast cancer, they were not, after all, to be taken too literally. Women, in other words, could dress up in military uniform and answer to a military chain of command, but the tasks they were expected to perform had little to do with the battlefield.

Physicians, anxious to protect their authority, argued that it would be all right to allow women to encourage others to seek medical help, but not for them to volunteer any advice or information that they were not qualified to give. In other words, they could facilitate the work of physicians but they could not materially interfere with that work. Doc-tors, in reality, were probably less alarmed by the possibility of their patients being misinformed than they were by the prospects of their becoming more informed. After all, the educational aspects of the Women's Field Army opened the doctor-patient relationship to outside interference, giving women patients just enough knowledge to come to their doctors armed with questions, about treatment as well as about disease. This consequence was not openly addressed either by the can-cer society or by the AMA but it was obviously an unwelcome threat to the nature of medical practice.

The status of women volunteers as unpaid workers meant that they had no professional territory to defend. Active at a time before national health care debates had divided the country along clear ideological lines, the volunteers were in a position to cultivate a more disinterested response to the problems they encountered. Inevitably, in carrying out their work, they saw that few clinical services were available to poor women, either for diagnosis or treatment. Most radical mastectomies were performed on fee-paying patients in private hospitals. A comparative study of breast cancer surgeries performed over a six-month period in Detroit in 1926 revealed that 39 breast amputations had been carried out in one private hospital but only *one* had been performed over the same period in a city hospital of comparable size where the treatment had been free. The author of this study acknowledged that "the poorer classes come much later for treatment and hence are more frequently in an inoperable condition."[20]

The response of some of the women volunteers to this widespread inequity was to assume responsibility, where possible, for the financing of cancer treatment, covering the costs of care for women too poor to pay. For those who were not indigent but still had insufficient money on hand, they helped to set up loan funds. In the days before large-scale government intervention in the provision of health care (well before Medicaid or Medicare) this gesture of solidarity seemed suspiciously like an underhanded redistribution of wealth.[21] Physicians accused women of "advocating State Medicine" which, ironically, they often described as "a menacing cancer of the body politic."[22] Not surprisingly, the AMA also opposed a Congressional bill to establish a National Cancer Institute at the same time, warning that "the danger of putting the government in a dominant position in relation to medical research is apparent."[23]

The ASCC supported the legislation and gained support for the measure by recruiting Eleanor Roosevelt into the Women's Field Army. In the meantime, Women's Field Army Commanders attempted to reassure their medical colleagues that the "women of America have proved their faith in the American way," emphasizing their participation as individuals rather than as members of any socialist cabal. "Individual responsibility has been the keynote of the movement," wrote the

Commander of the WFA in New York, "as it is the keynote of democracy."[24]

But if the WFA was a thorn in the flesh of many physicians, for women at risk its work was arguably the most important source of information about breast cancer in the first half of the twentieth century. The surgeon general, addressing the 1938 convention of the General Federation of Women's Clubs, remarked that the WFA's campaign against cancer had "started an avalanche of public interest and public understanding."[25] *Time* magazine called its "2,000,000 women operating in 39 states . . . the largest evangelistic movement ever loosed against a disease."[26] Although it lasted for barely a decade and in a few states never operated at all, it did manage to involve many hundreds of thousands of women as direct participants. Each of the enlisted volunteers had direct contact themselves with hundreds more, passing on, at the grass-roots level, the message of the parent organization. For the first time, a national organization not only permitted but encouraged women to discuss the disease with each other. They believed that their interaction could be life-saving, that just talking about it was fortifying in itself. Public exhibitions gave the disease a name, elaborated its symptoms and its statistics. All these activities helped to lay the groundwork for the crucial development of public awareness, and, down the road, for national organization.

Early detection: public relations and pragmatism

Underlying the education drives for early detection was the conviction that not all breast cancers were incurable. The earlier a tumor was detected, the smaller it was likely to be and, given immediate treatment, the greater the chances for survival. That treatment, of course, had to be surgery: "if any doctor offers you [other choices], run, do not walk, to the nearest exit." Hidden behind this uninflected rhetoric was a more complex truth, one the American Society for Cancer Control never owned up to. This was the fact that some cancers, no matter what their size, were going to kill the patient no matter when she turned up for treatment.

Public relations broadcast the fact that the number of deaths from breast cancer could "be greatly reduced by using the known means of preventing them—early discovery of the disease and proper treatment." A poster widely circulated in the late 1930s by the ASCC in conjunction with the Public Health Service broadcast the slogan, "70 percent of the 35,000 women who die annually of cancer of the breast and uterus could be saved if treated in time." But what about the other 30 percent? (And, following the logic of the discussion in the previous chapter, was this 30 percent of those treated or 30 percent of all women with breast cancer?) While neither the poster nor any other campaign claimed that all breast cancer deaths could be eliminated, the ASCC did not face this issue head on. If early detection saved some lives, why didn't it save all of them?

The ASCC, of course, couldn't supply an answer to this question. But its failure to admit to the limited effectiveness of treatment was not lost on American women. Even in the days before talking about breast cancer became acceptable, most women knew someone who had died of the disease after being treated. Personal experience, in other words, had taught them that early detection was not a panacea. By choosing to evade this difficult truth, the Society weakened its credibility. Playing down the more painful aspects of the disease was admittedly a conscious choice. An early in-house publication acknowledged that "the incurable nature of advanced cases is never stressed; the great suffering which follows neglect is not described; the repulsive features are not detailed. The Society's slogan is, 'In early treatment lies the hope of cure.' "[27]

But a parallel admission of the limited effectiveness of treatment was never forthcoming. Any disclosure of the actual survival rates following surgery, not to mention the risks of the procedure itself, was felt to be counterproductive. Public relations consistently adopted an upbeat posture, emphasizing the benefits of treatment, relying heavily on misleading associations between treatment and "cure." Telling women the whole truth, rather than a cleaned-up version of it, might discourage too many women from ever seeking a doctor's advice. The belief that women would be scared off by the truth no doubt rationalized the use of half-truths by those drafting promotional materials for distribution by the Women's Field Army. But the use of half-truths could sometimes shade into pure misrepresentation as well. An article in the AMA's *Hygeia,* a popular health magazine distributed through doctors' waiting rooms, argued that cancer "almost invariably has its starting point in some simple, feelable, and often visible thing, as a lump, an abrasion, an ulcer or a common sore which persists and refuses to heal. This early stage is *not* cancer but an ordinary condition responsive to treatment."[28] The expectation here is that a woman will only submit herself to treatment for cancer if everyone agrees that what she is being treated for is *not* cancer.

The same dilemma faced the physician confronting a newly diagnosed patient. How much tolerance did she have for the unadorned truth? All the issues surrounding the problem of disclosure that so distressed Rachel Carson (described in Chapter 4) applied with equal force to the early cancer education campaigns. Twenty-five years later, Rachel Carson was told, after having a radical mastectomy, that she had "a condition bordering on malignancy."

In allowing its armies of volunteers to circulate a sanitized rendering of the disease rather than an unvarnished one, the ASCC was throwing its weight behind the interests of the medical profession. It generated a great deal of business for surgeons without ever publicly questioning the validity of the treatment that they had to offer. On the contrary, it helped, if inadvertently, to solidify the monopoly position of radical surgery in the treatment of breast cancer. For the ASCC, the widespread availability of unpaid labor (including significant fundraising capacity) came at a time when the resources of the society were quite modest. Economic constraints may have made the slant of its educational campaign irresistible. With no funds to underwrite large-scale research and no desire to alienate the medical profession, the decision to use the volunteer labor of women to educate the public and to advertise the benefits of radical surgery may have seemed the best option. But the dynamic set in motion by this campaign cast a long shadow.

The ASCC did not confine its early detection campaigns to women. General practitioners were targeted as well. Their sluggish response to the Society's appeals reflects, in part, the legacy of ingrained fatalism.

No medical (as opposed to surgical) treatment for breast cancer had ever appeared to cure it. This endemic failure had no doubt contributed to the reluctance of doctors to treat breast disease at all. Most family physicians practicing in the 1930s would have had little training in distinguishing benign from malignant tumors. The ASCC understood this. Periodically, it published monographs on breast and other cancers that were distributed through medical journals to physicians. It also financed a range of postgraduate training programs to bring nonspecialists up to date. But where a doctor might admit in private that "it is very little use in educating the public until the general practitioner knows more about cancer than he does," the public face of the ASCC's programs for physicians was always respectful of medical professionals.[29]

Over time, as the campaign to alert women to the danger signals of cancer broadened, a more strident, even punitive, voice crept into the public discourse. There was a clear suggestion that women who failed to avail themselves of treatment in a timely manner were themselves to blame for the consequences. In this construction, the focus is on women and how they respond, not on treatment, which is taken as a given. A 1947 article in the *Journal of the American Medical Association* (*JAMA*) insists that the failure to reduce cancer mortality "is not due to inadequate therapeutic measures . . . [but to] the prolonged delay between the time when the patient has first symptoms and the time when definitive treatment begins."[30] Medical science, this seems to imply, has done its job, held up its side of the bargain. If women fail to take advantage of it, then who is to blame? Women may no longer be dying from disease, suggests one commentator, but from "ignorance, fear, carelessness, neglect." There are occasions, in fact, when even the disease is "not guilty." " 'Cancer' is written on many a death certificate when 'suicide' would be far nearer the truth."[31]

Taken to this extreme, it becomes easier to see the campaigns for early detection as part of a much older and much broader American tradition. The insistence on personal responsibility that dominates so many aspects of American life infects our approach to illness as much as it inspires our approach to politics. A culture that has always valued the virtues of self-help finds it hard to escape the self-blame that accompanies failure, whether that failure is expressed as a loss of health or a loss of income, employment, or faith. The dynamic in each case is the same: to internalize the problem, and the search for its solution. If the source of disease was a woman's body, so, then, must be the remedy.

In this closed system, there was no incentive to seek elsewhere for either the cause or cure of breast cancer. The individual remedy—radical surgery—and the social remedy—early detection—reinforced each other. Both kept alive the ideas of personal sacrifice and responsibility. Of course, this also lay at the heart of military discipline, whose language and accouterments the ASCC was so eager for the Women's Field Army to adopt. A woman, following instructions, sacrificed her breast in the war against cancer and was rewarded with life. A surgeon performed a radical mastectomy and became a hero. Both played a role in a code of behavior based on a set of mutual obligations.

Anything that threatened to interfere with this response would be shunned. The idea, for instance, that breast cancer might be triggered by genetic damage caused by environmental insults originating outside the body was as unwelcome as the idea that it was a systemic disease rather than a local one. Both threatened to sabotage the exclusive relationship between a patient and her surgeon that the Women's Field Army did so much to cement. Both, in fact, suggested a disease whose complexity had to be addressed by social and scientific expertise that lay outside this central dyad. But the prescribed pattern set in motion by the mass-based campaigns did not foster much productive exchange between surgery and the emerging fields of biochemistry, epidemiology, medical oncology, and radiology either. Surgery was not yet ready to make any concessions to these newer disciplines and, before the Second World War, it never had to.

The success of the ASCC in mobilizing women by their thousands set a precedent in the national approach to breast cancer that remains in force to this day. Women had answered the call. They had absorbed the information fed to them on the "danger signs" of breast cancer and had acted responsibly when encountering any symptoms of the disease in themselves. They were, in other words, a public health success story.

They had proved themselves to be a valuable and cost-effective resource in the fight against breast cancer. Given the competition for limited resources, it would be hard for the American Cancer Society, when
planning its next round of expenditures, to look an apparent gift horse
in the mouth. If women themselves were willing to participate in
tracking down breast cancer, as they seemed to be, it would be folly not
to make good use of their acquiescence.

In this way, the very availability of women both as volunteers of the
ACS and as potential patients may have influenced the direction of the
Society's overall policy. Their compliance with the program enabled
the ACS to push early detection to its limits. As long as women were
willing to be patients, ACS campaigns could emphasize treatment
with a hope of cure rather than prevention. As the techniques grew
more sophisticated, moving from breast self-examination to screening
mammography, the survival rates did improve but the underlying bias
of the strategy remained unchanged. The emphasis on early detection
shifted attention and accountability away from the medical profession
and toward the patient, away from the inadequacies of treatment and
toward the inadequacies of personal behavior.

Early detection in the postwar era:
breast self-examination and screening mammography

Despite the impressive work of the Women's Field Army in most states
across the country, deaths from breast cancer continued to rise. Although the number of participating volunteers had grown to about
300,000 in the late 1930s, by 1948 the work of the Field Army had
either ceased or been absorbed into other departments of the American Cancer Society. In that year, breast cancer deaths rose to almost
19,000, the highest number ever recorded. The mortality rate per
100,000 women had risen almost threefold, from 10.9 in 1901 to 26.9
in 1948.[32]

Cancer education campaigns had achieved their objective; many
women did discover breast lumps when they were smaller and did go
promptly to consult a doctor. The average size of primary tumors did

decline. But as we now know, by the time any tumor is palpable at all, there is a good chance that it has already spread to the lymph nodes or other parts of the body. In 1948, however, no one in the United States had ever seriously challenged the prevailing belief in breast cancer as a local disease. If women had demonstrated that early treatment enhanced their chances of survival, then getting the word out to more women would surely help to stem the tide of rising deaths. In other words, the message brought home from the experience was that the drive for early detection should not be abandoned; it should be intensified.

The first enhancement of early detection was the encouragement of breast self-examination (BSE). In 1948, Alfred Popma, a radiologist from Utah, produced a 16mm film in his own house using a woman volunteer he trained himself to demonstrate the proper technique for carrying out a breast self-exam. He knew he was treading on thin ice. "Many people thought this would be immoral, photographing a woman's breasts. . . . They didn't think we could show it without creating trouble," he recalled.[33] But after testing the film on a local audience of women volunteers, it was screened for state divisions of the ASC and then for the ASC National Board of Directors. With their approval, and an agreement from the NIH to pay half the costs, a professionally made film was produced and circulated throughout the United States.[34] While rating the film "excellent for physician and layman alike," *JAMA* criticized it for its "use of the term 'cure.' There are those who hold that 'arrested' is preferable to 'cured' with respect to carcinoma."[35]

Whatever its limitations, by 1953 the film had been shown to more than three million American women. But breast self-examination, no matter how conscientiously performed, still failed to catch tumors early enough. Even the most skillful fingers in the world would find it hard to feel a lump that was much smaller than about half an inch in diameter (about one centimeter). But even a tumor this small might already have been growing for years.

By the early 1950s, many breast cancer researchers were well aware that a primary tumor could still be undetectable at a time when there were already clear clinical indications that it had spread to another part of the body. This apparently anomalous finding threw into doubt the established belief that early diagnosis followed by radical mastectomy would result in almost universal control of the disease. The combined forces of improved public education and physician awareness that were expected to make this utopian dream a reality were based on the assumption that breast cancer was *one* disease that invariably displayed "progressive local tumor growth and dissemination in *a linear relationship to time*, with surgical intervention representing *the* critical variable in relation to survival."[36] Now researchers were beginning to discover that, contrary to accepted dogma, breast cancer showed considerable biological variability; and that it was the nature of these biological factors, rather than the speed with which the disease was detected and treated, that was more likely to determine survival. Rather than its being a matter of urgent concern, the differential impact on survival between a delay of a month and a year could, in fact, be quite small. And so might be the curative power of radical mastectomies.[37]

These findings, even if confined to obscure medical journals, nevertheless struck at the heart of the medical response to breast cancer and the public education campaigns it controlled. There were two possible reactions to these first shots across the bow. The results could be acknowledged as suggestive and worth pursuing even if this put the entire rationale underpinning existing breast cancer treatment at risk. Or they could be ignored altogether, and attention could be switched to the search for better methods of detection. Given the level of investment propping up the professional and financial status quo, and given the implications of being wrong, it's not surprising to learn that no sign of this controversy ever ruffled the composure of the men in white throughout the 1950s or 1960s. It remained business as usual.

Finally, an improved method of detection did come along, in the form of screening mammography. But despite the fact that this new diagnostic tool helped to refine and sustain the surgical approach to treatment, surgeons played very little role in bringing it forward. They were, in fact, the last medical professionals to come on board. The research and development for mammography came from other quarters entirely, but surgeons controlled its final acceptance as a standard component of clinical practice.

By anyone's account, the development of screening mammography in the United States was exceptionally slow. Europeans were much quicker to exploit the diagnostic possibilities of this new technology. In the United States, although several independent researchers had carried out experiments demonstrating its potential value and had published their results, they failed, individually and collectively, to generate much excitement among the American medical community.

The use of x-rays, or roentgenograms as they were then called (after the German physicist, Roentgen, who discovered them), was first reported in 1895 and was used shortly afterward in the treatment of inoperable breast cancer. Radium was isolated soon after, in 1899, by the Curies. In Germany, postoperative radiation was used routinely in the first decades of the twentieth century. Subsequent experiments in the use of radiation as a primary therapy for breast cancer occurred only in Europe. In the United States, where surgery dominated the management of the disease, radiation was altogether less acceptable.[38] Surgeons obviously had little incentive to explore a new technology that might threaten their own dominance in the field. They were unlikely to welcome research that attempted to compare the results of surgery with those following treatment by radiation alone. Very few American studies, in fact, were ever carried out to evaluate the impact of radiation therapy on established disease. This exclusion protected the primacy of surgery. But in rejecting any possible competition from radiation used as therapy, American medicine also discouraged support for the development of radiation used as a diagnostic tool. Interest in the latter was tainted by indifference or even hostility to the former.

The delayed American response to the potential of x-ray technology seems to have been part of a larger pattern of unconcern. According to one government-sponsored history, "the steadily increasing breast cancer mortality rate in the early decades of this century apparently was not considered noteworthy by American physicians. Thus, the investigation of breast disease was not pursued with diligence until the late 1930s."[39]

In the 1920s, a lone researcher in Rochester, New York, took x-rays of the breast before surgery, and was able to demonstrate a close correlation between his preoperative findings based on his reading of the films and the results of tissue analysis carried out after surgery. His observations, published in 1930, met with apathy.[40] But even twenty years later, mammography remained largely untested. Another independent researcher, Jacob Gershon-Cohen, carried out a five-year screening program in 1956 for women with no symptoms. His promising results met with the same lack of enthusiasm. Finally, in the late 1950s, a physician working at the M. D. Anderson Hospital in Texas, Robert Egan, used mammograms to diagnose (correctly) 238 out of 240 tumors that were later confirmed by biopsies. With federal support from the Cancer Control Program, Egan's results were successfully reproduced by other researchers.

Most physicians and researchers understood early on that the success of mammography depended on its somehow winning the support of surgeons. It could "only be developed by demonstrating that 'quality management' of breast disease requires mammography."[41] To achieve this end and to prove the value of the new technology, several large-scale trials were conducted, beginning with the well-known Health Insurance Plan (HIP) study in New York in the early 1960s. This study enrolled 62,000 women members of the health plan between the ages of 40 and 64. They were randomly assigned either to a group receiving clinical exams and screening mammograms or to a control group whose members were not screened. The study demonstrated a significant reduction in breast cancer deaths after five years among women over the age of fifty in the group that had been screened. Its findings put screening mammography on the map.

This was the first intervention of technology into programs designed to promote the early diagnosis of breast cancer in asymptomatic women. Until then, the "success" of early detection programs had depended largely on the behavioral response of women. Now, the results were mediated by technology. But the burden of responsibility on women remained undiminished. If anything, it was increased. Mammography was not intended to replace breast self-exams but to supplement them, adding an annual ritual to the sequence of monthly ones. It added a layer of complexity to the process of early detection, opening up new sources of confusion and potential conflict between women and their health care providers.

Screening mammography represented an enormous advance on all earlier methods of detection. It could spot evidence of disease while it was still microscopic, years before it grew into a tumor large enough to be felt. This gave doctors a tremendous head start. If there was a period when breast cancer behaved exclusively as a local disease, and mammography allowed doctors to intervene during this narrow time frame, then perhaps treatment could actually cure. Undoubtedly, the use of mammography has facilitated the cure of many thousands of women.

But the very real advantages of mammography have made it much harder to come to terms with its equally real limitations. As with all the earlier breast cancer campaigns, the first campaigns for mammography concentrated exclusively on its potential benefits. The primary objective of the American Cancer Society and other public health organizations was to encourage women to make use of the new technology, to present themselves at the appropriate time for a baseline mammogram and then to take responsibility for returning, at regular intervals, for the rest of their lives. This goal was already difficult enough to achieve without admitting to any complicating factors. Public commitment to mammography had to be optimistic and unqualified.

But by the last quarter of the twentieth century, early detection campaigns were already long in the tooth. Echoes of earlier slogans promising breast cancer cures in exchange for a woman's prompt cooperation were still circulating in the culture while the number of deaths continued to rise. Organizations like the American Cancer Society were, in effect, having to fight a war of attrition against the cumulative impact of their own prevarications. Women began to weary of the glaring gap between rhetoric and reality.

Screening mammography, alas, came to offer many opportunities to express this growing disaffection. As a diagnostic technique, it turned out to be seriously flawed. Even under optimal conditions, screening mammograms could miss up to 15 percent of breast tumors. Under less than optimal conditions, they could be easily misread or misinterpreted. The potential for error, in other words, was not negligible. The legion of misdiagnosed women grows annually and so does their anger, expressed in the steady rise of medical malpractice suits.[42]

The reception of early detection campaigns has clearly changed within the past few decades. The controversies surrounding mammography are now shared with the public. The question, for instance, of whether a woman should have a first mammogram at 40 or 50 is one that has raised many tempers and consumed many thousands of column inches in the national media. Earlier campaigns did not broadcast their internal disagreements or difficulties, only their successes. This makes it much harder to assess the kind of response that women actually had to successive waves of anticancer propaganda. It is at least certain that the response was probably as varied from region to region as it was from one campaign to the next.[43]

As the century progressed, women's response to breast cancer was filtered through many other social changes that have influenced their awareness of their bodies and their health. Women over 60 today witnessed the virtual elimination of diseases such as polio, smallpox, and pneumonia following the introduction of vaccines and antibiotics in the early postwar period. But they rarely made a connection between these acute infections requiring immediate attention and the more chronic disease of breast cancer, which permitted women to procrastinate with apparent impunity. There was nothing in the postwar culture that might encourage women to make this link, to consider breast cancer another disease that science might reasonably be expected to cure. On the contrary, many women experienced the prefeminist postwar years as a throwback to a more sexist culture than their wartime experience may have led them to expect. And one of the clearest signs of the retrograde shift was a change in the status of breasts themselves.

Marilyn Yalom has described "the American breast fetish of the war." "In your face bosoms" appeared on the noses of bomber planes and in millions of pin-ups distributed to G.I.s to "raise the morale" of U.S. troops. According to Yalom, men "looked to the female bosom as a reminder of the values that war destroys: love, intimacy, nurturance."

Breasts were beautiful, the bigger the better. "Bombshells" like Marilyn Monroe, Jayne Mansfield, and Anita Ekberg flaunted them. After the war men needed to be reassured "that the breasts they had dreamed of were now available to them." The message was clear: "your role is to provide the breast, not the bread."[44]

There was other postwar fallout from the G.I.'s obsession with big breasts. Japanese prostitutes, in an attempt to gratify the tastes of American soldiers in the occupation forces, injected liquid silicone or paraffin directly into their breast tissue. The practice of breast enlargement quickly spread to the United States where it was first adopted by Las Vegas showgirls whose livelihoods could be directly enhance by the treatments. The first modern silicone implants, manufactured by Dow Corning, were available from the early sixties on; breast augmentation soon became one of the most popular cosmetic procedures ever.[45]

If success as a suburban housewife depended upon being visibly breasted, as Yalom suggests, then the consequences of losing this emblem of respectability became much more complex after the war. Breast cancer now became a threat to one's social standing as well as to one's private self-image. The potential loss of a breast became doubly dangerous at a time when modern technology promised to boost the efficiency of early detection. Given the enhanced status of the breast, women might understandably be more reluctant to look for symptoms that could lead, down the road, to a mastectomy.[46] And in the absence of symptoms, they would be even less likely to answer the appeal of any public health campaign to sign up for a mammogram. It is hard to imagine their husbands encouraging them to do so, especially since the whole idea of a preemptive approach to health care was unknown to them as well.

From the late 1970s on, the availability of screening mammography squeezed American women between two alternatives in a no-win situation. They could either comply with mammography guidelines and submit to a screening procedure that might save their lives but also might miss an occult lesion altogether or give them a reading that was falsely positive or falsely negative. Or they could turn their backs on early detection, choosing instead to preserve their bodies, and possibly their marriages, at whatever cost to themselves. Both choices put them at high risk. Neither was a solution.

By the late 1950s, the promotion of early detection was so entrenched in American culture that most women probably took it for granted. As mothers of young children, they had ample exposure to the idea that vaccines could prevent some diseases (like polio and smallpox) but they didn't apply this logic to themselves. If they didn't grasp the distinction between cancer prevention and cancer control, it was partly because early detection campaigns had often confounded the two, referring to the practice of breast self-examination, for instance, as a "preventive" approach to breast cancer.

The introduction, in the early 1960s, of the Pap smear to test for the presence of cervical or uterine cancer only strengthened this confusion. Arriving well before screening mammography, it presented the first opportunity for women to be diagnosed with cancer well before any symptoms could appear. It was cheap and simple to use and produced results that were less ambiguous than those associated with any diagnostic test for breast cancer. And its acceptance and use by medical professionals did lead to a dramatic reduction in death rates, which, until about 1940, had been higher than those associated with breast cancer.[47] But although the Pap smear could prevent the appearance of symptoms, it still could not prevent the initial growth of any reproductive cancers. To most American women, this distinction was, for practical purposes, irrelevant. The two events (the moment of biological inception and the moment of detection) could not, in their minds, be separated very far in time. As long as treatment took place before the onset of symptoms, it could legitimately be thought of as preventive medicine.

The idea of prevention, in other words, lost its precise meaning and became a flexible concept.[48] At times, it almost came to mean the prevention of death rather than the prevention of disease. The muddle it became added yet another layer of difficulty for women trying to make sense of the medical messages that confronted them. They may easily have associated regular checkups with the prevention of disease. After all, the occasion of the annual breast exam and Pap smear was also the occasion when the doctor would repeat his or her warnings about all the other nonmalignant conditions (carrying excess weight, drinking excess alcohol, and so on) which the patient was deemed to have some power to prevent. Just the mention of any possible behavioral dereliction, any momentary lapse from rectitude, would conjure up the demons of responsibility and guilt. In this charged atmosphere, how could a woman be expected to separate out those illnesses which were preventable from those that were not? And who or what could be responsible for them if she were not?

That women could not begin to answer this question is evidence of their very limited access to information about breast cancer. The knowledge they did have was based largely on public health campaigns and on personal exchanges with their own doctors. Both released information sparingly, on a "need-to-know" basis, conveying just enough to gain a woman's cooperation but not enough to scare her off. They hoped to secure her compliance, not her active participation. A woman with breast cancer was, after all, to remain a patient, not a partner.

If magazine articles about breast cancer before the 1970s seemed to reflect the same bias found in literature from the ACS or in advice from a doctor, this was no accident. It remained one of the important tasks of the ACS to place articles in the national media that reinforced its overall campaign strategies.[49] Their heavy-handed presence in these stories was often obvious. In one early account written by an ACS officer in *Good Housekeeping*, a woman whose own life had been saved by a fortuitous reading of some ACS material was determined that "what she had learned should become the property of her friends. The pamphlet accomplished this for her naturally and without emotion."[50] A woman's experience here was hardly more than a vehicle for conveying the message of early detection.

The stories in women's magazines may have been personal (and hence more palatable to readers), but they were never subversive. They asked no controversial questions about rising death rates or inadequate or excessive treatments. For the most part they were cautionary tales of individual women who had responded (or failed to respond) early enough and had met with the expected consequences. Women who were members of "The Cured Cancer Club" recounted their personal experiences (a twenty-year survivor of breast cancer surgery talked about her case "as if it had been the 'flu' or a sprained ankle").[51] Doctors narrated exceptional case histories that provided yet another opportunity to beat the drum for early detection.

If women were not exactly suffering from an information blackout, they were certainly being fed intelligence with the gray areas deleted. What they got was a patient-centered picture of disease. The close, even claustrophobic, focus on the relationship between a woman and her symptoms, her doctor, and her treatment kept attention at an intimate scale. The wider world was absent. The disease, as a result, had no acknowledged social or political dimensions. It was a private experience. Nothing in this dynamic encouraged a woman to look beyond her own experience for answers to any of the many dilemmas posed by the disease. If she looked anywhere, it was more likely to be inward than outward.

Public health campaigns continued to exploit this ultimately passive response to breast cancer, relying upon women's enduring sense of responsibility to win their commitment to screening mammography. But just as this most powerful aid to early detection came on the scene, the rationale behind it lost some of its power. The belief that women could save themselves if they caught their symptoms early enough was now under assault from a new theory of tumor biology, first espoused by Bernard Fisher and others in the 1950s. They argued that breast cancer was not really a local disease at all, but rather a systemic one. Contrary to the belief that underlay the practice of radical surgery, breast cancer cells did not necessarily grow first into palpable breast tumors which then grew outwards along predictable channels at predictable rates. Instead, they might migrate almost immediately via the bloodstream to other vital organs in the body. In that case, survival would depend on the effectiveness of systemic treatment rather than on treatment of the breast alone.

There was, in fact, no method of early detection that could pick up this kind of lethal cancer in time. It could easily grow in the interval between one year's mammogram and the next. Even the most acquiescent women, therefore, could not be expected to preempt such a cancer's growth, no matter how rigidly they followed screening guidelines. But if this was commonly understood by health care professionals, it was not something shared with the women patients they served. Mammography may have been flawed but it was the best early detection method available and required the continued cooperation and good will of women, under whatever false pretenses were necessary.

This evasion of the full truth marked no new departure in the handling of breast cancer; it was simply an aggravation of a formula that had been in place since the earliest days of public health campaigns. It made use of the same ever-renewable supply of trust that doctors had always been able to count on. What dislodged this faith was not any sudden discovery by women that their well-behaved response had neither eradicated the disease nor prevented the rise in its death rates. Their slow-gathering awareness was more the delayed aftereffect of other upheavals in their lives, upheavals that disturbed the domestic peace at the center of their lives and then sent shock waves into every previously unexamined nook and cranny.

Women finally began to understand that their unvarying response to breast cancer over most of the century (and their loyalty to the principles of self-help) implicitly reflected a broader faith in the permanence of the social order that had regulated their behavior from birth to death. This turned out to be neither fixed nor God-given after all, but subject to fundamental shifts in direction, even complete reversals. Many women in the 1950s had themselves had personal experience of such a reversal. Hundreds of thousands of them had been stripped of their wartime jobs when men were demobilized following the armistice in 1945. The sympathetic rhetoric and social infrastructure that had accompanied their wartime employment (the provision of childcare, rations, moral support, and so on) had all disappeared in a flash with the return of peace.[52]

Equally ominous, the underlying trend toward greater equality had also turned out to be illusory. Following the success of the women's suffrage campaign, professional women as a percentage of total female employment had risen to 15 percent in 1930. By 1960, it had dropped back down to 11 percent. And even though more women went to college, they represented a smaller share of total enrollment. In their suburban isolation, women had plenty of opportunity to ponder these setbacks. And their discontent was brought into much sharper focus by the arguments in Betty Friedan's *The Feminine Mystique.*[53]

Perhaps it was the cumulative impact of these postwar reversals that, as much as anything else, brought home to women the cost of their own acquiescence. Their abrupt rise in society's estimation followed by their equally abrupt dismissal may have opened their eyes to the opportunism inherent in social upheaval. Their wartime cooperation was welcome; their postwar competition was not. But welcome to whom? Women began to understand that they had been instrumental in propping up a society that valued the ambitions and claims of some of its members more than (or at the expense of) others. The wartime propaganda that emphasized their commonality of interests may have been more an artifact of a society under threat than a reflection of its real beliefs. The postwar redrafting of women's approved roles as wives and mothers now seemed suspect, derived not from their own recent experience, but reworked to accommodate the needs of others, that is, of men.

These received ideas had a powerful impact, of course, on a woman's understanding of and response to her own body, and in particular to her own breasts. How she felt about them was as much influenced by male ideas of female sexuality as was the rest of her behavior. Whatever she chose to do or not to do with them (whether opting for medical or cosmetic treatment or no treatment at all) was influenced at some level by her expectations of male approval. This was one of the unexplored difficulties of the campaigns for early detection that, by its nature, could never be resolved. The battle for control of the breast, in effect, pitted the interests of husbands against the interests of doctors. Both relied upon a woman's passive submission to male authority but they were not always in agreement about what form that submission should take. The conflict this created for the woman in the middle could not be honestly addressed without exposing the underlying sexism of both husbands *and* doctors. Too close an inspection of her position would reveal that she was mediating between two male voices rather than expressing one of her own.

This sense of self-effacement that all medical encounters produced in women was about to be challenged. A younger generation of women was preparing another interpretation of a woman's body, one that made few concessions to male desire. But the first battles in the war that this evoked were not fought over the breast. Breasts were just too overworked, too powerful, and too visible a symbol of the culture's attitudes to relationships between men and women. They would take a back seat, for the time being, to other confrontations but would eventually return to center stage.

6

Breast Cancer within the History of the Women's Health Movements

WITH THE BENEFIT of hindsight, we can now see much more clearly the links between the postwar experiences of many American women in the 1950s and the social upheavals of the 1960s. The abrupt cessation of often liberating wartime employment together with the social propaganda that abetted it must have set off powerful reactions among many of those who found themselves suddenly banished to suburban isolation and Tupperware parties. Their bewilderment and discontent may have remained largely unspoken. But in 1963, they were finally given a voice by the controversial polemic of Betty Friedan's *The Feminine Mystique.*

Friedan turned upside down the central argument of nineteenth-century gynecological practice. This had given a commanding role to the uterus in determining a woman's physical well-being, mirroring the commanding role society had given to childbearing. Since all organs were thought to be connected to the womb, all medical complaints could be traced back to their source in some reproductive disturbance or failure. Betty Friedan described exactly the same set of symptoms to which women were thought to be especially prone—"emotional distress, depression, apathy, anxiety," and so on—but now attributed them to an *excess* of childbearing, rather than to a lack of or an inadequate interest in it. She cited hospital studies that found that women who suffered most intensely from these complaints were those " 'whose lives revolved almost exclusively around the reproductive function and its gratification in motherhood.' "[1]

This was an idea that many readers, even sympathetic ones, would find shocking. Sexuality and childbearing, defining wives and mothers, lay at the heart of the feminine mystique. To suggest that their blessings were not unmixed, that the lives they gave rise to were not wholly fulfilling, was inevitably threatening. The presumption that sexuality and motherhood might be uncoupled, that neither in itself need define a woman's life, was revolutionary.

With some trepidation women began to apply these ideas to their own lives. A retrospective review of their sexual and reproductive histories now recast many of their landmark events more as accommodations to male-dominated society than as choices freely made. Rewritten with women at their center rather than at the periphery, the stories yielded radically different versions of history that sometimes came flooding into consciousness on a wave of shame or anger. Ultimately, women came to realize that if they could reinterpret and reappropriate the past, they might also be able to influence the direction of the future.

The many women's health campaigns that emerged over the 1960s and 1970s drew upon the reconstructed and shared experiences of several generations of women—daughters, mothers, and grandmothers. Despite the wide diversity in their outward appearances and in the moderating influences of race and class, their stories were bound together by a growing sense that the control of one's destiny was indissolubly linked to the control of one's body. This expressed itself most clearly in the energy released by the new women's movement and directed toward birth control and abortion reform campaigns.

Within the longer history of breast cancer, the struggles over reproductive control in the 1960s and 1970s represent, in a sense, the overthrow of the uterus as the command center of a woman's life. As long as the womb remained captive, an agent of a male-dominated social agenda, it governed women's as well as men's reponses to their bodies, emotional and medical. Women's reluctance to pay proper attention to the rest of their bodies was abetted by a parallel lack of medical concern; male models of disease still dominated medical science. Before that could change, the issue of reproduction had first to be dealt with. It had to be reconceived as part of the normal rather than pathological workings of a woman's body. And its dominion over women's lives had to be reined in, leaving its authority still powerful but no longer absolute, and in the hands of women rather than men.

The evolution of the women's health movement that would achieve these objectives did not really begin to pick up steam until after Rachel Carson's death. Ironically, the feminism implicit in Carson's own response to disease, so transparent today, remained well hidden behind the more clamorous social mores of the early 1960s. The changes set in motion by the new world view unleashed in *The Feminine Mystique*, published just months before Carson's death, would eventually make it possible to recognize, in retrospect, the significance of Carson's extraordinary response to her disease and her doctors. But that hindsight awareness, with its public recognition of a private struggle, would take decades to develop. In 1964, the experience of an individual woman, no matter how remarkable, had no wider message for the culture at large. But the old order (with its conspiracy of silence between doctors and patients) was on the cusp of change.

Doctors in most states were still prohibited from providing any form of contraception or abortion to their patients. Now their visible resentment at this interference was beginning to gather strength, and support from their patients was growing. An impressive foundation for what would become the women's health movement had already been laid in the fifties and early sixties by individual activists, legislators, physicians, and journalists. The critical mass of involvement needed to secure national attention did not come together before the mid- to late sixties, but from that moment on, the pace accelerated.

Breast cancer, however, was not an issue that was swept up in these debates, not even marginally. It would take another twenty years before the public even began to think about the disease as a legitimate part of the women's health movement. To many, looking back, the delayed response now seems inexplicable. How was it possible for the women's movement to overlook the persistently high mortality levels associated with breast cancer? How did it come to be treated by the media as "Cancer: the issue feminists forgot"?[2] After all, breast cancer was not a new development; it had been claiming the lives of thousands of women every year for as long as records had been kept. Surely the liberating light of feminism could have focused its beam on the dark corner of breast cancer sooner than it did?

The explanation most commonly summoned to lay this charge to rest is that feminists caught up in the first generation of the women's movement in the sixties and seventies were simply too young and healthy to be concerned about breast cancer. If they thought about it at all, they considered it a disease of middle or old age.[3] To get to middle age at all, they had first to make sure that they would not die prematurely from septic abortions. Those veterans of the women's movement who survived the abortion wars would have moved into their forties and fifties (just into the higher-risk zone for breast cancer) in the 1980s and 1990s. Their spirit of injustice, already honed by their earlier political apprenticeships, would have prepared them for this next round of struggle against the entrenched paternalism of the medical establishment.

Of course there is more than a grain of truth to this story, even if its logic relies too heavily on the self-interest of activists. But the prehistory of breast cancer awareness and the influences on its development are much more complicated than this facile explanation allows for. To make a serious assessment of the connections between the first and subsequent generations of women's health care activism requires a closer look at the dynamics governing each of these campaigns. A better understanding of the factors at work in each case reveals the extent to which breast cancer was able to make use of the reform infrastructure put in place by the earlier movements. But it also reveals the areas of nonconformity, areas where the objectives of the earlier campaigns and the strategies that were pursued to advance them differed widely from those of the breast cancer movement. The way these paths diverged may help to explain the apparent head start that the reproductive campaigns enjoyed and the long interval between their coming to maturity and the first stirrings of breast cancer awareness.

The dynamics of social change

The movements for reproductive health were marked by their common passage through roughly similar stages of development. The movement for breast cancer reform recapitulated, in a more compressed form, these same stages of development, but lagged behind the others

by about twenty years. If this delay reflects some of the additional obstacles that faced would-be breast cancer activists, it was to some extent
offset by the cultural and technological innovations in communications that were introduced during the interim period. This made it
possible to mobilize mass support for an issue at greater speed and with
relatively fewer resources.

In all of these movements for reproductive control, lone voices in the
wilderness clamoring for change appeared at irregular intervals over
several decades. They all failed to generate much, if any, momentum.[4]
A review of the prehistory of contraceptive and abortion reform reveals
a startling amount of activity. For example, a nationwide chain of birth
control clinics had been established by lay advocates of reform by the
mid-1930s. At about the same time, the American Medical Association
(AMA) publicly announced its support for contraception.

It is difficult, in retrospect, to reconstruct with any accuracy the impact of either of these actions on the public awareness. Sixty years ago,
both the reach and coverage of what we would now consider national
media were extremely limited. Television had just been invented and
weekly magazines like the *Saturday Evening Post* and *Life* hardly ever
ventured into controversial waters. American society remained atom-
ized in a thousand isolated communities across the country. These
were all cut off from each other by cultural firewalls that served to for-
tify conservative values. Social change that required the mass mobiliza-
tion of public opinion would have to wait until more modern communications networks could break through these barriers. (Obviously,
breast cancer, being the last to arrive on the scene, has been well placed
to exploit the advantages of these technological innovations.)[5]

In the absence of national television news networks before the mid-
sixties, one of the best ways to attract attention was to focus on specific
cases that were exceptional or sensational enough to be newsworthy.
Real dramas could be tracked via print media on a daily or weekly basis
for months. Such was the case with Sherri Finkbine, who was willing
to undergo a very public ordeal in order to get the abortion she wanted
in 1961. She had taken Thalidomide during her pregnancy before discovering its possible link to birth defects. When she failed to obtain

legal clearance for a therapeutic abortion in the U.S., she was forced to go to Sweden. Her unfolding drama was picked up and reported on an almost daily basis in all major U.S. newspapers.[6]

The coverage of individual dramas was set in context by the work of investigative reporters. An extended series on birth control in 1957 in the New York *Post* won for its author the Albert and Mary Lasker Award in Medical Journalism.[7] Advances in medical science gave an additional spur to the pro-reform camp: In 1960, the FDA approved the use of oral contraceptives for the first time.

Gradually the frequency of media coverage intensified and began to cluster. Early in 1965, the *New York Times* published what was probably the first editorial to endorse the liberalization of abortion. Later the same year, *Atlantic, Time, Redbook*, and *Look* magazines all published major pieces on abortion within one three-month period.[8] Radical feminists appeared on the scene and carried out a series of political protests, calling for national demonstrations ("Days of Anger"), invading AMA conventions, distributing instructions for do-it-yourself abortions, free contraception, or referral lists of doctors willing to terminate pregnancies. Political action, whether carried out in the streets, in doctors' offices, in state courts, or in state legislatures, became more focused and more capable of drawing media response.

For birth control and abortion, all roads led ultimately to the Supreme Court. In 1965 (*Griswold v. Connecticut*), the Court struck down a state law forbidding the use of contraceptives by married couples. In 1972 (*Eisenstadt v. Baird*), it declared unconstitutional another state law forbidding the sale of contraceptives to people who were not married. Finally, in 1973 came the famous *Roe v. Wade* decision which acted to repeal nearly all the existing laws restricting abortion.

This same year witnessed the first public expressions of discontent written by survivors of breast cancer.[9] Because this followed so closely on the heels of *Roe v. Wade*, it might look, in retrospect, as though the seasoned combatants of the reproductive rights battles were passing along the baton to the raw recruits of breast cancer activism, suggesting a smooth and continuous transition from one social movement to another. This kind of continuity had, after all, been important in shifting attention and resources, as well as momentum, from birth control to abortion reform. Both these issues had shared a primary focus on the control of reproduction and relied upon similar tactics to promote their interests. Both birth control and abortion reform counted on similar support from the legal and medical professions and faced similar opposition from the Catholic Church and other religious organizations. So not only was the infrastructure for social change already in place, but the players were already lined up and rehearsed. The supporters and opponents of birth control, for the most part, became the supporters and opponents of abortion rights.

But breast cancer, as a developing issue of concern to women, could not be so tidily slotted into the preexisting framework. It could make only limited use of the foundations for reform put in place by these earlier campaigns. What it could and did exploit were the feminist principles that the campaigns first brought into the public arena and legitimized. The idea that women have "the right to choose," to determine every outcome that might affect their own health, had itself become deeply engrained in the culture. It has, to varying degrees, underwritten almost all subsequent women's health campaigns. The emergence of the Boston Women's Health Collective in 1969 (and its publication of the first edition of *Our Bodies, Ourselves* in 1971)[10] was the first concerted attempt by women to speak the "unspeakable," to appropriate medical terms and knowledge for the practical use of women readers.

For its ability to enable women to reconceive their understanding of the female body and their own relationship to it, the women's movement, in its response to the challenge of contraception and abortion reform, provided an essential spur to breast cancer activism. But beyond this fundamental support, the consequences for breast cancer of either birth control or abortion reform were neither immediate nor clear-cut.

To disentangle those aspects of the earlier campaigns that benefited the incipient breast cancer movement from those that did not requires a closer look at some of the distinctive characteristics of all of them.

What follows below is not a comprehensive outline of any of these initiatives but a review of some of their defining features, selected for their relevance to the dynamics of breast cancer reform.

The sexual politics of reproduction

If the culture's response to breast cancer helped to perpetuate women's oppression in the nuclear family, its response to birth control and abortion provided a strong counterweight. Where breast cancer bred inertia, reproductive issues, *always* threatening to traditional family values, triggered a dynamic response. Women's efforts to control their reproductive lives probably constitute the oldest form of resistance to the basic inequalities of Western marriages. Well before legalization, women found their own solutions to family planning. The fact that they were often willing to put their own lives at risk to carry out their plans reflects the strength of their determination. Legal access to contraception and safe and affordable abortion made it much easier for a woman to act unilaterally, without her husband's permission, even without his knowledge. While this obviously did not eliminate all the inequalities between husband and wife overnight (a wife still might not control her sexual availability or the family finances), it did at least begin to undermine the traditional model of marriage in which a wife submitted to her husband's authority on all matters. Here was at least one important matter on which a wife's authority could not be summarily dismissed. The abolition of legal restrictions on birth control and abortion sanctioned her resistance to male supremacy.

The social ramifications of this change were significant. The move toward reproductive freedom extended potentially to all women, even to those who would never choose to exercise any of its powers. And since the role models reproduced within the family formed the basis for many other relationships in society at large (in schools, in the workplace and, most significantly for this discussion, in the doctor's office), any dynamic that altered the balance of power in women's favor at home would eventually come to make itself felt in other male/female encounters.

The first birth control pills and intrauterine devices approved for use in the early 1960s provided a great—and immediate—boost to the reproductive health campaigns, levering them out of their own backwater and into the limelight. Easy access to apparently safe and effective contraceptives helped to trigger both the demand for these products and the moral outrage that their availability occasioned. Contraceptives unleashed all the demons associated with human interference in the process of conception. If medical science made it possible to intervene at one point in the reproductive cycle, why could it not be used to intervene at other points as well, after conception as well as before? The very availability of birth control pills, in other words, enhanced the medical justifications for abortion.

The explosive arguments created by the ability to regulate reproduction, whether before or after conception, had little bearing on the issue of breast cancer (except in the rare case of a diagnosis made during pregnancy). But for those caught up in the movement to legalize abortion, the passionate responses evoked by defenders of the fetus inevitably brought the subject into the much larger arena of public opinion. Out of the woodwork emerged an extraordinary range of activists, many of whom had convictions (philosophical, ethical, religious) and financial resources, but neither professional nor personal experience of abortion. The widening (some might say "hijacking") of medical issues by outsiders had the effect of bringing the discussion of both birth control and abortion before a much larger audience, where it has remained. As a subject of general rather than narrowly special interest, it multiplied opportunities for media exploitation. Inevitably, the very visibility of birth control and abortion as issues made them hostages to electoral politics, issues over which votes were gained or lost.

The debates over the control of reproduction attracted national interest at a level of intensity that made breast cancer advocacy seem parochial by comparison. Of course the number of those caught up in reproductive issues far outweighed those affected by breast cancer. Each year in the mid-seventies the estimated number of abortions performed in the United States was about ten times higher than the number of women newly diagnosed with breast cancer.[11] No wonder the early reports back from the breast cancer front made so few ripples in the national consciousness. Throughout the 1970s, the discontent expressed publicly by a few brave breast cancer survivors attracted some local interest but still failed to generate the kind of national attention that seemed to accompany every abortion skirmish, however small. The issues were simply deemed to be too narrow and too self-enclosed. Neither the Pope nor the Supreme Court, after all, was ever moved to express an opinion on the overuse of radical mastectomies.

The failure to generate interest among society's "decision makers" left breast cancer in a public relations blackout. There were seven times as many articles on abortion in the *New York Times* in the first three months of 1970 as there were for the whole year on breast cancer. And although breast cancer has appeared in its columns with increasing frequency in the years since then (the *New York Times* Index lists 76 entries for 1997), the coverage of abortion still outstrips it by a ratio of almost three to one.[12]

The role of professions: ally or adversary?

Beginning in the nineteenth century, every state in the nation enacted its own laws prohibiting the practice of abortion under any circumstances. By the early twentieth century, control over reproductive issues had been comprehensively captured by the state. Antiabortion legislation had been a preemptive strike to contain the growing practice of abortion by converting it from a medical to a legal issue. This was a transformation that denatured it permanently. No longer was abortion a private transaction between a patient seeking medical care and a doctor delivering it. Incorporated into common law, doctors and patients became plaintiffs and defendants and their behavior became a matter for public concern and public regulation.

Before legalization, physicians in private practice who flouted the laws prohibiting birth control and abortion could be arrested and prosecuted. By the 1950s, some hospitals allowed therapeutic abortions to be performed but only if a doctor had successfully argued the case before a hospital committee (whose lay members were sometimes more concerned with the possible impact of their decisions on future funding than with their human consequences). Physicians, in other words, were not in charge. Their autonomy was compromised by law and by regulations subservient to that law. By restricting access to treatment, both set limits on the doctor/patient relationship.

Physicians, then, and the legal counsellors who represented them, mounted the earliest challenges to laws restricting abortion. From the beginning, well before they were joined by feminists, both the medical and legal professions were extremely active in pursuing the reform or repeal of these laws. A national conference on abortion organized by Planned Parenthood in 1955 prepared a statement urging abortion reform. The model abortion statute that was later used as the basis for legislation in several states had been drafted in 1959 by attorneys, judges, and law professors from the American Law Institute. These were the weapons of a professional movement and they were duly accorded the attention and status that professionals could command. Of course the opponents of abortion had access to equally respected and influential networks of professional organizations.

If professional engagement with abortion reform played a critical role in laying the foundations for a mass movement, the alliance between feminists and professional advocates also had its drawbacks. The interests of doctors did not always coincide with those of their patients. At the Planned Parenthood conference mentioned above, for example, doctors focused narrowly on their right to make decisions without interference from either the law or hospital committees. But they did not demand this right for their patients. Interference by meddling outsiders may have violated the doctors' sense of professional integrity but it did not necessarily dislodge their ingrained belief in their own superior authority. The conference's final statement, in fact, reflected the enduring paternalist bias by advocating birth control "in the name of the family rather than female freedom."[13]

It is tempting to ask whether the fate of breast cancer might have turned at this juncture if gynecologists had taken a more active interest in the treatment of breast disease. Because the threat of cancer loomed over all irregularities in the breast, women with any suspicious symptoms were (and still are) immediately referred to a surgeon. As Chapter 2 laid out, gynecologists thus lost the incentive to treat benign breast conditions as well as malignant ones. The consequences of making a mistake were just too great. Malpractice suits were not just expensive; they could end a career. But if this split had not occurred and gynecologists had retained a more active involvement with conditions of the breast, perhaps their greater experience with the implications of a "woman's right to choose" might have carried over from reproductive issues to breast cancer. As intermediaries between patients and their cancer specialists, gynecologists might then have been in a position to add their collective weight to their patients' individual expressions of anger at the inadequacies and serious consequences of treatment.

For the most part, the relationships between women breast cancer patients and their doctors could rarely be described as partnerships. Doctors were, if anything, more likely to be feared than loved (obstetricians and to some extent gynecologists were at least associated with the blessings of childbirth). Medical authority over all aspects of breast cancer treatment was absolute; treatments, where they were standardized at all, were regulated by an unwritten consensus rather than by law. Death from mistreatment was no more accountable than death from disease. Unlike the position of gynecologists performing abortions, breast cancer physicians faced no legal constraints on their capacity to act. They were subject to no outside interference. The law, consequently, had no natural oppositional part to play, no locus in the debate. It did not, therefore, play any significant role in the mediation between doctors and patients.

The legal disputes over breast cancer that did eventually arise in the 1980s were more transparently adversarial. Women promoting informed consent legislation were actively opposed by physicians fighting to retain their professional authority and freedom from outside interference. This was cast as a battle between proponents of lay and professional control, not as a fight over the interpretation of legal doctrine. Although in the 1980s women, as patients' rights activists, did succeed in winning passage of informed consent laws in sixteen state legislatures, the laws they passed did not seriously curtail the power of doctors. The new regulations required that patients be informed of the risks and benefits of recommended treatments and medically viable alternatives, but they carried few penalties for noncompliance.[14]

While the issue of breast cancer remained largely a contest between women and the medical establishment, the battle for abortion was a conflict that attracted a much broader spectrum of players. Women and doctors were joined by lawyers, religious activists, and civil libertarians, among others. At any one time, the status of the contest could be gauged from the prevailing mix of legislation (at both state and federal levels), public policy (governing, for instance, funding of abortion and and public health campaigns) and the shifting equilibrium of values governing public opinion. The relative importance of each of these components was itself the result of fierce competition and political maneuvering by an extraordinary range of interest groups.

Many of these groups, or their more numerous offspring, continue to operate. A record-breaking 78 "amicus" (friends of the court) briefs were filed in a challenge to *Roe v. Wade* in the late 1980s.[15] They represented more than 300 different organizations and alliances based on clashing interpretations of law, history, science, philosophy, and medicine. As long as the balance of power between them continues to fluctuate, with some growing stronger (gaining prestige, public presence, political clout, financial strength, and so on) and some growing weaker, the status quo will never be fixed. The culmination of one campaign inevitably precipitates another. If one legal argument is vindicated in court, its opponents will pursue another. In the year after the *Roe* decision, for example, state legislatures introduced over 200 abortion-related bills of their own; 39 passed.[16] If one elected representative or other public figure changes his or her stance on abortion, another will be targeted for conversion.

The future of breast cancer, by comparison, is neither so uncertain nor so unstable. In the end it will be resolved by science, not by sociology. What is at issue is not the final outcome of medical research, but the pace, direction, and intensity of its progress. These are the variables that are controlled by public policy (through the allocation and distribution of research funds). So breast cancer activists must lobby for dollars, scrambling for their share of public monies. The expectation of increased funding is that it will bring forward the date when breast and other cancers can be cured or, better yet, prevented. It is a battle to save more lives sooner. The real opponents are invisibility and inertia; there is no *pro*-cancer lobby in Washington to compete with!

As a result, the battle to eradicate breast cancer, unlike abortion reform, moves forward in one direction only. However slow the pace of change has been, the progress that has been made is irreversible. The disease has entered the public realm; it will never again be treated as "untouchable." There will be no going back to the days of frozen sections, when women submitting to a biopsy often woke up to discover that an entire breast had been removed without their explicit permission. Nor will radical mastectomies ever again become the "gold standard" treatment. These reversals are now unthinkable.

The right to privacy: a help or a hindrance?

So dominant was the clash of belief systems in national debates on abortion that the actual medical aspects of it played only a minor role. The appropriateness and risks of medical intervention carried out by licensed personnel in a hospital setting were never at issue in the early days of the movements for reform. They were certainly not a catalyst for activism as they would become for women with breast cancer.

The procedure then most commonly used to terminate early pregnancy (typically a D & C, or dilation and curettage) was, in fact, known to carry far less risk of complications than a pregnancy taken to term. What interested activists and legislators was not the safety of the procedure used to carry out an abortion but its legal availability. It was the denial of legal access to a simple and safe procedure that put women's lives at risk, not the procedure itself. This essentially reverses the problem facing women with breast cancer. They were confronting high-risk and unproven medical treatments that were perfectly legal rather than low-risk treatments that were illegal.

Given these marked differences, it would not be surprising to discover that the legal arguments most commonly put forward in support of abortion reform would not work so effectively for breast cancer. Most test cases relied heavily on the defense of the right to privacy. Although the Supreme Court in the *Roe v. Wade* decision admitted that "the Constitution does not explicitly mention any right of privacy,"[17] it did identify the "roots of that right" in many of the amendments to the Constitution and used this interpretation to support a woman's right to choose.[18] In earlier cases the Court had presumed the existence of a "zone of privacy" that protected sexual relations of consenting adults, allowing them to make their own decisions about the use of contraceptives. It now offered similar protection to pregnant women wishing to make their own decisions about whether or not to bear an unplanned or unwanted child. The decision to uphold a pregnant woman's prerogative meant that any attempt by outside agencies, of whatever kind, to influence her decision-making could be construed as unwarranted interference.

Privacy is, however, a mixed blessing. Although it is universally cited as a single concept, its meanings vary widely with the context to which they refer, and those meanings are often in conflict with one another. Domestic privacy can be summoned to bar unwarranted intrusion or potential harm from the home, but personal privacy can be called upon just as easily to seal actual harm *in*, enabling it to flourish in secret. Where the exercise of privacy shades from protective use to dangerous abuse is impossible to define with any certainty. The variable interpretations that the concept gives rise to are reflected in our inconsistent responses to the threat of domestic violence, sometimes blaming social services for intervening prematurely and sometimes blaming them for intervening too late. Arguments based on privacy, therefore, remain inescapably controversial.

Some feminists believe that the distinction made between public and private has been instrumental in the oppression of women, that "the liberal ideal of the inviolability of the private uses the doctrine of privacy to protect the status quo." They would argue that "equality can only be achieved if there is public interference, not public abdication."[19]

Some of the legal briefs for abortion do illustrate potentially conflicting applications of the privacy argument and the way it can be used to shelter abuse. Lawyers in one successful constitutional challenge argued that the criminality of the law "violated the *physician's* right to privacy and freedom of speech" (italics mine).[20] This line of reasoning would obviously not be endorsed by the advocates of patients' rights, however instrumental it might have been in its original context. It grants to doctors the privilege to withhold information from anyone threatening to interfere with their practice of medicine. This includes patients as well as hospital committees.

Twenty-five years after the *Roe v. Wade* decision, we have much more ambivalent feelings about privacy. We are much more alert to the alarming frequency and varieties of domestic abuse, all of which are protected by the principle of privacy. But while we have become more aware of that abuse, our capacity to intervene to put a stop to it has been complicated by an increased respect for individual rights and legal safeguards to protect them. Our sense of social responsibility has been eclipsed by our apparent fervor for personal freedoms. This poses a dilemma we have not resolved.

Among those more injured than protected by 1970s-style privacy were women with breast cancer. Like any other taboo subject, the disease had to be hidden away from public view. Breast cancer, like leprosy, brought a terrible disfigurement that was thought to be a precursor of certain death. But unlike the deformities of leprosy (or the visible evidence of other amputations), signs of the disease could, in fact, be hidden away, not just within the privacy of the home but on a woman's body itself. So a woman recovering from surgery did not have to be literally shut away or banished to the equivalent of a leprosarium. Instead, as she dressed to preserve the necessary concealment, she became, quite literally, the living embodiment of denial. The appearance of wholeness that she presented to the outside world (and sometimes even to her relatives) may have been intended to protect her household from the stigma of disease. But it cruelly doubled her own affliction, encouraging her to disguise her pain and discomfort not only to the outside world but also to herself. And, paradoxically, it demeaned the value of privacy itself by allowing the public attitudes of shame and fear to penetrate and warp the intimacies of domestic life.

Virtually no woman with breast cancer was aware of anyone else suffering with it. And the language that would have enabled her to discuss her condition with a fellow sufferer, to exchange, for instance, information about symptoms and the side effects of treatment, was not available to her. The arcane lexicon of the disease (covering everything from axillary dissection to x-rays) was a secret code shared only by the brotherhood of physicians and available only to the exceptional patient like Rachel Carson with both the expertise and the determination to master it. Without it, women could not begin to describe their situation to themselves, let alone to others. But left to their own devices, physicians were unlikely to relinquish the exclusive command of medical knowledge that preserved their unassailable authority over the doctor/patient relationship.

Women with breast cancer were also placed at an additional disadvantage with their doctors by the very nature of their disease. Radical mastectomies were not seen as elective surgery but as life-saving procedures. Inevitably, this increased a woman's dependence upon her doctor and her subservience to him. Given her extreme vulnerability, it was highly unlikely that she would wish to jeopardize this relationship in any way.

Compare this with the nature of the relationship between a pregnant woman and her doctor. Whatever the outcome, whether the physician provided an abortion or delivered a baby, the decision had been made (after legalization) by the woman herself together with anyone she may have chosen to consult. The association between her and the doctor was not contaminated by the fear of death (except in exceptional circumstances). Nor was it a lasting one. Women's lives were not permanently medicalized by their pregnancies.

With breast cancer, there was no catalyst other than death to bring closure to the doctor/patient relationship. Nor was there any other internal trigger to instigate change, to disturb the status quo and expose medical practices to the scrutiny of the public. If anything, the existing dynamic worked in the opposite direction. In upholding the taboo against speaking out, breast cancer patients unwittingly helped to perpetuate the patterns of care that had been unchallenged for decades. Keeping silent about their disease kept them silent about their treatment as well. It allowed the practices they had endured to continue to stagnate in a kind of medical backwater. By minimizing leaks to the outside world, controversy was kept at bay. Privacy was a tool used not to protect the patient but rather to preserve inertia. Breast cancer, accordingly, remained secluded for much longer than many other women's health issues.

When it finally came, the shedding of breast cancer as a private and secret experience had a profoundly liberating effect. In the early 1990s, women quickly realized that the pooling of individual experiences— the sharing of their diverse emotional, medical, and political encounters with the disease—would forge a powerful tool. Underpinning the evolution of breast cancer advocacy, the demonstrated benefits of collective consciousness have been profound. They include the emergence of support groups, serving a variety of breast cancer populations (daughters of mothers with breast cancer, women with metastatic disease, women who have undergone bone marrow transplants, among others).[21] They also encompass the sharing of information on every conceivable aspect of the disease experience: on orthodox and alternative treatment options and their side effects, on clinical trials, and perhaps most important, on their interactions with doctors (how to talk to them, what to ask them, and how to evaluate the answers). There is, in short, now someone to ask anything concerning any aspect of the disease. The miserable isolation of the newly diagnosed woman has now become a thing of the past, at least for those who are well-educated and well-insured. For less privileged women, those whose access to information or quality care is limited (by income, geography, language, or other cultural barriers), the picture has hardly changed at all.

The parallel with hysterectomies

There was another reproductive health concern that surfaced in the late 1970s and early 1980s that may have done more than birth control or abortion to galvanize the attention of women with breast cancer. This was the growing awareness of the overuse of hysterectomies. Women in huge numbers appeared to be willing to undergo major surgery for what often turned out to be only minor medical complaints. Some studies suggest that up to a third of women who had hysterectomies had completely normal wombs at the time of their operations.

The history of the hysterectomy runs parallel to that of mastectomy. Both have been commonly performed since the last quarter of the nineteenth century. Both evolved, over time, from a procedure that removed a single organ to one that included the resection of a variety of other muscles, tissue, glands, or organs. In the case of hysterectomy, this might include the ovaries, vagina, or cervix as well as pelvic lymph nodes and other tissues. The labels attached by physicians to these escalating procedures were also the same: "simple," "radical," "total" (clearly words that reflect the surgeon's rather than the patient's perspective).[22] For much of this century, most women had little idea of the variable definitions of the procedures to which they submitted. For the most part, they agreed to what they understood as "standard" treatment that was universally recommended to everyone in a comparable situation. They simply trusted their doctor's judgment.

This sometimes meant that a woman's agreement to have an ovarian cyst removed could be extended without difficulty to cover the removal of her uterus as well, if her surgeon deemed it necessary to perform a hysterectomy once surgery was in progress. Like the woman submitting to a biopsy for a suspect breast lump who woke to find her breast amputated, the woman who discovered upon regaining consciousness that her womb had been taken away faced a terrible conflict. The wish to challenge the doctor's peremptory decision struggled with the need to be a "good patient" in a situation where death could be a punishment for disobedience. This was an acute form of the more pervasive conflict that emerged over time between a woman's prospective trust of her physician before surgery and her retrospective distrust of him (or her) afterward. Whether a breast or a womb was at stake, the same unresolved issues of dominance and submission were called into play.

By the 1970s the use of hysterectomies had skyrocketed to become the fourth most commonly performed operation in the United States, after tonsillectomy, hernia repair, and removal of the gall bladder. Figures supplied by the Center for Disease Control estimated that three and a half million women aged 15 to 44 had hysterectomies between 1970 and 1978. Between 1970 and 1975, the incidence rate had risen by 24 percent. Only about one-tenth of this total involved women with diagnosed malignancies. The rest had been carried out for a wide range of reasons, for instance, to alleviate backache or menstrual cramps, to remove fibroids, to provide guaranteed contraception.

The removal of a woman's uterus has much more in common with the removal of a breast than the removal of a fetus had with either. From a medical perspective, both the womb and the breast have long been considered primarily as reproductive organs with a usefulness that declines with the decline of a woman's fertility. For many doctors, once these organs had lost their reproductive vitality they were quickly demoted, first to the status of "useless" and then to the more sinister "potentially malignant." This provided the spur to their prophylactic removal.

As for women at high risk for breast cancer, the fear of a malignancy was often all that was needed to get a woman's agreement to the removal of a uterus that showed no sign of disease. In both cases, the presumed medical benefits of surgery overshadowed or ignored the psychological consequences. A psychiatrist writing about hysterectomy, but who could just as easily have been writing about mastectomy, objected to this disregard for women's appreciation of their own bodies. He argued that the surgery "is clearly and immediately visualized as an irreversible, drastic procedure, which removes an organ with high value in the woman's sense of identity and femininity."[23] This did not deter his colleagues from performing the procedure at phenomenal rates.

The operative mortality rate associated with hysterectomies was about 0.1 percent (12 to 15 deaths out of every 10,000 operations). The extraordinary volume of surgeries performed (over 600,000 every year through the 1980s) meant that up to a thousand women were dying annually from postoperative complications alone. Over the twenty-year period between 1965 and 1984 when 12.6 million hysterectomies were carried out, the procedure itself killed more than 12,000 women.[24]

Concerns expressed in the 1980s about the overuse of the operation echo those expressed in earlier reproductive health histories. Isolated studies appearing from the mid-1940s on revealed that up to a third of hysterectomies had been carried out for no apparent reason. Similar studies with similar conclusions appeared at roughly ten-year intervals.[25] Finally, in 1982, the gynecologists' own professional journal admitted that between 10 percent and 40 percent of all hysterectomies performed in the United States were probably unnecessary.

Comparisons of the patterns of surgical practice in England with those of the United States were made contemporaneously but independently by advocates of reform in gynecology and in breast cancer surgery. In the 1970s, studies pointed out that American surgeons performed proportionately twice as many hysterectomies as did their British colleagues.[26] In a similar vein, George Crile (who ten years after his patient Rachel Carson's death was still challenging orthodoxies) compared the low rate of radical mastectomies performed by British surgeons in a 1969 survey (21 percent) with the much higher figure found in a comparable American study (63 percent).[27] Critics of both procedures also drew attention to the different medical systems operating in the two countries. While surgeons working in the National Health Service in Britain had no financial incentive to perform radical rather than more conservative surgery in either case, the dominance of fee-for-service payments in the United States did provide such an incentive.

What separated these parallel discussions of hysterectomy and breast cancer was not their politics or their arguments, but twenty years of enhanced consciousness. Controversies about the abuse of hysterectomies tapped into a preexisting mass audience already primed by the earlier public debates on reproductive health. They were, of course, helped by the fact that for the majority of women involved, hysterectomies remained an elective procedure. However susceptible women were to their surgeons' warnings about potential malignancy, they were still at least minimally less vulnerable than women who were already dealing with an established cancer.

George Crile, on the other hand, was in the early seventies addressing a constituency that did not formally exist. He knew that the incidence of breast cancer was actually on the rise. More women were being diagnosed every year. Crile hoped to reach some of these women before they were diagnosed. His early book, *What Women Should Know About the Breast Cancer Controversy* (1973), attempted to popularize the subject of breast cancer, to make it a subject of general rather than specific interest. He wrote not as a feminist but as a professional advocate for change. Speaking as a lone voice, and vilified by his professional colleagues for doing so, he addressed an audience that had yet to be forged. Although he played a critical role in preparing the ground for the mass movement to come, the real catalysts for change in the public awareness of breast cancer were the voices of women themselves. These were just on the brink of making themselves heard.

Preparing for change

Many of the women who went willingly under the knife subsequently came to regret having agreed to a hysterectomy. There were many reasons to have postoperative misgivings. Besides the abrupt loss of fertility that could never be reversed, there were several serious health problems that could develop. These included urinary disorders, loss of bone density, loss of protection against heart disease brought on by premature menopause, loss of sexual desire, and joint aches and pains. But physicians had not warned their patients of any of these possibilities. They had told them of no risks or side effects. This made it much harder for women to describe or seek some kind of recognition for symptoms not acknowledged by the doctors they had trusted so completely.

Most of these women would not have described themselves as feminists. Yet bit by bit, they may have come to understand that their own best interests had not been served by their willing submission to the medical advice handed down to them. Even if they never consciously made a connection between their own behavior and any feminist theory of oppression, they became aware, perhaps for the first time, that there had been alternatives that had been kept from them. Some of them might even have realized to their dismay that they had colluded in preserving their own state of ignorance. By failing to ask any questions that might be interpreted as challenging, they had denied themselves access to a potentially different outcome.

Down the road, many of these same women would come to have another encounter with the same gynecologist, this time confronting a diagnosis of breast cancer. If one in three American women had a hysterectomy by the time they were sixty, then a large number of them were statistically likely to have to face another round of major surgery for breast cancer. But since the median age of women undergoing a hysterectomy was only forty,[28] well below the median age for breast cancer, there was probably a gap of several years between their first ordeal and their second. This was certainly long enough for a woman to reconsider the long-term impact of earlier surgery on her sense of well-being.

Even the most minimal sense of dissatisfaction could have planted a seed of retrospective doubt about the wisdom of having complied with her gynecologist's recommendation. And the popular media, in the interim, could well have abetted this yet unexpressed discontent. Magazines in the 1980s included widespread coverage of women questioning if not yet overtly challenging their doctors' advice. Even if a woman kept her reservations to herself and remained a well-behaved patient, by the time she had to face breast cancer, her outlook had changed. She knew, even if she didn't allow herself to act on this knowledge, that her doctor's authority was no longer unassailable.

This shift in awareness, however slight, sparked an important change in consciousness that would prove to be irreversible. Women began to see that their doctors' decision-making involved a much more complex mix of factors than they had ever appreciated. As it turned out, there were other issues besides their patients' "best interests" that physicians weighed in determining whether to perform surgery, and how radical that surgery should be. Some of these factors turned out to be financial, to reflect the structure of payment within various health care systems. Others seemed to be associated with the prevailing prejudices of the medical culture, which influenced the definition of a patient's "best interests." As late as 1971, a majority of those attending a conference of the American College of Obstetricians and Gynecologists endorsed the recommendation that *every* woman undergo a hysterectomy, once she had had all the children she wanted.[29]

Missing from the roster of concerns was any consideration of what a woman's uterus or breast might mean to her. This may also have been a question that no woman knew how to ask herself, since she had always been willing to take her doctor's evaluation for her own. The traditional assumption of an identity of interests was in fact a device that allowed the doctor to present his or her own views as a consensus. Packaged as an agreement between doctor and patient, it worked in practice to preempt any deviant views that might otherwise surface in the patient.

But where would those deviant views come from? In the case of abortion, an unwanted pregnancy provided a catalyst from outside the doctor/patient relationship. A woman seeking to have a pregnancy terminated in the seventies or eighties knew she was entering a zone of controversy, even after *Roe v. Wade* had legalized her search. Many doctors were not sympathetic to either the practice or the principle of abortion on demand. It was a direct affront to their practice of medicine as a male prerogative, which had allowed *them* to determine when and if medical intervention was warranted. Here were women who had made that decision independently, seizing authority for themselves. They anticipated a confrontation with their doctors but were either determined or desperate enough to make their choice known. They had, in other words, brought their own solution with them into the doctor's office and were asking not for the doctor's approval but only for his or her technical expertise.

Before the late 1980s, no such solution imported from outside the doctor/patient encounter was ever available to women facing either gynecological or breast surgery. As long as the public did not poke its nose into the medical rationale for either, patients would never think to question the treatments they submitted to. What they needed was as much medical knowledge as moral support. Without easy access to either, they remained alone in the doctor's office, without allies. Compare this with the massive support behind women seeking abortions, at least from the early 1970s on. Their battle had already been fought in the national media and, most important, in the state and federal courts. It was not the privacy arguments conjured up in *Roe v. Wade* but the enormous publicity given to the issue that ultimately emboldened women to act more assertively on their own behalf.

Most women seeking abortions, before or after legalization, had considered the implications of what they were about to go through *before* arriving in a doctor's office. They had discussed the matter either with the man involved or with a friend or relative. Whether painful or not, the decision-making process is itself a consciousness-raising experience, forcing some kind of evaluation of a woman's circumstances in life. The ultimate decision, whatever it is, is not primarily a medical one. And it has usually been made well before a woman enters her doctor's office. So a woman encounters her doctor in a state of emotional alertness, if not one of total certainty. This in itself plays a protective role and helps to redress the imbalance in power that governs other aspects of the relationship.

Again, this sense of preparedness was totally lacking for a woman with breast cancer. The disease literally struck her out of the blue. There was no natural reason for a woman to anticipate her response or discuss it with anyone before a diagnosis had been made. The media didn't discuss it; families didn't discuss it. And after a diagnosis, there was still no one to turn to. The resounding silence all round left a newly diagnosed woman in a state of terrified isolation; this could only reinforce her vulnerability to her doctor. She had few natural allies and a deadly natural enemy. The esoteric nature of the disease (as poorly understood by many doctors as by their patients, it turns out) and its high mortality kept the public at bay and the patient in thrall. Bringing aid to women immured in this relationship would prove to be daunting.

By comparison with breast cancer, abortion was largely a problem manufactured by the culture and would therefore always remain subject to its mutations. As Justice Blackmun pointed out in the *Roe v. Wade* opinion in 1973, "at common law, at the time of the adoption of our Constitution, and throughout the major portion of the nineteenth century, abortion was viewed with less disfavor than under most American statutes currently in effect."[30] If the pendulum had swung away from this position, it could always swing back. So the battle had to be fought continuously and on as broad a basis as possible. All sides had to appeal to the passions and pocketbooks of every thinking American. Like capital punishment or school prayer, abortion became ubiquitous as a public issue.

After the mid-1960s, no exchange between a newly pregnant woman and her gynecologist was ever really private. Even if abortion was never raised or discussed, it was still a hovering presence in the interview. Both the woman and her doctor brought with them into the encounter a history of massive exposure to the evidence and arguments of all sides in the abortion debate. Whether this knowledge was absorbed through the national press, television, professional journals, or personal experience, each side of this exchange understood that he or she was part of a larger discussion in which everyone had an interest. They were players in a recognized public drama.

Breast cancer was a problem that the culture had rejected. It was impenetrable. The encounter between a newly diagnosed patient and her doctor really *was* private, desperately so. Until the late 1970s, there were few breaks in the ranks of professional solidarity. Doctors presented as united and unruffled a front to their patients as they did to the world. Their dreadful knowledge of the disease remained a secret one. What finally broke through this frozen medical culture was the exasperation of the patient herself.

But those first few who did speak out were more truly on their own than most of the early reproductive health campaigners. There were no informal support networks of any kind behind them to break their fall—no sympathetic doctors willing to break the law, no civil liberties lawyers ready to take up their cases, no women's groups offering alternative treatments or do-it-yourself procedures. There was simply no infrastructure at all.

And what these women had to say was not always welcome, even to women with experience of cancer themselves. Although everyone knew about abortions, legal or not, not many people knew about breast cancer. Nor did they wish to know. Denial of the disease had been ingrained in the culture for so long that resistance to it had become second nature. Any woman drawing attention to her own cancer brought disgrace not just on herself but on everyone else with the disease as well. Shame itself proved to be contagious. Given these obstacles, the surprise may not be that it took so long for women to speak out but rather that they ever had the courage to do it at all.

7 𝔯►

From the Closet to the Commonplace, 1945–75

BEFORE THE EARLY 1970s, the literature of cancer had already passed through several distinct phases of development. The first generation expressed the determination of crusading journalists and physicians to reject the universal taboo against speaking out. Written exclusively by men, these early works adopted a no-frills approach to the subject, exhorting readers to reject quackery and to act expediently. "Most cancer, discovered early, is curable. The only cure is the knife," wrote Samuel Hopkins Adams in a widely quoted article in the *Ladies' Home Journal* in 1913. His sentiments were echoed by many others who drafted similar pieces for women's magazines over the next half century.[1]

Breast cancer narratives: the pioneers

First-person cancer narratives written by women began to appear in popular magazines in the late 1930s. These switched the perspective from the impersonal and sometimes hectoring tone of male authority to the more intimate voice of personal experience. They appeared to acknowledge the validity of the cancer experience from the viewpoint of the patient, rather than the doctor. But, in reality, they were performing the same job. Their purpose too was to inform women of the dangers of cancer and to impress upon them the need to consult a doctor as early as possible. They did not dwell on the pain and suffering involved. In fact, they didn't really offer a woman's perspective on the experience of cancer at all. More the instruments of orthodoxy than the voices of dissent, the well-intentioned authors of these accounts probably saw themselves as collaborators, in the best sense of that word. They were, after all, speaking out at a time when the word "cancer," uttered publicly, still had the power to shock. The willingness to attach that stigma to one's self clearly took courage. Most of the women willing to take this risk had to feel that they had the support of the professional cancer establishment behind them.

And, quite literally, many of them did. As wives or relatives of physicians active in cancer control programs, they understood the purpose of their narratives. Bearing witness to their own ordeals as well as to their survival, they intended to strip the experience of its more terrifying medical aspects and to recreate it as a personal or domestic issue. If this could reduce the aura of terror that surrounded breast cancer, more women would come forward sooner with symptoms. Getting the message out to the largest possible audience was critical. Their social connections worked wonders here; articles published in the AMA's *Hygeia* one month sometimes turned up in a condensed form in *Reader's Digest* just a month later.[2]

Behind most of these articles was the belief that fear alone kept women from seeking medical help. And for women like themselves, with immediate access to the best medical care then available, this assumption was probably true. For most middle- and upper-middle-class women, the primary obstacle to treatment for breast cancer was not a lack of money or connections but a psychological aversion to radical surgery and the prospect of dying. While these emotional responses were surely universal, they were probably the determining factor among only a minority of women. For the rest, the overriding consideration would have been the ability to pay; many would not have been able to scrape together even the modest fee for an initial visit.

Women who knew anything about the treatment for the disease understood that surgery was involved, and that surgery was expensive. In the 1940s, few women had health insurance. Those on low incomes, women and men, were significantly underrepresented in early Blue Cross plans of the 1940s.[3] Women poor enough to be eligible for free treatment as charity cases in public hospitals were unlikely to have known about the advantages of early detection; they did not, typically, attend public lectures or read national women's magazines. They often found out about breast cancer when it was too late, when the pain of their own symptoms finally drove them to seek medical help. By then, there was usually little that medicine could do for them.

The published accounts of breast cancer that began to appear in the interwar period, then, spoke to a specific cultural audience. They were clearly expressing the prejudices and privileges of a white middle-class elite. Preoccupied with the nature of the closed relationship between a woman, her physician, and her treatment, they kept the focus extremely narrow, following the format of a woman's magazine profile of the time. The question of a woman's access to treatment or how she was to pay for it did not arise. Nor was there ever any suggestion of patient dissatisfaction with the recommended therapy. To have aired in public any privately felt disappointment would have been as unthinkable for one of these women as exposing marital discord or infidelity.

Two "exposés" in the *Ladies' Home Journal* in 1947 effectively illustrate the cultural constraints at work.[4] Both are the stories of women married to physicians who lived extremely comfortable lives. One is a housewife, Marion Flexner, telling her own story, and the other describes the life of a well-known romance novelist from the interwar period, Mary Roberts Rinehart. Their narratives abound with details that betray a culture still at ease with the prerogatives of class. Rinehart is shown being served breakfast in bed by a maid in one photograph and chatting with her professional in-house chef in another. Flexner makes reference to her "houseman," "laundress," and "colored mammy." Both are able to travel to other cities to consult with internationally known surgeons.

Because breast cancer is involved, both articles take pains to establish the unimpeachable credentials of each woman as "housewife and mother." This is their primary defense against any presumed loss of femininity occasioned by their cancer—a defense used to cushion the impact of breast cancer stories since they first appeared. (The first modern account, presented explicitly as a cautionary tale, was published in 1914.[5] Like so many others that followed, it began on the evening of discovery with a woman "looking forward with the pleasure of an experienced hostess to the little dinner for the entertainment of three of her husband's business friends and their wives."[6] There is a whole world inside that one sentence; many women readers could have slipped inside it and felt completely at home thirty years later.)

Rinehart, we are informed, before becoming a writer, "became a model housewife." In a recitation of her domestic skills that would make Martha Stewart proud, she "made her own jams and jellies and refused ever to serve 'store bread.'" Her celebrity status, in other words, was not enough to excuse her from the compulsory demonstration of her wifeliness. On the contrary, her worldly success was another violation of the approved order of things, adding to the insult occasioned by her cancer. This makes the recounting of her domestic qualifications even more essential.

Cancer enters the profile of her life very late in the story. By the time it is mentioned, we are well aware of Rinehart as a powerhouse of energy, maintaining a furious pace of work, producing up to 5,000 words every day. Although a "tiny lump" is mentioned in a caption to one photograph, the text acknowledges only "cancer," not *breast* cancer, and goes to great lengths to emphasize Rinehart's speedy return to her normal life. Cancer, the article would seem to imply, played as "tiny" and insignificant a role in Rinehart's life as it did in the *Ladies' Home Journal* profile; it was just a minor interruption in an otherwise smoothly functioning and extraordinarily productive life. Only six months after her surgery, in fact, Rinehart, "began a new mystery novel. . . . She was never really out of harness."

Marion Flexner, more housewife and mother than celebrity, writes about her ordeal in the first person, using the format that has now become formulaic. She keeps her story simple and focused. Like the earlier account published by the ASCC in 1914, Flexner's discovery is precipitated by preparations for a dinner party. "I had stuffed the eggs, mixed the chicken salad, peeled the tomatoes and barely had time to take a shower. . . ." The fateful shower reveals a lump but its discovery does not disable her social skills: "there was dinner to be served, guests to be entertained." As soon as they depart, she informs her husband, himself a physician with whom she "had often discussed the subject of cancer."

From this point on, Flexner is, essentially, never alone. She portrays herself, in fact, as someone hardly able to make a move without the approval of either her husband or her doctor. This confirms, for the reader, the sense that women have their mens' permission to seek treatment for breast cancer, even if it compromises their sexuality. The idea that men, in any case, know more about women's bodies than do women themselves is reinforced when the husband in these stories is also a doctor; it adds credibility to his advice. The message seems to be that if women do as they are told, their men will forgive them for the harm that breast cancer inflicts on their femininity.

Everything Flexner knows about cancer she learned from a doctor husband who "had dinned into my ears the fact that all lumps were potentially serious." He "confirmed my findings" after she discovered her own lump in the shower. "What's the program? I wanted to know." He lays it all out for her and then reassures her, " 'It's a tough operation but I know you can take it.' I tried not to disappoint him." Later on, it is her husband who encourages her to face up to the truth. " 'Admit that you had cancer,' he told me. 'Call it by its right name.' " Her doctor is equally involved in her decision to go public. It turns out to be *his* idea for her to write an article, not hers. He even suggests the title. " 'I really think you could do a genuine service by telling others how you've met your problem.' . . . 'What shall I call it?' I asked. 'I have cancer?' He shook his head. 'Call it "Cancer. I've Had It." I think you're cured.' "

Even if women still had to be heavily chaperoned by men through these early, and presumably shocking, confessions of cancer, they did manage to get their stories into print. And their accounts did suggest that it was possible to survive breast cancer. This was a lesson not lost on contemporary readers. Every addition to the body of cancer literature contributed to a growing sense of confidence. And every survivor who had lived to tell her story was beginning to believe she was allowed to tell it, however guardedly.

The next spur to the unveiling of the disease came from contemporary revelations of cancer in other parts of the body (Babe Ruth died of nasal/pharyngeal cancer in 1948, Humphrey Bogart of lung cancer in 1957). The potentially erotic details that made the candid revelation of breast cancer so problematic did not complicate the experience of most other cancers. Malignancies in the liver or lungs were no less distressing, but they grew within organs that were invisible within the body and within the culture. Surgical intervention to remove or reduce them was primarily medical. It disturbed few of the bedrock elements of a patient's self-image, particularly those influencing gender. The association of some cancers, like those of the lung, more with men than with women was an effect of higher rates of smoking among men. Lung cancer in the 1950s in itself did not compromise the prevailing concept of manliness. (Prostate cancer did, and this was one of the reasons it remained invisible for so much longer.)

The underlying importance of gender certainly played a role in what was perhaps the most influential cancer story of the 1950s. This was the prospect of a death from rectal cancer that concluded the autobiography of Babe Didrikson Zaharias, the talented and popular American sportswoman. Zaharias managed to flout all the behaviors prescribed for her sex in the early postwar period. She was athletic and mannish rather than feminine, a high-earning professional rather than a nonearning housewife and, although she was married, deeply attached in her last years to a young woman golfer named Betty Dowd. Arguably, it was the very androgyny of her image and the indeterminacy of her life that made it possible to write such an open account of her experience of disease. Bolstered, too, by immense popularity, Zaharias could comfortably recount the entire story of her diagnosis and treatment, including the details of her colostomy.[7] For anyone else, this would have been unthinkable.

Zaharias did, however, stick to the prevailing rules of disclosure in some important respects. She did not challenge her doctors' advice, remaining, for the most part, a very well-behaved patient. She also kept her tone upbeat, emphasizing the narrative drive of the story rather than its emotional fallout and remaining optimistic throughout. When first diagnosed, she made it clear that she had every intention of returning to the world of competitive golf and she kept her word, winning a tournament a year after her surgery, in 1954. Even after the cancer recurred, she insisted, at the end of her book, that "my autobiography isn't finished yet" (she died in 1956).

Zaharias was an early media star and knew there was a mass audience out there eager to read about her. She would have written her autobiography whether she had had cancer or not. Her expectation of an early death may have brought this task to fruition much sooner than expected, but it didn't supply the motivation to write about it in the first place. The cancer was an adjunct to the main event; it merely rode the coattails of our fascination with celebrity.

Cancer, in other words, had been inadvertently brought into the limelight. But the link with celebrity, which Zaharias's autobiography established, became a useful tool in prying open the closed world of breast cancer. Popular figures in American culture have always been excused for violating conventions, for "pushing the envelope." It has, in fact, become one of their responsibilities to give voice to issues that are forbidden to the rest of us. Where we would be punished, they can speak with impunity. And it's not only celebrities themselves who carry weight with the public. Edward Bok, an early editor of the *Ladies' Home Journal*, reveals "the amazing discovery that the name of the wife, husband, daughter or niece of a celebrity was a lure to the feminine heart almost as potent as that of the celebrity with which it claimed kinship."[8] This celebrity-by-association was to play an important role in the unveiling of breast cancer.

Underpinning our adulation of the famous, at some superstitious level, is the belief that their larger-than-life status may grant them immunity, not just from social codes of behavior but from the laws of nature themselves. They may, in other words, actually manage to outwit death as well as disgrace. Life does not always discourage such irrational beliefs. The history of women with breast cancer who have fallen under the protective power of the presidency is a case in point. All have shared the knowledge of their disease with the public (beginning with Alice Roosevelt Longworth and moving through Betty Ford and Nancy Reagan). But only one has so far died from it (Bill Clinton's mother, Virginia Kelly). Alice Longworth died at the age of 96, in 1980, from other causes. The long-term survival of First Ladies Ford and Reagan, and of Happy Rockefeller and Shirley Temple Black, has only confirmed the mantle of immunity that public power seems to confer.

But the path toward the full disclosures that many of these women would make in the 1970s was really laid out for them by unknown women such as Marion Flexner who took the earliest steps in overcoming the taboos against speaking out. For the next 25 years after her article appeared in the *Ladies' Home Journal*, women's magazines would remain the most important source of information, consolation, and debate on breast cancer.

Throughout the 1960s, male medical authority continued to set the terms of the debate in published articles. The *Ladies' Home Journal* ran a regular column called "Tell Me Doctor," which, as its title implies, perpetuated the supplicant role of women patients. The temptation among doctors to adopt a priestly condescension toward their parishioners must have been hard to resist. They still held all the cards, the power to heal and the power to absolve. In a 1962 issue of the *Journal*, a doctor tells a woman recovering from radiation treatment that he has "especially high hopes of a cure in your case . . . because of your temperament and courage. For instance, look at the calm way we are talking this over. So often a conversation of this kind is a ghastly ordeal."[9]

"Tell Me Doctor" disappeared from the *Journal* by the mid-sixties, when the magazine began to publish articles by writers such as Betty Friedan and Pearl Buck (with titles like "Woman: The Fourth Dimension," "The Sexual Revolution," "The New Political Power of Women," and so on). When a new medical column was introduced, it carried the more neutral heading "Medicine Today." This time out, personal accounts alternated with news stories that addressed issues that were pertinent to all women facing the disease. These articles (and others like them in other women's magazines) probably constituted the only source of information about cancer for most readers.

As early as 1965, the new *Ladies' Home Journal* column raised the question of the possible overuse of radical mastectomy, citing "studies that were widely circulated in the newspapers [that] have cast doubt on the value of radical surgery." At roughly the same time, it drew attention to the low take-up rates for the Pap smear; in New York State, only 11 percent of women were being tested for cervical cancer while in

South Dakota it was as low as 4 percent. The potential usefulness of screening mammography was also raised and the difficulties surrounding both false positive and false negative results discussed. But if these small changes were slowly and quietly advancing a revolution in consciousness among the magazine's politically conservative readership, their significance was lost on younger women newly radicalized by Women's Liberation. One of the token "instruments of torture" that feminists tossed into a Freedom Trash Can in protest against the Miss America contest in 1968 was a copy of the *Ladies' Home Journal* along with bras, girdles, and high-heeled shoes.[10] This was as clear a sign as any of the separate but coexisting strategies for social reform; both acknowledged that change was afoot but each represented a different set of concerns as well as demonstrating radically different approaches to their resolution.

If different generations and classes of women did not yet seem to be speaking directly to one another, what they wrote in the seventies betrayed their common exposure to a real upheaval in ideology. All the writing on women's health from the early seventies on, by men as well as women, bears the marks of those who had lived through the sixties, even if the experience has been refracted through very different lenses. Where attention in the earlier decade had focused primarily on the reproductive concerns of younger women, by the early seventies it began to extend its reach to other female health issues and to all who were involved with them. Male doctors, for instance, still did most of the talking about breast cancer in women's magazines, but their tone had begun to soften. Their approach to their readers as potential patients began to reveal a distinct shift in attitude.

Dr. William Nolan, writing in *McCall's* in 1971, confessed that "choosing between simple removal of the lump and radical surgery may often be a philosophical rather than a scientific matter. When we surgeons try to make this decision alone, we weigh many factors. I believe women have every right to know what these factors are, and to join in the decision." That power-sharing between doctor and patient remained only a radical proposal is evidenced by the response that Nolan's article evoked from another member of the medical brotherhood.

"The surgeon abdicates his responsibility," wrote Dr. Edward Apen, "when he allows a patient to help him decide which operation to perform, especially on such an emotionally charged area of the human body as the breast."

But some patients were now not only ready to help their doctors decide which procedure they wanted to have performed but to make that decision unilaterally. In 1971, Rosamund Campion, a fiction editor at *Seventeen*, refused to sign a consent form permitting her surgeon to carry out an immediate radical mastectomy if a biopsy he was to perform proved to be malignant. As she reported in *McCall's*, her surgeon's response was not pretty: " 'You are being a very silly and stubborn woman. You ask too many questions. I could have performed the mastectomy while you were under, and you would not have to go through this trauma twice and everything would have been fine. . . . Now with a radical mastectomy you'd have a nice clean area.' Urban renewal I thought. Or a pleasant place to picnic. A nice, clean, empty, useless area."

Campion had decided that what she wanted was a simple rather than a radical mastectomy. She had learned about this alternative from an article in *McCall's* written by the ubiquitous crusader George Crile, Jr. When she called the American Cancer Society asking for its support, the ACS declined to give it. Her own doctor told her that "she must put her faith and trust in her surgeon—he knows best." Campion, however, had the determination to disobey, and made the then-remarkable decision to document her doubts in print. In the end, she flew to Crile at the Cleveland Clinic where he performed the surgery she wanted.[11]

Women's magazines often found themselves occupying a vanguard position by default. The unorthodox physicians who published articles in their pages were pleased to address a mass readership, but some of them also had little choice. In the 1970s, many mainstream medical journals continued to reject articles submitted to them by researchers whose work challenged the established pattern of treatment. There were always statistical inadequacies that could be cited as grounds for dismissal—study samples were often too small or biased in some other way that rendered their conclusions invalid. Underlying the clinical reservations expressed by the medical establishment was a determination to suppress the implications of these new studies, to keep their message at bay. So the publication of their heretical ideas within more popular media contributed to a kind of breast cancer *samizdat*, a growing underground literature disowned by the medical establishment but eagerly consumed by readers. If most mainstream physicians turned a cold shoulder to the ideas these unorthodox physicians represented, then the interest of women could be engaged directly, bypassing the professional gatekeepers entirely. This direct appeal to women as an end run around the medical establishment of course compounded the betrayal of those who risked it.

George Crile was not the only conspirator, but he was a member of a very select group.[12] William Nolan was able to admit in *McCall's* in 1973 what would never have passed the censors at *JAMA*, that "if more members of the medical profession had been women, research into the results of more conservative operations for breast tumors—research that has started only recently—would have gotten underway years ago."[13] Actually there were a few women doctors who did play a significant role in testing alternative treatments. Both Vera Peters in Toronto and Eleanor Montague in Houston were involved in trials that explored the use of radiation as an alternative to surgery.

Oliver Cope, a surgeon at Massachusetts General Hospital and a member of a family of Philadelphia Quakers, had, by the early seventies, been a supporter of more conservative breast surgery for many years. He attributed his disaffection with the more radical procedure to his patients, claiming that he had first been made aware of his own prejudices when faced with a patient in 1956 who simply would not consent to radical surgery. "I had done over 200 radical mastectomies and nobody had told me how it affected these women psychologically. The surgeons didn't pay attention and the women didn't dare tell them. It has proved hard to convince the medical profession that a woman's desires should be considered. As for myself, I had not realized how chauvinistic I had been." Cope stopped performing radical mastectomies altogether in 1960. Having repeatedly failed to get his own case study results approved for publication in the New England Surgical Society, he was invited to publish his views in the *Radcliffe Quarterly*. The article that appeared there in June 1970—"Has the time come for a less mutilating treatment?"—was subsequently reissued in *Vogue*.

The beginnings of respectability: clinical and political shifts

The time had certainly come for an overhaul in the medical approach to the disease. The first randomized, controlled trial of mammography screening exams published its five-year follow-up results in the early seventies.[14] These revealed that the mortality rate for women who had undergone screening together with a physical exam was almost a third lower than for those in the control group. The findings gave another powerful spur to early detection, a trend that was encouraged by the development in the sixties, of new biopsy techniques that made it possible, for the first time, to pick up lesions preclinically, that is, before the appearance of any symptom.

Both of these changes—promoting the earlier discovery and the earlier confirmation of breast cancer—prolonged a woman's survival after diagnosis. Where once the length of time between diagnosis and death could be measured in months, it was now likely to be a matter of years, if it happened at all. In some cases, very early intervention did catch the disease before it had a chance to spread so that treatment did effectively offer a "cure." But even in cases where the cancer was simply too virulent to overpower, its earlier discovery (what is called "lead time bias") significantly extended the treatment period. Women were now caught up in the process much earlier on. They had a great deal more time to live with, think about, and adjust to the disease. Although this did not necessarily alleviate their distress (women whose tumors were going to kill them now had time to undergo many more desperate remedies), at least it provided them with breathing space between rounds of treatment in which to reflect on their experience and gather their thoughts.

In the half-century leading up to this point, the appearance of breast cancer had undergone a radical change. The successes of early detection campaigns in bringing forward the date of discovery meant that fewer and fewer women actually suffered from the symptoms of disease *in the breast*. If grotesque, painful, and ulcerating lesions had not yet disappeared entirely, they had at least become rare. Women, as a result, were less debilitated by the disease in its early stages. They no longer had to take to their beds, to withdraw from the world and lapse into illness. Most did not even feel ill but thought of themselves as completely healthy. In other words, a diagnosis was no longer a confirmation of illness but an advance warning of disease.

This downplaying of both the signs of illness and its site in the breast helped to make the disease more culturally acceptable, and made discussion with a newly diagnosed woman more approachable. Paradoxically, as the disease itself became less and less visible, the public recognition of it grew. As friends and relatives were relieved of the obligation to confront breast cancer manifested *as a disease*, they became more willing to take it on *as a medical problem*.

Unfortunately, the incremental changes in perception brought on by earlier and earlier diagnosis did not meet with any equivalent changes in treatment. Radical mastectomies still monopolized the field, producing an ever more anomalous contrast between an apparently healthy woman before surgery and an often permanently disabled patient postoperatively. The starkness of this contrast must have played some role, however gradual, in altering the awareness of women themselves, some of whom came to see themselves as victims of treatment rather than of disease. Of course many of their physicians had already begun to suspect that activity in the breast was no longer the main event. But the time lag between any such suspicions and a change in clinical response would be measured in decades, not years. Still, by the early seventies, medical research had shown unmistakable signs of a shift, like the behavior of the disease itself, away from the breast and toward the system as a whole.

A great many strands had begun to come together at roughly the same time. There were signs of clinical advances in detection and diagnosis, if not in survival rates, that transformed breast cancer into a more presentable disease in its early stages. It was becoming less an illness (with women in visible distress) and more a disease (with science and statistics at its command). The issue of women's health and the growing determination of women to take an active role in promoting it had begun to be taken more seriously as a social issue. The theory that had rationalized standard treatment for three-quarters of a century was under attack from inside the medical establishment.

The links between all of these issues may still have remained fairly tenuous. But even if they were still only dimly perceived by most Americans, they were all contributing nonetheless to a redrawing of cultural boundaries. However poorly understood, the very multiplicity of issues invoked helped to fashion a three-dimensional image of the disease. Whatever its exact components, the elusive process that raises an issue from obscurity to familiarity had now begun.

Newpapers played an important role in fostering this sense of breast cancer as a topic of substance, drip-feeding the public a slow but steady stream of news stories on the subject. For readers of women's magazines, articles in the press added stature to the arguments written by mavericks that were circulating in the pages of the *Ladies' Home Journal*, *McCall's*, and *Vogue*. For everyone, breast cancer now began to take shape as a respected if formidable disease with habits and a history of its own.

The broadening of interest conveyed through the press in articles focused on incidence, research, methods of detection, treatment, and so on, hinted at the changing dynamics within the medical establishment itself. Even if the ranks of professional solidarity had still not been breached and the public remained unaware of the medical controversies that were brewing, the fact that clinical studies and experimental programs were underway was in itself a sign of dissatisfaction with the status quo.

In 1971, interest in breast cancer and other malignancies was given a tremendous boost by the passage of the National Cancer Act, which made the conquest of the disease a national and highly visible priority. Within a year, funding allocated to the National Cancer Institute almost doubled. The details of a five-year plan mandated by the new legislation were announced in the summer of 1972. Beginning with an annual budget of $500 million, the new program would emphasize basic biomedical research but would also oversee the establishment of specialized cancer centers within existing hospitals. By the end of 1974, more than 100 million Americans would have access to one of them. The first eight of these centers were set up by January 1973 in hospitals across the country (from the University of Miami to the Fred Hutchinson Research Center in Seattle).

One of the beneficiaries of this surge in resources were clinical trials set up by the NSABP (the National Surgical Adjuvant Breast and Bowel Project), under the direction of Bernard Fisher. These were designed to test the validity of an alternative theory of tumor biology, one that, if proven, would refute the hypotheses underpinning the Halsted mastectomy. Fisher himself remarked that while "the Halstedian hypothesis, contrary to usual scientific practice, was readily accepted without test of its validity, it was realized that a competitive theory would of necessity require the attainment of credibility before it would attract most of the next generation of practitioners."[15] The new breast cancer trials were the first step toward establishing that credibility. Financial support from the National Cancer Institute suggested a new openness on the part of the cancer establishment toward at least the possibility of change. If breast cancer turned out to be a systemic disease rather than a local one, then the primary emphasis on local treatment, that is, on radical mastectomies, would be misplaced. It might turn out that conservative surgery (removing the breast but leaving the underlying muscles and axillary nodes intact) would yield survival results that were just as good. In the early seventies, newspapers began to describe the newly funded trials that were testing this possibility. Although they were still referred to as "studies" and the NSABP was never mentioned by name, their objectives and methods could be explained.[16]

Meanwhile, the promotion of early detection, the one strand of publicity with a well-established lineage, continued unabated. In the early seventies, newspaper articles described the plans for over twenty breast cancer detection centers sponsored jointly by the American Cancer Society and the National Cancer Institute. Set up as demonstration projects, they were designed to provide free examinations and mammograms to thousands of American women. A careful monitoring of results would, it was hoped, confirm the value of screening mammography. The first three centers were located in Atlanta, Louisville, and New York City. The *New York Times*, in its coverage of the program, even supplied its readers with the telephone number of a local screening facility to make it easier for women to make an appointment.

All of these news stories, covering the often concerted activities of the National Cancer Institute, the American Cancer Society, the NSABP, and other research projects suggested the beginnings of an infrastructure dedicated specifically to breast cancer. The disease now commanded the interest and funding resources of the medical research establishment. It was beginning to acquire respectability.

More breast cancer narratives: a gentle acclimation

The pace of media interest did not suddenly accelerate in the early 1970s but neither did it diminish. The modest rate at which articles continued to appear gently acclimated readers to a subject that many still found shocking. Regular, unsensational news stories helped to build up an alternative view of the breast, one that viewed it dispassionately in a context that was plainly medical rather than erotic. The shift in perspective was given a boost by contemporary feminist campaigns protesting the use of sexist imagery in advertising. The traditional representation of breasts in print journalism had served, almost without exception, to titillate male readers and to remind female readers of their own physical shortcomings. *Ms.* magazine, from early 1972 on, included a regular section called "No Comment" which reproduced some of the more egregious examples of sexism in print. It drew attention to the use of suggestive breast images to promote products of all kinds.

In the context of scantily clad women selling everything from plumbing to pot roasts, stories of breast cancer were obviously subversive, cruelly undermining the very associations that the ad agency's art department had worked so hard to encourage. That there was conflict between the different representations of the breast portrayed by newspapers is clear. Whether any editor ever consciously worried about the impact that breast cancer stories might have on advertising revenue is unknown. One journalist wrote that her editor wanted to place her breast cancer piece in the wrong section of the paper, "sprinkled amongst ads for denture adhesives and trusses." He didn't "think nipples should appear in the staid old" section of the paper devoted to serious thought and editorials.[17]

In these early days of public discussion, the press served as a critical intermediary between the closed world of medical science on the one hand and the equally sequestered world of breast cancer patients it was deemed to serve on the other. But the two worlds still remained at arm's length from each other, not yet communicating in any productive way. The terror surrounding the disease may have left many women reluctant to find out any more about it than they had to. The dry and impersonal nature of breast cancer stories, full of science and statistics, made it easy enough to turn the page and move on to something more palatable.

At the fringes of the medical issues that formed the core of newspaper coverage were a very few stories that pursued the "human interest" angle, openly investigating the social impact of breast cancer. Stories appeared documenting the discrimination faced by cancer patients in the job market. They described the employment policies of organizations like the United Nations that prohibited the hiring of cancer patients for five years following "successful" treatment. A few surgeons began campaigning against this discrimination, with support from the American Cancer Society.[18] Women's pages began to run articles on the fashion implications of mastectomies. One paper ran an interview with a woman who had just opened a shop (called Regenesis) for those like herself, who had found it almost impossible to ask for or receive help in buying suitable clothes after undergoing radical surgery. The new boutique sold clothes designed for just this group of women. The description of their special features—all dresses and tops with sleeves, necklines cut not too low, and loose armholes—was as close as the papers had yet come to an admission of the physical consequences of mastectomies. It was one thing for news or science stories to list the tissues and muscles removed by radical surgery but quite another for stories on the women's page to hint at the impact of their removal on the daily lives of women. This was a clear step in the appropriation of the disease by those most affected. As one of the new customers put it, with a recognizable whiff of group consciousness, "We want to be able to buy what other people buy . . . there are a lot of us walking around."[19]

Finally, a story came along that arrested everyone's attention and merited front-page coverage. Betty Ford's breast cancer, picked up in a routine physical checkup, hit the headlines in early October 1974. The announcement came just months after Nixon's resignation, following the most egregious demonstration of presidential nondisclosure that Americans had ever witnessed. Although not the first celebrity to go public with her diagnosis (Shirley Temple Black had come forward with her own story two years earlier), Betty Ford's revelation seemed to reverberate through the culture in an unprecedented manner. Her breast cancer was front-page material.

The news, however, was not released to the public until Ford entered the Bethesda Naval Hospital, after completing a full round of official duties performed with all the composure expected of a First Lady. The following day, she submitted first to a biopsy and then, when the results showed the presence of a malignancy, to a radical mastectomy. Coverage of this event was universal. *Newsweek* featured Betty Ford on its cover; coverage inside included a long sidebar that set out to explain the four different surgical options used in the treatment of breast cancer (Ford's had been the most radical). Unusually, this was accompanied by diagrams of the breast. Despite the candor inside the magazine, the banner headline stamped across Betty Ford's photograph on the cover failed to give a name to the procedure that she had actually undergone, identifying it only as "The Operation."

Rose Kushner and the rise of breast cancer activism

An immediate and important consequence of Betty Ford's breast cancer was its propulsion into the limelight of a woman who would become the first nationally known breast cancer advocate, Rose Kushner. She had been diagnosed with breast cancer herself in July of the same year. A medical journalist, she had written an account of her own experience for the *Washington Post* shortly afterward. The newspaper sat on her piece, waiting for some "news peg" to hang it on. Betty Ford provided that opportunity.

Kushner's first breast cancer article, like all her work, was a heady brew of personal experience mixed with wide-ranging medical and sociological data, and it overflowed with indignation at the way women with the disease had been treated. She took aim at the Halsted mastectomy, refused to have one herself, and had a great deal of trouble finding someone willing to perform a modified radical instead. After learning of Betty Ford's diagnosis, she tried to get through to the White House to encourage Ford to consider the more conservative surgical option, but she was too late. The message came back to her through an intermediary that "The President has made his decision." Kushner felt that Mrs. Ford had been "butchered unnecessarily," the inevitable consequence of going into the operating theater uninformed. She wrote in a private letter, "Most women know nothing when this calamity strikes and there is apparently an enormous education and information gap everywhere about what to do when it does. Mrs. Ford didn't know either. She could have used this article a month ago."[20]

For perhaps the first time, Kushner made it clear that the more a woman herself understood about the disease *before* a diagnosis, the less traumatic her experience of illness would be. This was a radical departure from the message conveyed by articles of the 1940s and 1950s. Behind the voices of the earlier breast cancer survivors was the voice of the medical establishment. In speaking out, women like Marion Flexner hoped to persuade others with early symptoms of disease to come forward as soon as possible and put themselves in the hands of their doctors. At that point, judging by the lack of further details documenting her actual experience, a woman's responsibility seemed to end. The physician took over, worked his magic, and released her back into everyday life.

Breaking completely with this tradition, Kushner opened up a wide space of her own from a position inside her ordeal and filled it with the complex mix of reactions that diagnosis and treatment had evoked in her. She refused to be rushed through it but insisted on hanging around long enough to take stock of the inconsistencies and illogic that seemed to be part of the standard approach to therapy. The eclectic nature of her writing, its rough edges and inconclusiveness, reflect an unresolved but nevertheless clear attempt to break up the standard narrative of the breast cancer experience. If she could not single-handedly put all the pieces back together again, she could at least draw attention to the extraordinary number of pieces that there were. Each of them, she insisted, had to be held up to the light and examined on its own.

Her story became both living demonstration and advocacy of the role of the informed patient in the experience of breast cancer. The subtitle of her pioneering book, *Breast Cancer: A Personal and an Investigative Report* (1975) reveals the author's intention to transform her personal experience into a public platform. This was really an act of daring. None of the earlier writers had made any attempt to relate their own experience to those of other women with disease, to move, in other words, from the specific to the general.[21] Kushner used the reconstruction of her own ordeal to expose, at every turn, the entrenched medical practices that had remained unchallenged and unproven for more than half a century. What made her narrative so compelling was not just the graphic descriptions of the physical and emotional trauma she endured but the rendering of her change in consciousness as she passed through the maze of treatment. She emerged from it all a breast cancer activist, and remained one until her premature death from the disease in 1990 at age 60.

Kushner's book was really the first attempt to use a personal narrative of breast cancer as a springboard to a much broader discussion. A memoir, a comprehensive handbook, and a manifesto all rolled into one, it opened up an extraordinarily rich debate. High on Kushner's list of targets was the enduring "one-step" practice of carrying out a biopsy on a woman while she lay unconscious on the operating table and then, if the results were positive for cancer, proceeding directly to a radical mastectomy, without conferring with her at all. She argued fiercely for the introduction of a "two-step" procedure that would give doctors more time to stage the disease correctly and women more time to make up their minds about the best course of action for them to pursue. "Separating biopsy from mastectomy," she argued, "gives women *a voice in controlling their own destinies*" (italics hers).[22] In 1979, Kushner made sure that a recommendation for a two-step procedure was presented to an NIH Consensus Development Conference by delivering it herself in person. The positive response, which effectively put the NIH's seal of approval on the practice, sent an unequivocal message to surgeons across the country.

Kushner also accused surgeons of being overeager to operate and of being driven by the economic rewards of their practices. She would be surprised to discover, 25 years later, that the economic incentives driving the allocation of medical resources had passed from doctors to health insurers. They too are interested in the costs of breast surgery but from a perspective that now includes hospital costs as well as surgeons' fees.[23] Kushner knew that conservative surgery had the potential to lessen the traumatic effects of a breast cancer diagnosis but that its negative impact on the incomes of surgeons might delay its adoption.

The conflict of interest that surgeons faced in recommending treatment to their patients was a subject pursued by George Crile, Jr., as well. Crile connected the fact that American surgeons performed twice as many operations per capita as their British colleagues with the prevalence of the fee-for-service system in the United States. He pointed out that Blue Shield's reimbursement for a radical mastectomy was as much as three times that paid for a simple mastectomy at a time when most European surgeons, operating within state-sponsored health services, had more or less abandoned the practice altogether.[24]

The fight against excessive treatment was for Kushner, as it was for Crile, just one of an extraordinary range of battles she fought on the breast cancer front. She urged women to seek counseling before they were treated, and to find specialists with experience in breast cancer, rather than putting themselves in the care of general surgeons. She argued for better and more widely available prostheses and for greater sensitivity in fitting women with them. She fought for health insurance

coverage for mammograms. Her courage in criticizing medical practices she disagreed with was much less common then than it has since
become. Not afraid to contradict the arguments of individual doctors,
including her own, she went around the world interrogating them, always on the lookout for alternative approaches that American doctors
might have disregarded.

In keeping with earlier breast cancer narratives, Kushner's book-
length account of her own experience carried a medical seal of approval in its forward, written by her own doctor. But she is no longer
speaking under the armed guard of the medical establishment. In what
is a departure for the genre, her doctor gives the necessary imprimatur
but then qualifies it, distancing himself to some degree from her assess-
ments. Kushner, he says, "is harder on general surgeons than I would
be and what she says about the 'economic incentive' in the diagnosis
and treatment of breast cancer is not what I would say—but the value
of her discussion far outweighs any differences we may have."[25] Here,
then, is the first suggestion of a dialogue between physician and patient. They might not agree on everything, but both are allowed to have
their own opinions and to air them.

The extent to which American women were ready in the early 1970s
to accept the responsibilities that Kushner recommended can be
gauged by the response her book evoked. One TV interviewer told her,
"I would never have read your book if I hadn't been assigned to do it."
Another reporter told her, "I put another jacket on it so I could read it
on the subway."[26] While most reviewers welcomed the exposure of the
subject to broad daylight, the objections raised by some read today as
expressions of false consciousness. Their defense of the prerogatives
of male surgeons could be fierce. One writer, dismissing the idea of a
"two-step" procedure as likely to cause "mental and emotional agony,"
made clear her faith in her own surgeon's ability to decide what was
best for her. "In 1973 I gave my surgeon the order of, 'Do the job that
has to be done, doctor.' " She believed that it was "a gross disservice to
women that the subject of breast cancer has become another toy of the
Women's Movement."[27]

That the Women's Movement was not yet poised to give a proper answer to this challenge once and for all was evidenced by the insistence of Kushner's publishers a few years later that she change the title of her book for its second edition. In that and all subsequent editions, the words "breast cancer" were deleted from the title. The title *Why Me?* replaced it in the reprintings of 1977 and 1982 and *Alternatives* took its place in 1984.

Kushner's willingness to tackle so many of the obstacles she had encountered herself, and her ability to bring the public's attention to them, laid the groundwork for what eventually would become the modern culture of breast cancer. At its most basic, this was the recognition that the disease had a continuous presence within the culture, independent of its victims. Breast cancer was no longer viewed as a string of isolated events, surfacing for a moment each time the news of a friend or relative's death was passed on and then scurrying back to its hiding place. It now began to acquire staying power, a kind of cultural depth.

Its regular (if still uncommon) appearance in the national press was itself a sign that the disease had a claim on the attention of the general readership. Included in that coverage was news of the rise in breast cancer incidence; it was clearly not a disease that had been conquered. The introduction of stories about the national investment in hospital cancer centers, in mammography screening facilities, in clinical trials, were as much public health announcements as they were news stories. Even if it was information that women, in their dread of treatment, chose to ignore, they could still discern the outlines of a national network of biomedical and clinical involvement. All of this was indirect evidence of the huge numbers of women affected. Hospitals from around the country were participating in the same clinical trials, enrolling thousands of participants; mammography screening facilities were pooling the results of many tens of thousands of x-rays.

Should any readers down the road have cause to bring this vague perception into sharper focus, they would now have a sense that a diagnosis of breast cancer no longer branded them with a unique stigma or banished them from the world, particularly from the modern medical world. Rather than being whisked away under cover of darkness and forced to submit to an ordeal cloaked in secrecy, they would be ushered instead into well-lit medical corridors where the no-nonsense clinical atmosphere and multidisciplined approach of hospital staff conveyed a confidence based on years of experience with the same dread disease.

Breast cancer on television

While Kushner and others like her (Betty Rollin, Rosamund Campion, Helga Sandburg, and others)[28] were bringing breast cancer to life on the printed page, television also began to take some risks. Television broadcasting considerably extended the public's awareness of the disease, reaching out to what would become, by the sixties, a truly mass audience. Although coverage before the mid-seventies was rare, there was enough early programming to suggest a pattern of development similar to the process visible within print journalism and books.

One of the earliest programs about breast and other cancers actually predates most of the magazine and newspaper coverage. In 1959 (when five out of six American homes already had television), the National Broadcasting Company, the American Cancer Society, and the Educational Television and Radio Center collaborated on a six-part series called "Tactic," designed to improve the public's attitudes toward early diagnosis and treatment. The show's producers had invited "creative" input from the country's artists, including screenwriters, actors, and dancers, to help find imaginative solutions to the problems of fear, procrastination, vanity, and shame.

To kick off the series, the president of the American Cancer Society introduced the film director Alfred Hitchcock, who clearly knew a great deal about the dramatic manipulation of fear. His view was that "it's not fear that keeps people from doing what they should about cancer. It's the avoidance of fear. Fear is a perfectly normal response to a real threat." To demonstrate ways in which a sympathetic doctor might encourage a newly diagnosed patient to express that fear, he "decided to stage an impromptu drama, a technique," he said, "that anyone can use—the PTA or a drama class." With the help of two actors, both preposterously young, he directed a semi-improvised sketch of a woman receiving and reacting to a diagnosis of breast cancer delivered by her doctor. Interrupting now and again to tease a more realistic and human response from one or the other of his volunteer actors, Hitchcock drew from them a portrayal of this exchange that was actually quite moving.[29]

"Tactic" may well have been the first broadcast on the subject to reach a television audience. The show's purpose was unabashedly didactic. Its messages were explicit, and delivered first by the president of the ASC and then reinforced, each in his or her own idiom, by the various artists who contributed to the series. Cancer had to be confronted head on. As the comedian Steve Allen put it in one of the episodes, the word "cancer" had to be brought into the common language so that we would use it the way we would "use a word like baseball or bread or streetcar."

But if we were encouraged to name it, we were not encouraged by this series to find out much about the disease itself. Candor stopped abruptly at the gates of scientific knowledge. None of the programs encouraged curiosity about the science involved; there was no mention of malignancies or metastases, a reminder that the medical profession in 1959 was still a long way from being willing to share its trade secrets with the layman, not to mention the laywoman. Nevertheless, the shared assumption behind this series, that cancer was a public enemy that could be fought collectively and that everyone had something valuable to contribute, was an important idea to broadcast.

By the time the first soap opera ran a story line on breast cancer fifteen years later, that sense of public commitment had begun to disappear. Public health messages about cancer were now more often delivered by indirect rather than direct means; they were embedded in the scripted dialogue of characters set within the structure of a dramatic narrative. The era of broad-brush documentaries like "The Killers" broadcast in 1974, which had a separate episode on cancer, gave way to more intimate, personalized dramas written for day and nighttime series. At the same time, responsibility for the cure or management of the disease began to move away from being a concern of society at large (and the subject of optimistic documentaries), as it became apparent that cancer was going to be much more difficult to control or eradicate than anyone had suspected.

CBS's "The Young and the Restless" was the first soap opera to broadcast a fully realized version of a breast cancer saga on television. Reaching millions of regular viewers, the story, broadcast in 1974, followed a woman through all the stages of breast cancer treatment. According to Bill Bell, creator of the series (who still works today on "The Bold and the Beautiful"), the original idea for the plot line came from his wife, who had done some research on breast cancer for her own radio talk show. The story line drew an enormous mail response, mostly positive.[30]

Jennifer Brooks, estranged from her husband Stuart, discovers a lump in her breast. She is shown in her hospital bed (fully made-up, of course) struggling with her urge to flee. As with many of the narrators of the early magazine sagas, Jennifer is primarily concerned about the threat to her sexual attractiveness. "The thought of being disfigured this way. How could I ever be with a man again? I'm not going through with it." Her daughters prevail upon her to at least agree to a biopsy, citing the statistics and probabilities of its being malignant. Ultimately she agrees and the clinical adventure begins. . . . For the next several months, the soap follows her treatment story, interwoven with other plot lines, through all stages of her subsequent treatment.

The significance of this first televised portrayal of the disease is hard to overestimate. For the millions of women who were reluctant readers, daytime drama offered an intelligible demonstration of what was involved. Although it generated no critical perspective, it did present the step-by-step ordeal of one woman going through all the prescribed paces, emotional and physical. It made clear to its audience that breast cancer was something that could be both named and discussed. The continuation of the story week after week made the point that the disease was a drawn-out process rather than a crisis, that women had time to consider what options to pursue, and that they could change their minds. The chronic nature of the disease could, in fact, be extremely well conveyed in a soap opera whose most characteristic dramatic feature, was, after all, its open-endedness and lack of closure.

Just a year later, at the end of 1975, two breast cancer stories appeared on television within three weeks of one another. The first, a documentary called "Why Me?," aired on public television in late November and was advertised in *TV Guide* under the heading "Breast cancer patients tell what it was like." Hosted by the actress Lee Grant, it recounted the experiences of women who had undergone mastectomies and was followed up by a discussion among doctors of the different types of surgery available and their reputed effectiveness. This was followed in early December by an episode of "Medical Story" which featured another breast cancer story.

Over the next decade, television incorporated a personal experience of breast cancer into many dramatic series, among others, "Lou Grant," "Cagney & Lacey," "Thirtysomething," and "St. Elsewhere." In addition to fictional stories, the networks also produced made-for-television movies based on published accounts of breast cancer written by or about celebrities. So, for example, CBS broadcast a movie version of Betty Rollin's book *First You Cry*, ABC broadcast "The Betty Ford Story," and NBC, "The Ann Jillian Story." (Later transfers from the book to the television screen include "Reason for Living: The Jill Ireland Story," in 1991 and "My Breast," based on a book of the same name by Joyce Wadler, made in 1994.) All these stories relied upon the same formula, that is, they all followed the path of an individual woman from diagnosis to recovery (death on the TV screen is rare).[31] For the most part, they emphasized the impact of the disease on a woman's self-esteem and on her personal relationships. They did not document the transformation of personal experience into political consciousness, following the experience of Rose Kushner.

In producing movie adaptations from books, television was clearly following the lead of the print media. But television, in reaching what are truly mass audiences, had access to a much broader range of the American public and exercised a much more pervasive influence over the definition of cultural issues. In adopting the perspective of the early breast cancer testaments, television certainly helped to create and then to reinforce a national awareness of breast cancer as a *personal narrative*. This emphasis on the intimate, individual struggle between the disease and its victim, with its focus on breast cancer as predominantly a domestic drama, has colored every aspect of its social history until quite recently. Even if it has now taken to the streets and legislative chambers, the terms of debate in which it is now embroiled still show the unmistakable signs of this early and persistent bias.

8 ≈

At the Close of the Century

IF THE breast cancer experience of Betty Ford marks a boundary between the "before" and "after" of our breast cancer consciousness,
something similar might also be said of Franklin Delano Roosevelt's
experience of polio 40 years earlier. The national perception of polio
after F.D.R. was, like the perception of breast cancer after Betty Ford,
indelibly altered. Both understood their extraordinary influence on
the public's acceptance of disability. Before F.D.R. and Ford, physical
perfection was still a requirement of membership in the presidential
pantheon; any impairment in a president was thought to compromise
his capacity to lead; in a presidential wife, to threaten her image as the
figure of idealized American womanhood.

The parallels between the two really stop there, with the basic association between a White House name and a turning point in the history
of disease. Much more revealing is the striking contrast in the nature
of the dynamic that each set in motion following his or her diagnosis
and public disclosure. The differences between them, in fact, reflect
not simply the expected differences between a president and a First
Lady in their command over resources and their ability to act independently but also clear differences in ideology prevailing in the country at
the times the two were prominent. The contrasting political and social
environments of the 1930s and 1970s, in other words, also contributed
significantly to the fate of the two diseases that these national figures
brought into the limelight.

Essentially, the mechanisms that F.D.R. set in motion in response
to his own disease led to the eradication of polio as a national health
emergency within twenty years. From the time of his trial rehabilita-

tion in the waters of Warm Springs, Georgia, Roosevelt was always engaged with the experience of others suffering from the disease. As he knew only too well himself, they were as much the victims of prejudice as they were of disease. Anyone so afflicted was deemed to be "a menace and burden to the community . . . only too apt to graduate into the mendicant and criminal classes."[1] Roosevelt, by his own example, did a great deal to dispel this view of those who were then called "cripples." But he did much more than that. Deflecting attention away from his own illness toward a confrontation with the disease itself turned out to be extremely productive, as well as politically expedient.

When Roosevelt established the National Foundation for Infantile Paralysis and the March of Dimes in 1938, neither government nor the medical profession had come to monopolize the control of disease. So while the new Foundation drew upon the services and expertise of physicians, it was never controlled by them. It remained in the hands of appointed volunteers. As a result, it could announce its intention to fund the high cost of patient treatment for those who needed it. Roosevelt, who had set up a patients' aid fund at Warm Springs in the 1920s, insisted that he didn't want "anyone to be sent away for lack of money."[2] To many medical professionals, this, of course, set a dangerous precedent.

By 1938, physicians, not volunteers, had already gained control of the privately funded American Society for the Control of Cancer. In the same year that the polio charity was set up, the ASCC's newly formed Women's Field Army, designed to bring the message of early breast cancer detection to women across the country, was operating according to guidelines provided by physicians. A few volunteers, acting unilaterally, had begun to use some of the funds they had raised themselves to help lower-income women pay for their treatment. This was not a self-conscious attempt to sabotage the fee-for-service arrangement that dominated American medical practice but a pragmatic response to a growing awareness that only women who could afford to pay for treatment would be able to reap the benefits of early detection. But most doctors who treated cancer patients were less concerned with access to treatment than with the narrower issue of payment for it. The women who had charted this unauthorized venture into the waters of "socialized medicine" were taken to task and their activities reined in.

Polio volunteers represented a much broader cross-section of the American population than did breast cancer volunteers, reflecting the diversity in the disease population itself (in age as well as gender). The money they raised was also more evenly distributed across the country as a whole. While about 70 percent of the funds raised by both charities remained in the communities in which they were raised, the March of Dimes reached all areas of the United States while the early benefi-ciaries of ASCC outreach efforts were confined largely to the north-eastern region of the country.

More important were differences in the structure of the two organi-zations. The ASCC was built upon the classic paternalist relationship between the almost wholly male medical establishment in charge of policy and the almost wholly female army of volunteers willing to im-plement it for them. Clarence Little, the director of the ASCC, at-tempted unsuccessfully throughout the 1930s to increase the represen-tation of lay members on the board of directors. But physicians feared a takeover. With the prospect of "womb-to-tomb" health services cir-culating freely in the later years of the Depression decade, many were fearful of the politics that lay members might bring to the table. They resisted any dilution of their own monopoly position, either on the board or in the activities of the organization itself, noting, for the rec-ord, that "the profession is inclined to view with a good deal of antago-nism, national organizations which have as their objective the educa-tion of the laity."[3]

F.D.R. himself inadvertently helped to legitimize this restrictive point of view. In 1937, in addition to setting up the privately financed polio foundation, Roosevelt also signed into law the first National Can-cer Institute Act. This called for the appointment of a six-member Na-tional Advisory Panel to develop strategies to combat the disease. Four of the six members selected to serve on the first council were directors of the American Society for the Control of Cancer, the forerunner to the American Cancer Society. At a stroke, all the prejudices of the can-cer charity were imported wholesale into the new government organi-

zation. From its inception, then, the federal cancer infrastructure incorporated both the disdain of medical professionals for the laity and
a male chauvinism that, as expressed in the workings of the ASCC,
paired the skilled and well-paid work of men with the unskilled and
unpaid work of women. This may have reflected the domestic lives of
upper-middle-class white culture, but as the foundation for a national
perspective on a disease that struck all races and classes of society, it
had considerable shortcomings.

The overriding concern with research, for example, rather than
with access to or payment for treatment, reflects the long-term perspective of the affluent for whom the costs or availability of medical care
were never at issue. This attitude in itself is a luxury to the poor, for
whom the exigencies of illness are brutally short-term. The preference
for research that emphasized treatment rather than prevention also reflected the enlightened self-interest of those at the helm. Putting the
money into a search for better therapies could only enhance the reputation and incomes of doctors, drug companies, and equipment manufacturers. At the same time, it served to keep the government well away
from the direct provision of health care. Efforts to win Medicare coverage for screening mammograms, for example, were not even discussed
until the 1980s. The debate, even then, originated not with the National Cancer Institute (NCI) but with Congresswomen like Mary
Rose Oaker (Democrat-Ohio) in the House. It took several false starts
before legislation was finally passed in 1991.

The new legislation passed in the 1930s enabled Congress for the
first time to appropriate funds to build the research arm of the cancer
operation. But the money raised on behalf of the NCI paled in comparison with the funds raised by the March of Dimes. This national fundraising campaign, which drew on the support of celebrities ranging
from Eddie Cantor to the Lone Ranger, raised twice as much money in
its first year ($1.8 million) as had been allocated to the NCI. Roosevelt
wanted to "make the country as conscious about polio as it is about
TB." In 1948, the year the American Cancer Society celebrated its
thirty-fifth birthday, the number of women who died of breast cancer
was more than ten times higher than the total number of deaths from

polio.[4] Yet by the early 1950s, the March of Dimes was raising over $50 million every year, reaching a level of funding that breast cancer research would not attain for many decades to come. Out of these funds came fellowships to support the work of scientists like Jonas Salk and to pay for the vast experimental vaccination programs whose eventual success led to the eradication of the disease.[5] But between 1938 and 1956, the March of Dimes also dispensed an astonishing $203 million to defray the costs of medical treatment.[6]

The March of Dimes was a maverick operation that answered to no outside authority, medical or federal. Breast cancer was, by comparison, caught up early on in the doubly binding prejudices of its ranking charity and the government agencies whose policies it came to influence. In the mid-forties, Mary Lasker, doyenne of the American Cancer Society, did succeed in replacing many of the physicians on the board of the ACS with members of the corporate elite. But the new board, still all white and all male, was no more enlightened about the sexism of the cancer establishment than its predecessor had been. The repercussions of second-wave feminism took a great deal longer to percolate through to this inner sanctum than it did to most other "old world" redoubts. But since the ACS was far and away the most prominent nongovernmental cancer organization, the consequences of its delayed response have been critical. Its failure to grasp (or to accept) the long-term implications for cancer research of its lack of serious female representation played a major role in what Robert Proctor has termed "the social construction of ignorance."[7]

It's not surprising then that Betty Ford's unquestioning submission to the decisions made on her behalf by her doctors and her husband recalls the much earlier experience of women like Marion Flexner (whose stories convey the impression of an ordeal endured under the armed guard of men). That Betty Ford's surgery took place in the Walter Reed military hospital rather than in a hospital associated with the nearby NCI serves only to strengthen the image of the First Lady as under White House arrest.

Betty Ford herself would probably have felt right at home among the ranks of the Women's Field Army. Her brave disclosure of her breast cancer to the American public belongs to no tradition of radical feminism, but to a quieter strain of social change introduced by largely conservative women. These women drew less on political theory and more on political influence to implement what were sometimes radical changes. Exploiting the protection offered by their husbands' privileged positions, women like Mary Lasker and Betty Ford stuck their necks out in the right direction.

Most of the foot soldiers of the Women's Army had little familiarity with the objectives of the progressive women's movements of their day, and little sympathy for them either. Because they were largely unemployed housewives and mothers, they were not caught up with the reforms of the New Deal that enhanced the rising participation of women in the workforce, intervening, for instance, to set minimum wage and maximum hour standards at work. Nor were they likely to have been intimates or supporters of New Deal appointees such as Frances Perkins, who became secretary of labor, or Mary McLeod Bethune, who was named director of the Office of Minority Affairs of the National Youth Administration. Women committed to volunteerism did not always support the entry of professional women into traditional male preserves. Their interests outside the home were more likely to be an expression of their interests inside it. And their volunteer efforts reflected this bias, extended as they were to issues surrounding the health and education of women and children.

What was new about Betty Ford's response to breast cancer was the change in relationship between a private diagnosis of breast cancer and a public acknowledgment of it. It did not imply any change in the interaction between a patient and her physician. As news coverage made perfectly clear, Betty Ford acquiesced in all the decisions made for her by her husband and doctors. Her open acknowledgment betrayed no hint of anger on behalf of others suffering along with her and certainly no finger-pointing. It reinforced the experience of the disease as an essentially private affair. The outpouring of breast cancer literature that followed Ford's disclosure took her as a model rather than Rose Kushner, whose activism, more overtly feminist and challenging to the medical status quo, did not find such an immediate sympathetic following.[8]

The rise of a national breast cancer consciousness, in other words, occurred, for the most part, outside the progressive feminist tradition. Although Betty Ford, like every other American woman, was inevitably influenced by the myriad changes in thinking that feminism had forced into the culture, her disclosure to the public was prompted by neither theory nor a political agenda. This was both its strength and its weakness. An important piece of consciousness-raising, it made her experience palatable to all Americans. But lacking any wider perspective on the disease, it opened no productive dialogues. For Betty Ford, breast cancer remained a force of nature, beyond the reach of human intervention.

For feminists as well, breast cancer remained an untouchable enemy. Women activists of all stripes had shown themselves eager to participate in the battles between patriarchy and biology, when biology signified normal reproductive processes. But when the battle joined patriarchy with pathology, a different dynamic arose. Where male authority and expertise were believed to be tied up with life-saving skills, the habitual female response of total surrender was much harder to dislodge. If the physician was all that stood between a newly diagnosed woman and death, it would be not just foolish but possibly suicidal to put sexism over survival. Who would risk it, for the sake of principle?

The only way out of this quandary was to demonstrate, as a few of the early campaigners tried to do, that medical intervention had had much less of an impact on the course of the disease, individually or collectively, than its practitioners wanted women to believe. It was not just the political or moral authority of the doctor that had to be brought into question, as it was with birth control and abortion issues; it was his or her medical authority as well.

This was not only a much harder argument to make but a harder argument to make convincing. It was one thing to elaborate the details of women's oppression in the doctor/patient relationship. But to question the accumulated expertise of Western medicine, as a lay outsider and potential patient, was not something that most feminists felt qualified or encouraged to undertake. It was, on the contrary, a course fraught with risk. This helps to explain why so many feminists become breast cancer activists only after their encounter with the disease, not before. There is, alas, no more effective way to learn firsthand about the limits of medical knowledge and the intractability of the disease it hopes to control (and no better way to acquire command of the arcane language involved). Once a woman has been through treatment, she has much less to fear from her doctors; they have already done their worst, or their best. In either case, she is fired with the sense of empowerment that accompanies her liberation back into the "real" world. At this point, the power of her retrospective enlightenment or her anger may at last be sufficient to galvanize her into action.

For a brief period in the late 1970s, corresponding to the short-lived reclamation of the White House by a social liberal, Jimmy Carter,[9] there was, in fact, a surge of protest about the handling of disease that conveyed a great deal of anger, as evidenced by the exigent *First Do No Harm . . . : A Dying Woman's Battle Against the Physicians and Drug Companies Who Misled Her About the Hazards of the Pill* by Natalie Greenfield, published in 1976. The first of Audre Lorde's passionate diatribes against the benevolent paternalism communicated in treatment, *The Cancer Journals,* was another important departure dating from this period; it remains the best-known description of the experience of breast cancer from the perspective of an African American. These accounts, like Kushner's, made connections between the experience of disease and wider social concerns (in Lorde's case, the patronizing and sexist behavior of the medical establishment and all those who represented its interests; in Greenfield's case, the profit-maximizing behavior of corporations). But society still had little tolerance for attacks of this sort, particularly when their messengers were women. However dispassionately presented, social criticism directed at male institutions was inevitably construed as an expression of female anger. And, in the 1970s, taboos against female anger were still very much in place. "To express anger—especially if one does so openly, directly or loudly," as the psychologist Harriet Lerner has written, "makes a woman unladylike, unfeminine, unmaternal, and sexually unattractive."[10] Since breast cancer itself conjured up a terror of these very adjectives, it was only the most brazen or desperate of women who would be willing to lay herself open to a double dose of them.

So it's not surprising to discover that the broader perspectives opened up by these early writers could not, on their own, survive. The flurry of interest and activity—and, yes, anger—that cropped up in the 1970s did not provoke a groundswell of breast cancer activism. And with the return of a Republican administration in 1980, the incipient sense of shared responsibility for social ills, with its promise of remedial action, lost its welcome in the culture.

The retreat this engendered is reflected in the breast cancer literature that followed. While the earlier cancer journals were memoirs with a mission, front-line dispatches, the breast cancer literature that has emerged since the 1970s has been based more on the Betty Ford template than on the Rose Kushner one. It has turned inward, becoming ever more introspective and idiosyncratic. Connecting with a long-established tradition of "women's" literature, it holds the world at bay, while exploring in minute detail the emotional reverberations of a life-threatening illness.

The proliferation of this literature of pain and sorrow helps to explain, at least in part, why the breast cancer experience of Nancy Reagan in 1987 caught so many people off guard. Reagan was an ideal candidate for a lumpectomy; she had a lesion that was tiny, just seven millimeters, and still confined to the ducts. Physicians refer to this kind of tumor as "noninvasive" or "precancerous" because it has not yet entered the bloodstream and so cannot spread to distant sites in the body. For this kind of tumor, a modified mastectomy offered no better chances of survival than a lumpectomy, according to the results of a large study that had been widely reported two years earlier in 1985. Yet Reagan opted to have a modified mastectomy. Although the NIH by now had given its blessing to the "two-step" approach, the unbundling of the traditional practice of moving straight to a mastectomy from a positive "frozen-section" biopsy, Reagan rejected the offer of this procedure, which would have allowed her time to review the test results with her doctors and family.

In saying no to this option, Nancy Reagan lost another opportunity to participate in the discussion of her own treatment: "If you get in there and find out that what you expect to find is true," she said she told her doctors, "don't bring me out to talk about it. . . . I've made up my mind. I want it over and done with. . . . It won't take you long, because I was never Dolly Parton." She told Barbara Walters that in the recovery room she repeatedly apologized to her husband, saying, "I'm sorry, I'm so sorry, I'm sorry for you."[11]

If Nancy Reagan's response disappointed feminists, she was at least willing to share her thoughts with the public. And there were now many others, medical professionals as well as feminists, who were at last willing to speak out, even if some still felt obliged to cloak their identities. One anonymous cancer specialist objected to Reagan's dismissal of the two-step procedure. "Most who are really knowledgeable would view this as wrong," he said. Rose Kushner said that Nancy Reagan's decisions had "set us back 10 years" although she did add that she had the right to make her own choice, however unpopular that might be. Breast cancer specialists at the NCI had not been consulted and had been forbidden even to discuss the general subject of breast cancer with reporters. "We've been frozen out," said an NCI press officer.[12]

Putting an embargo on the dissemination of current medical thinking was a draconian response, one that could only have been initiated by a president determined to protect his wife's privacy at whatever cost to the nation. In the place of a productive exchange of information that the event might have sparked, there was silence. No more than his wife did Ronald Reagan understand or take an interest in the consequences for others of decisions they deemed to be private.

But the consequences of Nancy Reagan's choices were significant. Between 1983 and 1985, the choice of lumpectomy among women with Stage I or II breast cancer had risen from about 15 percent to about 30 percent of the total population of newly diagnosed women. Between 1985 and the time of Mrs. Reagan's diagnosis, the rate remained stable. But in the six months following that diagnosis, there was a 25 percent reduction in the use of breast-conserving surgery as women opted for the same treatment that Nancy Reagan had chosen. Those making that choice were women who, like their role model, were white and over fifty years old; there was apparently no decrease in the use of lumpectomies among African American women. The drop was not associated with any publications during that period in either the medical literature or popular press that questioned the effectiveness of the less radi-cal surgery.[13]

This setback in the steady decline of radical surgery was the clear consequence of the way breast cancer consciousness had been shaped in the culture. Most women's understanding of the disease was limited to the knowledge that could be gleaned from personal narratives, col-lected either from direct experience with friends or relatives, or from published accounts in magazines and books. No generalizations could be made from the disconnected assortment of experiences they de-scribed; with a disease as unpredictable and as variable as breast can-cer, no experience could be representative. Yet women resolutely turned their back on this fact, preferring instead to put their faith in the exemplary power of celebrity.

What is invariably played down or missing from an approach that ignores the forest for the trees, is the range or depth of controversies that infect every aspect of contemporary breast cancer, from the ratio-nale behind various treatments, including the use of high-dose chemo-therapy and bone-marrow transplants, to the explanations given for the wide discrepancies in the use of radical surgery between one part of the country and another. Women need to appreciate this lack of con-sensus; it keeps the handling of the disease in a state of dynamic ten-sion. But it is just this lack of certainty that they hope to avoid by opting decisively, if irrationally, for someone else's solution.

In 1987, there were, in any case, few alternative sources of advice. News stories hinted at changes that were underway but it was often hard for women to relate these to their own predicament. The National Alliance of Breast Cancer Organizations, which would grow into an organization ideally suited to just this sort of challenge, had been in existence for just a year at the time of Nancy Reagan's surgery. Set up by four women with a $5,000 grant, it still had little visibility. In the absence of any other national or representative voice, it is not surpris-ing that some women would make their decisions based on information they had at hand. If Nancy Reagan had access to state-of-the-art treat-ment, they reasoned, how could anyone go wrong following her ex-ample?

In the years following Nancy Reagan's surgery, the public's appetite for breast cancer narratives did not abate but grew by leaps and bounds. It could no longer be satisfied by celebrity cancers. In answer to the demand, a new breed of cancer diaries began to appear, written by relatively unknown victims of the disease. In the first generation, it was established writers like Rose Kushner or Betty Rollin who had carried the disease into print. In the second, it is often the disease that carries the writers. Musa Mayer (author of *Examining Myself: One Woman's Story of Breast Cancer Treatment and Recovery*) had a career as a community mental health counsellor. Rosalind MacPhee (*Picasso's Woman: A Breast Cancer Story*) was a paramedic and a committed outdoorswoman. Juliet Wittman (whose *Breast Cancer Journal: A Century of Petals* was nominated for the National Book Award in 1993) was a writer and teacher. Although each of these journals reflects the perspective (and the metaphors) of their authors' chosen métiers, they remain individual and highly personal accounts.

There can hardly be anyone over 35 today who has not had personal experience of breast cancer, whether directly or indirectly. The impact of the disease on a woman's body, on her personal and family relationships, on her expectations of life are all well known. The motivation for so many of the earlier writers—the need to bear witness, to enlighten an otherwise ignorant public—has disappeared. What, then, explains the proliferation of these newer books?

For a start, every generation is characterized by its own pattern of disease treatment. High-dose chemotherapy and bone marrow transplants, for example, were not features of the cancer diaries of the 1970s. So there will always be a need for updated versions of the basic story. But more significantly, breast cancer diaries have been caught up in the larger trend toward the public observance of private trauma. Upgraded to prime time and center stage, the media now gives to revelations of familial abuse, suffering, and survival the status and attention once reserved for worldly accomplishments. Candid personal exposés have never had such high literary value. First-person accounts of every disease and disorder from back pain to manic depression find sympathetic readers. In most of these stories, the external world is taken as given, a backdrop against which the personal drama is played out. Treatment failures or their uncertain outcomes are interpreted through the narrow prism of individual personality rather than viewed more dispassionately through a broader historical frame. But, as Anne Hawkins has written in *Reconstructing Illness*, although these books "may be read as 'true stories'. . . the emphasis must be as much on the word 'stories' as (on) the word 'true.' . . . As autobiographical writing, they may be less a chronicle and more an interpretation of a life."[14]

Creatures of the nineties, these more recent tales are really more "a thousand points of light" than a concentrated beam aimed at the inadequacies or failures of the health care system. They bear the markings of our contemporary view of suffering, one that views the solutions to personal afflictions as the responsibility of the individual rather than of society. Even if it is nowhere acknowledged, the rise of the self-healing movements of the 1980s and 1990s is evident in these memoirs in their almost ritualistic patterns of self-interrogation and sometimes self-incrimination. The popularity of books by Bernie Siegel and Deepak Chopra attest to our loss of faith in collective responsibility. This does not mean that we can no longer derive any comfort from sharing our experience of disease. For many women writing about their experience of breast cancer, including many African American women, the experience of breast cancer strengthens both their church involvement and their religious faith. Prayer is a daily comfort as is the support of the church community; both play an important role in the healing process.[15]

But the journey chronicled by cancer diaries can also express a darker side of religious fervor. Some of them, in their reconstruction of the steps from discovery through denial to enlightened acceptance, are more self-punishing in outlook, uncomfortably reminiscent of the scripted programs of the recovery movement or of spiritual rebirth as experienced by born-again Christians. Both revive an ancient connection between illness and sin or spiritual disorder that effectively reduces the battle against disease to a matter of personal redemption. Given the right attitude, their stories imply, women can take charge and overcome disease by themselves. By implication, those who fail in this pursuit (that is, those who die, or those for whom the experience was simply not uplifting in some way) demonstrate a lack of moral courage, perseverance, and general grasp of all those virtues associated with a "go-ahead" attitude.

With this tendency to be bullish if not downright Pollyanna–ish about breast cancer, it is not surprising to find most of the diaries published over the past ten years with upbeat endings. The Rosalind MacPhee book typifies the attitude. "Life was full of endless possibilities," she writes at the end of *Picasso's Woman*, "and I was eager to live as fully as I could for the rest of the sweet life that was given to me. Because now I was not dying of cancer—I was living with it." This is surely what most readers want to see. The newly diagnosed patient (in a specialized reading market that grows by 180,000 *every year*) desperately needs proof that survival is possible. The more the better.

But despite this bias toward the optimistic outcome, the depressing truth remains that breast cancer continues to outsmart medical science, behaving insidiously and unpredictably. One in four American women with breast cancer will still die of the disease within five years of diagnosis, and the other three will not be out of the woods. For those with many other kinds of cancer, arrival at the five-year benchmark triggers a final rite of passage, this time back into the world of the well where they are welcomed as "cured" and their cancers forgiven. But women with breast cancer are not so lucky. Their death rates remain elevated for as long as 25 to 30 years after the original diagnosis.[16] In other words, breast cancer remains a killer, however unpopular it may be to say so. Most personal accounts evade this central issue.[17]

A rare exception is Christina Middlebrook's *Seeing the Crab*, subtitled *A Memoir of Dying*. A Jungian analyst diagnosed at 50 with a cancer that had already spread to her spine (stage IV), Middlebrook takes up her story well past the point where most other diaries end; she knows she is going to die, sooner rather than later. She knows that for her, treatment will be palliative, not curative. Nonetheless, she is able to give a wonderfully written and often humorous account of her passage through the desperate remedies of high-dose chemotherapy and bone marrow transplant. The catalog of side effects is staggering—she loses her appetite, her ability to swallow, her fingernails, her capacity to walk unaided, to urinate, to defecate. The collective impact of this roll call is to make us realize how various are the tasks of the body that, when in working order, not only constitute our notion of health but also contribute to our definition of self. Middlebrook loses not just her head hair, but her eyelashes and her underarm and pubic hair as well. With them go all the bodily odors by which she implicitly recognizes her animal existence. One of the pleasures of her recovery from treatment is the reappearance of these odors.

Woven in and out of Middlebrook's gruesome medical saga are speculations on the use of metaphor as an aid to comprehension—whether, for example, images of war and the companionship of an imagined soldier enrich or distort her own expectations of dying or whether, ultimately, any metaphors of war, cancer, or death compromise their reality. These meditations are provocative. They remind us that we are witnessing a battle royal between a mind that is fully alive, alert to the powers, pleasures, and betrayals of language, and a body that is determined to destroy it. What is impressive, and what distinguishes the book from so many other diaries in the genre, is that while we are under its spell, we believe this to be a contest of equals.

At every step of the way, Middlebrook challenges the bromides, evasions and denials of others that express their own dreadful discomfort with her situation. Despite their resistance, she chooses to take an active interest in the prospect of her own death, to become what she calls "a dier" and accept that her "only ally is surrender." Cutting through the self-destructive advice served up by avatars of "New Age tyranny," she rejects their suggestion that "if I have cancer I must have 'needed' it in order to resolve some previous life issue that lies rotting beneath the surface of my life." Many chroniclers of breast and other cancers do in fact argue that the emergence of disease is an expression of a deeper failure to reconcile emotional conflicts and tensions. Even Gloria Steinem, whose *Ms.* magazine has done so much to open up the discussion of breast cancer, treated her own bout with the disease more as a welcome corrective to her denial of aging than the straightforward invasion of a potentially lethal disease.

This willingness to accept responsibility for a life-threatening illness can double the burden on the newly diagnosed patient. If she feels that she has brought the disease upon herself through some form of personal inadequacy, then it becomes her responsibility, rather than that of medical science, to provide a cure. As we have seen from the promotion of early detection campaigns, it has been extraordinarily easy to persuade women to take upon their own shoulders the liabilities that properly belong to society at large.

Their vulnerability continues to be exploited. Without much fanfare, campaigns in support of early detection have, over the past decade, shaded into campaigns for prevention. But prevention in its new context no longer refers to the global eradication of breast cancer from the face of the earth but to each woman's individual ability to prevent the disease *in herself* alone. Prevention, in other words, has been privatized. This approach taps into the same guilt-inducing response that has fueled all the campaigns for early detection but now broadens its scope to encompass many more aspects of individual behavior. The emphasis has shifted from taking responsibility for the warning signs of breast cancer to taking personal responsibility for its recognized risk factors as well.

Gathered loosely under the rubric of "lifestyle," these are crudely assumed to be under a woman's direct control. But even the very few that are (the age at which a woman first has a baby, the number of children she has, her educational attainment, her level of alcohol consumption) are really heavily influenced by her socioeconomic status and her cultural environment. This new approach to prevention ignores the social context in which women live their lives, dismissing at a stroke all the additional constraints they might already face. Women on low incomes in poor neighborhoods, for example, are less likely to have access to either critical information about breast cancer or to have health insurance that might pay for the costs of screening mammography. They are more likely to live downwind of incinerators or factories emitting toxic chemicals into their air and water supply. These are "lifestyle" failures that are hard for individual women to correct. The fact that many of them have their babies early may offer them some protective benefit against the disease but this might well be more than off-set by the impact of early motherhood on the rest of their lives.

Of course the scientific community looks favorably on risk factors that individual women are presumed to control and which can there-fore be modified by changes in individual behavior. If a suspected link can be scientifically proved, then responsibility for eliminating that risk or for reducing its impact on disease passes from the medical es-tablishment to women themselves. But even most of the *known* factors that predispose a woman to breast cancer lay beyond her reach alto-gether (the age of first menstruation, of menopause, a family history of breast cancer, and so on). Lumping them altogether and dumping them in the laps of women deflects attention away from the more intrac-table and still unknown causes of the disease. The hard fact remains that a woman with none of the known risk factors still has a lifetime risk of about one in sixteen through the age of eighty.

Perhaps the clearest expression of this recent trend is the *Harvard Report on Cancer Prevention*. Published in 1996 by the Harvard School of Public Health, it argues that "prevention offers the best hope for significantly reducing the suffering and death caused by breast can-cer . . . this hope can be realized only if the public is adequately in-formed about . . . what measures they can take *as individuals* to reduce that risk" (italics mine). In this formulation, government and corpo-rate responsibilities for disease prevention virtually disappear. They are transferred from society at large to individual women. The buck no longer even passes by the chemical and power plants, incinerators, dry cleaners, sprayed fields. These days, it stops at home.

The radical slippage that has occurred in our perception of breast cancer, which redefines both early detection and the pursuit of low-risk lifestyles as prevention, not only reveals a willful disregard for the truth (which would have to include the fact that many aspects of breast cancer remain unexplained). It also reveals the extent to which the whole approach to the disease has been distorted by an economy con-trolled by powerful economic interests. Corporations driven by the need to maximize profits will naturally fight off any attempts to inter-fere with this process. Efforts to regulate the waste products of production, no matter how toxic, are obviously unwelcome. But the threat of regulation, whether by labor or by government, can often be pre-empted. Large corporations do not simply react passively to public views of accountability; they help to create them. Contributions to the Harvard School of Public Health by some of the largest chemical pol-luters in the country can be seen as efforts, however indirect, to influ-ence the climate of opinion. And, sure enough, the activities of the Harvard Center for Cancer Prevention do not feature campaigns against corporate irresponsibility.

The corporate response to cancer is, in any case, no longer simply a defensive one. That newly diagnosed women have become "medical consumers" as much as "victims" of disease attests to the rise of mul-tiple treatment providers in place of the solitary surgeon. Playing an increasingly prominent role in the therapeutic scramble are multi-national corporations dispensing powerful pharmaceuticals.

The acceptance of breast cancer as a systemic disease inevitably stimulated the development of potent chemical agents. Decision-making about early chemotherapies used as adjuvant treatments was firmly in the hands of physicians; the drugs were also administered in a hospital setting and supervised by hospital staff. The newer genera-tion of drugs include many that are packaged as pills, marketable prod-ucts that can be taken orally by patients at home without medical over-sight. They may be regulated by the FDA and require a doctor's prescription but they are owned by private corporations that are keen to establish an independent relationship with their customers. Adver-tising, once prohibited for use by the medical professions, now gives drug companies direct access to the American public, bypassing medi-cal opinion altogether. Recent changes in the scope of permissible tele-vision advertising greatly extends the potential reach of some propri-etary products into the home. This too plays down the role of the medical intermediary and plays up the consumption of highly toxic drugs as just one more among hundreds of other domestically con-sumed products. Advertising, of course, is not known for its accuracy. But its common use of evasions, half-truths, and hyperbole have more serious consequences when the product it sells is a potentially lethal drug.[18]

The potential market for a drug or a vaccine that could really deliver a clean form of prevention with no side effects is, of course, vast. Drug companies, in the meantime, seem to have few qualms about capitalizing on the fear that drives this market, even if the products they are flogging may be potentially quite harmful.[19] In mobilizing their public relations campaigns, they are, in a sense, reviving and trading on age-old beliefs in women's inherent physical deficiencies. But the modern incarnation of this anxiety is even more sinister than its ancient manifestation. Still fixed upon the reproductive functions that distinguish a woman's body from a man's, such marketing campaigns have replaced a general sense that a woman is inherently weak with a darker underlying assumption that she may be innately carcinogenic.

Drug companies with vested interests in broadening and sustaining their product markets have, of course, an incentive to perpetuate this view of a woman's body as an endless font of treatable symptoms. (In a similar vein, the promotion of antidepressants like Miltown in the 1950s and 1960s depended upon a comparable belief in innate depression among middle-aged middle-class white women—at least until Betty Friedan came along to set them straight.) But as Cindy Pearson, director of the National Women's Health Network, has pointed out, the need for renewable sources of profits yields a dynamic that substitutes one disease (or set of symptoms) for another rather than searching for any true preventative.

The fact that women are vulnerable to the propaganda put out by drug companies is a reflection of their desperation. For more than a hundred years now, they have been promised a cure, and they have obediently lined up for whatever treatment they were offered, however punishing. Throughout the century, their complaisance has been bought by promoting the same sort of negative body image that drug companies continue to rely upon today. It is still a culture of fear that determines women's response, just as it was a hundred years ago.

Medical men, of course, have been equally deceived by the false promises of therapies they pursued. Their own record of persistent failure, particularly their overuse of radical surgery, has made them, too, vulnerable to the promises of wonder drugs. In a sense, physicians and women have been partners in the same *danse macabre* for centu-

ries, with the important difference, of course, that when the music
stops, the doctor may suffer a loss of hope or self-esteem but his patient
most often loses her life.

But if a newly diagnosed woman is just as tightly bound to the medical establishment as ever, both the typical scenario and the cast of characters she encounters within it have radically altered. A hundred years
ago, the management of breast cancer passed from the hands of family
physicians and gynecologists into the hands of surgeons. Accompanying this change was the transfer of treatment from the familiar setting
of home, where relatives were never far away, to the clinical atmosphere
of the hospital, beyond the immediate reach of family and friends,
where the authority of the surgeon in charge was absolute. Today, even
if the experience of disease remains hospital-bound, the authority of
the surgeon as healer-in-charge has been much diluted. After a century
under surgical command that witnessed not the eradication of disease
but its marked increase, the medical management of breast cancer is
moving on once again, this time away from surgery and toward oncology.

A surgical detour

This does not mean that surgeons have retired from the fray; far from
it. There are now more opportunities for surgical intervention than
ever. The emergence of breast reconstruction for women who have
chosen mastectomies has kept surgeons extremely busy. There is some
irony in the fact that Halsted's own strong objections to the use of plastic reconstruction delayed the development of this late-blooming specialty, which has given mastectomies a new lease on life.[20] Halsted believed that any covering of the mastectomy site with muscle taken from
another part of the woman's own body should be "vigorously discountenanced"; such a procedure, he believed, would conceal the recurrence of tumor and increase the possibility of its spread to other parts
of the body. Halsted's radical mastectomy, in any case, did not make
breast reconstruction easy. It removed the chest-wall muscle, and removed so much skin that a skin graft was often required to close the

wound. During his lifetime, a few intrepid European surgeons had begun to experiment with modified mastectomies that enabled them to
relocate some of a patient's own skin and muscle to reconstruct a breast
mound at the site of surgery. But faced with continuing Halstedian opposition, most of these pioneering efforts soon withered on the vine.

It has really been only in the past twenty years—since the general
decline of the radical mastectomy, in fact—that surgeons have finally
mastered the use of combined skin-and-muscle flaps to achieve good
cosmetic results in immediate reconstruction.[21] The shift from radical
to modified radical mastectomy (which removed less skin and left the
chest muscle intact) opened up new possibilities for the surgical replacement of a breast. The later shift to the even more conservative simple mastectomy, which left the axillary nodes undisturbed as well as the
pectoral muscles, provided an additional spur to the development of
new procedures. The timing and actual development of "postmastectomy" breast surgery, then, can be seen as an integral part of the Halsted legacy.

The new surgical specialty that has developed over the past twenty
years has attracted as much controversy as the older battles over mastectomy. There is, as yet, no single preferred solution. Several con-
tenders have their own bands of advocates. The new operations fall
roughly into two camps, chronologically and technically. The first generation of procedures relies upon some kind of prosthetic device such
as an implant or a tissue expander.[22] The second, more recently developed approach (of which the so-called TRAM flap[23] is the best-known
example) uses the patient's own skin and muscle. Those in the latter
group are referred to as "autogenous" to distinguish them from the
"nonautogenous" procedures in the first group. Autogenous procedures involve more major surgery and more serious complications but
they avert the problems associated with the potential rejection of foreign bodies that the use of implants creates.

Running parallel to differences inherent in the procedures themselves are differences in the professional profiles of those who perform
them. Plastic surgeons in private practice tend to endorse prosthetic
breast reconstruction while those working in universities and cancer

centers are more likely to specialize in flap procedures. The former are more interested in "the most practical and least complex solution" to the problem while the latter are "looking for the most innovative or technically challenging approach."[24] The pattern of use of these different procedures, therefore, would seem to reflect the preferences of clinicians as much as those of patients.

Implants have been around for over thirty years. For most of that time they were filled primarily with silicone gel. Despite all the problems of infection, leakage, and possible connective tissue disease that came to be associated with the substance, silicone implants were extremely popular. Introduced to breast cancer patients in 1965, only a few years after they were first used in breast-enlargement procedures, they were quickly accepted by mastectomy patients, rising from an estimated 10 percent of the total number of implants in the late 1960s to about 30 percent in 1991.[25] Controversy surrounding the use of silicone led eventually to its withdrawal from the market in 1992, but the use of implants continued unabated. The silicone filling was simply replaced by saline solution (essentially salt water). Although there is still little information about the long-term effects of this substitute filler, implants have become more popular than ever. The number of surgical implantations following mastectomies in 1998 approached 50,000, almost four times the number performed in 1992.[26] The use of TRAM flap and similar autogenous procedures has also increased. One major study of postmastectomy surgeries found that autogenous procedures accounted for just 13 percent of all reconstructions over the period 1979 to 1983, but ten years later their share had risen to 37 percent.[27]

All these procedures together add significantly to the sheer volume of surgery associated with breast cancer. Surgery is more intensive: a mastectomy followed immediately by reconstruction can take up to eight or ten hours. It is also more extensive: reconstruction can involve many more operations all together. The actual number of procedures depends on the original method chosen by the patient, and on its success. With any of the approaches, a woman might require "revisional" surgery to correct for complications or failure (like the removal or replacement of an infected, deflated, or otherwise damaged implant). The TRAM flap procedure normally requires a separate operation for the reconstruction of the nipple.

Pursuing any of these methods leaves a woman "medicalized" over a much longer period. More procedures mean not just more time in the operating theater, but more time in hospitals (pre- and postoperatively), more tests, more follow-up visits to doctors' offices, and more time convalescing. Of course they also mean more pain and morbidity, adding considerably to the complications of mastectomy and any adjuvant treatment that might be involved. All the procedures involve additional scarring, inside the body as well as out, some of which may create difficulties in interpreting the results of follow-up screening for recurrence. The TRAM flap reconstruction also carries postoperative risks of pneumonia, pulmonary embolism, and hernia as well as pain and muscle weakness at the "donor site" on the patient's body.

The need to make some decision about postmastectomy surgery in advance of primary treatment (even if this is just to make *no* decision) also complicates an already overburdened process and requires the acquisition of yet more medical concepts and jargon. A woman already reeling from the difficulties of sorting out complex concepts of breast disease is further challenged by an introduction to yet another surgical specialty with its own esoteric language, risks, and alternatives to absorb. It does not help that the description of reconstruction relies upon alien imagery that transforms a woman's body into an abandoned field where tissue or skin-and-muscle flaps may be "harvested" or, more ominously, after surgical failure or recurrence, "salvaged."[28]

Although many of the risks of these surgeries are rather serious, they are often quickly overshadowed by the cosmetic concerns that reconstructive surgery stirs up. Aesthetic imperatives, in other words, can easily overrun medical considerations. Plastic surgery can now achieve results that are truly astonishing, both in terms of their aesthetics and their verisimilitude. The appeal is seductive. The albums of "before" and "after" photographs that surgeons share with prospective patients can be very persuasive. Held out to a woman at precisely that moment when she is most vulnerable, the promise of a return to the status quo ante—the almost instantaneous restoration of her body before diagnosis—may be very hard to resist.

The appearance of the breast, in this emotionally fraught setting, can easily become entangled with a woman's hopes for survival. In a curious, unexamined way, the preoperative pacts a woman may make with her own gods or demons, drawing on private beliefs or superstitions, may actually endow the image of a restored breast with magical properties, including the power to ward off recurrence down the road. (In an age still unaccustomed to bionic body parts, these replacement breasts may seem truly "miraculous.") It is the rare plastic surgeon who can acknowledge the exceptional powers that irrational thinking may bestow, or who can refrain from exploiting them. A silent participant in the decision-making process, which admits only "rational" and "scientific" discourse, the mix of illogical hopes and fears can only make a woman even more dependent on the Pygmalion-like judgment of her surgeon. As a result, the extent to which the cosmetic results of reconstruction reflect the surgeon's aesthetics rather than the patient's remains unexplored.[29] So too does the wider influence these aesthetics may come to exert on the culture's changing concept of the ideal breast.

Once a woman has been enticed into this arena, the potential loss of a breast may be transformed from an impairment into an opportunity, that is, less an occasion for introspection and more an opening for unlimited self-enhancement. Suddenly, it becomes possible not only to obliterate the signs of illness but also to fulfill long-held but unspoken fantasies about the appearance of *both* breasts. The postmastectomy reconstruction may be only the beginning. The new breast may no longer match its mate; its size or shape may be preferable to that of the older one, highlighting the latter's imperfections and resurrecting past insecurities about one's breast and body images. In other words, what may be a deeper anxiety associated with loss (of a familiar body, of a sense of wholeness or well-being, even of symmetry), now finds expression as a cosmetic crisis.

Whatever the reasons, about a quarter of women undergoing reconstruction surgery choose to undergo additional, follow-up surgery on the other breast, adding tissue (or another implant) here, removing it (or deflating an implant) there. The process is now open-ended. The patient can undergo as many operations as she chooses. This unrestricted access to elective procedures has altered the perception of surgery. Once considered a life-saving intervention, in which a woman participates reluctantly if not involuntarily, it has become an ongoing process of bodily enhancement in which a woman is a willing and active partner. The long-term commitment to cosmetic adjustments, then, with all its medical drawbacks, has helped to give back to a breast cancer patient some semblance of control.

The marked appeal of these newer operations makes it easier to forget—and to forgive—the fact that they no longer represent any direct assault on established disease. Operating instead at one remove, breast reconstructions are attempts to disguise the consequences of treatment rather than the consequences of disease. The recent addition of prophylactic mastectomies to the surgical repertoire shares this indirection; they are preemptive strikes against a high *probability* of disease, not against confirmed malignancy. Neither gets us one whit closer to a cure or prevention. Both keep alive the idea of breasts as negotiable body parts, bargaining chips in the fight for survival. The willingness of surgeons to perform these procedures confirms both the belief that real breasts are expendable and, at the same time, that substitutes for them are essential. In this light, the immediate reconstruction of the breast following mastectomy seems a latter-day parallel to the immediate performance of a radical mastectomy following a positive biopsy (the old "one-step" practice that Kushner fought so hard to stop). Both practices seem to accelerate and to complicate the experience of disease, depriving women of a necessary breathing space between one step and the next that might allow them to absorb the impact of disease on their bodies and on their lives. Instead, they are forced to contend with a host of secondary demands and consequences that are every bit as exacting of their physical and emotional resources as the diagnosis or the primary treatment itself. The quick succession of treatments, eliding one stage of the experience of breast cancer with another, seems to insinuate that women must not be allowed to dwell on the reality of their illness but must be distracted by an appeal to their vanity.

In truth, the popularity of these procedures may simply be a reflection of the fact that surgery has had markedly greater success in achieving its cosmetic objectives than accomplishing its therapeutic ones.

The aggressive marketing of breast reconstruction inevitably recalls the earlier promotion of the radical mastectomy. Just as the latter was once enshrined as the "gold standard" of treatment, so the TRAM flap now bids fair to occupy a similarly commanding position. The same confidence that once characterized the surgeon's presentation of the Halsted procedure (minimizing its risks, maximizing its alleged benefits) now forms part of the sales pitch for the TRAM flap. The fact that many breast surgeons share offices or close affiliations with plastic surgeons suggests the operation of a well-oiled strategy to increase the efficiency of medical practice by accelerating the pace and intensity of the decision-making process.

But the streamlined presentation that results obscures the real complexity of the issues involved, making a careful consideration of choices virtually impossible. The mutually reinforcing recommendations of two surgeons delivered one after another to an already bewildered patient might be almost impossible to resist. They certainly make it difficult for a woman to ask the right questions about a procedure that may seriously compromise other parts of her body as well as her breast. The lymphedema and loss of arm movement that lay in wait for the woman recovering from a radical mastectomy have their contemporary counterpart in the loss of critical pelvic muscle taken at the donor site of a TRAM flap procedure, to take just one example. In neither case does a surgeon dwell on the details of physical impairments that follow surgery. These are secondary considerations, longer-term consequences for the physiotherapist or occupational therapist to manage. The immediate objective is to gain the patient's approval for the surgery itself, and then to get on with it. Perhaps what is needed here is a revival of the old "two-step" philosophy that, however surgically inefficient, shows some respect for the real difficulties facing *the patient*. The clear separation of treatment surgery from reconstruction surgery would help immensely to disentangle the risks and benefits of one from the risks and benefits of the other.

Ultimately, all these newer surgeries bear the same relationship to the prevention of breast cancer as the introduction of gunshot wound units in city hospitals do to gun control. Both responses are more accommodations to the underlying problems than real solutions. Both use expensive science and technology to mount rescue operations that keep attention focused on the individual drama. All efforts are directed toward the immediate outcome fueled by the desperate hope of a return to normal life, and to a normal body.

The impressive results that can now be achieved seem to generate their own dynamic. If cosmetic surgery can re-equip women with passable substitutes for their own breasts, then their loss is no longer as threatening as it once was. Mastectomies, whether for established or anticipated disease, may lose some of their sting.[30] Never mind the risks of surgery or its possible side effects. More important than these risks, the surgery seems to imply, is the restoration of femininity that it appears to offer. With the promise of ever-better cosmetic results, the supply of sophisticated science and technology and the skills that put them to use have created their own demand. The prevention of disease is not, however, a part of this dynamic; it remains completely outside the loop.

Back to the future

Inside the loop, where treatment of established disease occurs, the transition from one medical paradigm to the next, that is, away from surgery and toward oncology, has been facilitated by a team approach that brings together representatives of all relevant therapies, radiation and social work as well as surgery and oncology. With the patient herself an active participant, the team puts together a course of action. The increasing frequency in treatment plans of high-dose chemotherapy, bone marrow or stem cell transplants, chemotherapy for node-negative patients, and hormonal therapies are a clear indication of the expanded role now played by systemic treatments and, correspondingly, by the oncologists who administer them.

This is, of course, a double-edged sword. The chemical arsenal now in the hands of prescribing physicians gives them every bit as much power over the life and death of their patients as the heroic surgeon wielding a knife at the turn of the century. In an attempt to improve survival rates, drugs of unprecedented toxicity are routinely prescribed. These can take patients to the brink of death, as Christina Middleton has so compellingly described, subjecting them to physical pain and degradation every bit as terrible as those imposed by the disease itself. Some critics of high-dose chemotherapy have, in fact, likened the use of ever more dangerous drugs to an earlier tendency toward extremism in surgery. In the latter case, some surgeons, hoping to improve survival rates, began removing ever more muscle, tissue, and lymph nodes, taking patients to the brink of death. In both surgical and oncological cases such behavior may be a sign of desperation, expressing a reluctance to confront the evidence of diminishing returns for a mode of treatment that may have reached its therapeutic limits.

In a curious way, then, breast cancer at the end of the twentieth century recalls the status of the disease a hundred years earlier. In both periods, the medical consensus accepted forms of treatment that were known to carry high risks in pursuit of uncertain outcomes that could offer no promise of cure. The enduring failure to prevent breast cancer or even to cure it (in its metastatic forms) has given it a reputation for deadliness matched by few other cancers. Over the past hundred years, breast cancer has killed more than two million American women.[31] The prospect of subjecting women to suffering on this scale for yet another century is unimaginable.

Perhaps the best guarantee that no comparable lament will be forthcoming in 2099 is the determination of American women themselves to prevent it. Over the past decade, women have at last begun to respond en masse to the enduring iniquity of breast cancer. Grass-roots organizations began to spring up in the late 1980s, following the clarion call of manifestos like Susan's Schapiro's "Cancer as a Feminist Issue."[32] The earliest of these groups, like the Women's Community Cancer Project in Cambridge, Massachusetts, and Breast Cancer Action in San Francisco, were set up exclusively with volunteer labor. Operating for many years on shoestring budgets, they have had an impact that far exceeds their resources. Many other groups gradually appeared on the scene, across the country, eventually drawing together into loose coalitions at both the regional level (like the Massachusetts Breast Cancer Coalition) and the national level (like the National Alliance of Breast Cancer Organizations). Among the best known of the umbrella groups is the National Breast Cancer Coalition (NBCC), set up in 1991, that today draws upon a network of more than 500 organizations representing close to 60,000 individuals. Activity coordinated by the NBCC has been at the heart of the sixfold increase in breast cancer research funding, rising from less than $90 million before the coalition got underway to more than $600 million in 1999. National signature campaigns succeeded in raising awareness of the disease and gathering support for another escalation in research activity (collecting 2.6 million signatures in 1993 in support of a budget of $2.6 billion dollars by the year 2000).

These achievements, unthinkable even ten years ago, are certainly impressive. And they have been accompanied by massive education campaigns directed at politicians, scientists, and the media, as well as at women. And yet, despite the clear departure that all these new activities represent, there is a sense in which today's breast cancer activism still belongs within the tradition established by the Women's Field Army half a century earlier.

Despite the visible presence of professional women serving on powerful government committees at the highest levels, of spokeswomen whose views are well represented in the media, and of levels of funding that seem astronomical compared with the expectations of just a few years ago, something redolent of the earlier generation of cancer crusaders remains. This may be partly because the great majority of women who have now become active have entered the movement through the classic channels of the ladies' auxiliary: volunteering and fundraising. Of course many professional women have also risen to well-paid positions working within or alongside the cancer establishment. But for the most part, the movement continues to rely upon the goodwill and generosity of unpaid women supporters. At least this time around, these duties can be performed without white gloves.

Women can now demonstrate their support by engaging in distinctly unladylike activities, in distinctly unladylike gear, breaking a sweat by running, bowling, swimming, even in-line skating for breast cancer research. And the results of these exertions have been extraordinary.

But what of the fruits of their labors? Here is the difficulty. How many of these modern-day Amazons would be able to follow the trail of the money they worked so hard to raise? How much influence do they really have on what happens to it after it is collected, dollar by dollar, from friends and neighbors too out-of-shape to participate themselves? Many of them would surely be dismayed to discover that the foundations they have sweated so hard to support accept financial contributions from the very drug companies whose eagerness for profits may put their own health in jeopardy. Nor would they be reassured to know how little of the massive breast cancer research budget was actually invested in projects aimed explicitly at prevention rather than at treatment or cure, or how few projects are designed in any way to investigate the impact of environmental toxins released as by-products of industry.

Prevailing biases in the research agenda reflect the influence of powerful interest groups in society at large. It is impossible to acknowledge one without the other. The scarcity of research into the role of manmade chemicals in cancer causation, for example, is not an innocent oversight of otherwise "objective" science. It reflects at best the indifference and at worst the active opposition of pharmaceutical and chemical industries to any research that might threaten to interfere with their operations. Many women are uncomfortable with this. Despite all the evidence provided by the history of the tobacco industry, they do not want to accept that corporations could put profits before women's lives. They do not welcome the prospect of confrontation. They want, instead, to be left to believe that science will indeed bring them "better lives through chemistry" (as DuPont used to promise them), if only enough money is poured into it.

This is why the NBCC's efforts to draw women more closely in to government research programs has been so important.[33] Educating breast cancer activists to participate directly as informed consumers on peer-review panels exposes them as much to the politics surrounding the awarding of research grants as to its science. What these women will learn from their first-hand experience of government decision-making may prove to be invaluable in the next generation of breast cancer activism.

The future of breast cancer may, ultimately, be held hostage as much by political and economic interests as by the continuing slow pace of research. The problem, in other words, may be as much an ideological one, which asks women to re-evaluate their wider views of society, as one that allows them to focus narrowly on questions of research fund allocation. After all, changes in the delivery of health care that have nothing to do with research could significantly and immediately reduce the toll of breast cancer deaths. More than 40 million Americans have no health insurance. Making comprehensive cancer screening and treatment available free of charge to all uninsured women and men would undoubtedly save many lives. In this underserved population, an estimated 30,000 women are newly diagnosed with breast cancer every year, many of them too late to benefit from available treatments.[34]

Some of the national spokeswomen for breast cancer are reluctant to address the thorny issue of health care provision, mindful of the Clintons' failure to make any headway in this arena and fearful of being dismissed as "radicals." They may not want to stick their necks out when that might antagonize other vested interests in the cancer establishment, including potential sponsors or donors. So, for instance, there has been little criticism of the American Cancer Society, which refused to support informed consent legislation in the 1980s or to join with the March of Dimes and the American Heart Association to endorse the Clean Air Act.[35]

Challenging the power structure may prove to be almost as difficult for today's activists as it was for their grandmothers in the Women's Field Army. It's not just diffidence or inexperience that keeps women from adopting a more far-reaching critical stance. Many of them do not want to look too deeply at the real roadblocks in the path to prevention. They still see breast cancer as their grandmothers did, as somehow *separate* from society, not compromised by its overriding economic imperatives. They fervently hope that it is an issue that can be resolved without open conflict (particularly open conflict with their husbands, fathers, or other familiars at work in corporate America). Behind this hope is a suspicion that commitment to the eradication of the disease may be acceptable only as long as it does not threaten the status quo.

Inevitably, the culture of breast cancer has brought us face-to-face with its politics. It is, in the end, impossible to have a clear-eyed view of the disease that overlooks the wider workings of society. Economic and political concerns bear on it as surely and as relentlessly as does medical science. All will have a hand in the experimental solutions that emerge over the next decade. It may be that, in order to bring us closer to the ultimate goal of prevention, women will have to be willing to accept more wide-ranging roles in society and to create broader coalitions within it (across divisions of industry and science as well as race and class). They have, after all, already demonstrated themselves to be in full possession of all the necessary skills. In fact, it is precisely because the breast cancer movement has already accomplished so much that we forget how very young it still is. Perhaps a shift to a more exacting perspective would simply represent a natural progression of its development so far. Based on the evidence gathered for this book, it could be a life-saving one.

The Last Word: Obituaries

My MOTHER grew up believing that women never died. After all, she claimed she never saw an obituary of a woman in a newspaper. Men, on the other hand, lived heroic lives in the public arena and were cruelly cut down by old age, disease, and, occasionally, by other men.

At their deaths, men's lives, like their bodies, were tidied up for eternity. Like epitaphs cut into tombstones, they were built to last, to be the Last Word. Distilling the messy raw material of life into a streamlined story, obituaries reflected prevailing ideas of the virtuous public life. Airbrushed out of the picture were all the complicating factors of character, temperament, family and personal connections, all those features that help to animate a life story. So assiduously did obituaries strip away all flesh-and-blood details, in fact, that their publication often marked a kind of second death, leaving the reader with a lifeless portrait of sanctified achievement, purified of all personal entanglements.

This traditional emphasis on male self-mastery and the obituary's uninflected roll call of life events made it very hard to accommodate women; they lived much of the time in a domestic world that obituaries never acknowledged. Women themselves had no expectation of any such recognition. "Anonymity runs in their blood," wrote Virginia Woolf in the 1920s. "The desire to be veiled still possesses them. They are not even now as concerned about the health of their fame as men are, and, speaking generally, will pass a tombstone or a signpost without feeling an irresistible desire to cut their names on it."[1]

Their lives, in any case, were not easily adapted to the requirements of the obituary format. They did not move forward in an unbroken line of worldly accomplishments but followed their own, less linear paths. These often strayed off the page altogether, looping in and out of view at unpredictable intervals. With apparent disregard for the tyrannies of chronology, women's lives mixed the "productive" with the "reproductive" in combinations that defied easy categorizing. To attempt to condense them into a simple summing up would inevitably compromise the obituary's simplified story line.

The poor fit between the life and the life story helps to explain both the historic delay in reporting the deaths of women and the curious denaturing of those women's lives once they were covered, reconfigured as they often were to fit the male model. Even now, some obituaries still give off a whiff of the gentleman's club. But if we don't expect to see many women's portraits lining the walls of these establishments, we do at least recognize that membership in the club has now been extended to them.

The admission of women to obituary columns has, like the admission of women everywhere else, altered the nature of the beast. Traditionally, obituaries have been slow to reveal the cause of death. The perennial use of the euphemism "after a long illness bravely borne" made it possible to keep the intimacy and the messiness of death at arm's length. It preserved the idea of dying as a controlled event, with its own rules of decorum. A good death ran parallel to a good life; both required manly and orderly behavior. For men in particular, any disclosure of actual suffering would violate the formality of the occasion, undermining the illusion of a dying man presiding over his death in much the same way he had presided over his life. Any show of emotional distress or pain would also be out of step with the more upbeat portrayal of the life that the obituary enters into the record. And it is the life that matters. Death may provide the occasion but it is not the obituary's true subject. After passing on the bare mortal facts, an obituary quickly sets them aside, retreating at once to the much safer ground of biography.

Women's obituaries have forged a closer connection between life and death. As caretakers of the sick and dying, women are presumed to be familiar with physical ailments and less likely to be squeamish about the body. There is an expectation that their greater intimacy with the process of birth, the beginning of life, somehow bestows on them an easier acceptance of its end as well. Or maybe their presumed familiarity with the so-called life forces is just a projection of the male writer, who hopes to insulate himself from his own inevitable end by recasting death as a female adornment. Whatever the reasons, whether these responses are simply unexamined prejudices or legitimate observations, they have made a mention of dying more acceptable in women's obituaries.

This hasn't come upon us all at once but reflects incremental changes over a long period of time. The gradual disclosure of breast cancer in the columns of obituaries over the past century reveals the slow shift toward a more open accommodation of disease and death. It also offers, in miniature, a summary history of the changes in cultural awareness that I have begun to outline in this book.

For the evidence of this progression, we are indebted to those women whose lives were just too exceptional to exclude from newspaper obituaries. As it turns out, it is not just their lives that have taught us something of value; it is also their deaths. And though probably only one of these women would have considered herself a cancer activist, the end-of-life experiences of all of them have nonetheless enlarged our understanding of the social history of the disease.[2]

Our general awareness of breast cancer is of relatively recent origin. What we know of its nineteenth-century impact comes from late twentieth-century scholarship. No newspapers, for example, reported on the death in 1892 of Alice James, diarist and smart sister of William and Henry. Yet we know, from a recent biography, that she was completely aware of her own breast cancer. She had discovered a lump herself and understood that her refusal of treatment would hasten what she called her "mortuary moment."

The first public discussion of cancer occurred about twenty years after James' death, in an article published in the *Ladies' Home Journal* in 1913. Early campaigns to increase awareness of the "dread disease" did not distinguish between cancers at different sites in the body. This made it much more sinister; cancer could strike at random anywhere in the body and kill. With this kind of power, it's not surprising that the disease became demonized. So dangerous was the Hydra-headed monster that even referring to it by name could attract the "evil eye"; any approach to it had to be veiled behind the "c-word."

The gradual isolation of breast cancer as a separate disease in its own right has obviously had an enormous impact on every aspect of the illness from basic research at one extreme to the everyday consciousness of women at the other. But even before it acquired independent standing, there was already a tendency to view cancer as a woman's disease. Promoted by education campaigns in the 1920s and 1930s, widely circulated slogans claimed that "more women die of cancer than do men" or that "cancer afflicts women in a very much larger proportion than it does men."[3] This early depiction of cancer as a disease of women (contrasting with heart disease as a male affliction) may help to explain why references to it, even if still quite rare, do begin to appear in women's obituaries before the Second World War.

One of these exceptional references appeared in the obituary of Charlotte Perkins Gilman, the social reformer and writer (*The Yellow Wallpaper, Herland*). Diagnosed with breast cancer in 1932, Gilman refused to undergo a mastectomy and determined to kill herself when her illness became unbearable. Three years later, she carried out her plan. Newspapers reporting her death made great play of the fact that she had taken her own life and quoted liberally from her suicide note. "Public opinion," she had written, "is changing on this subject. The time is approaching when we shall consider it abhorrent to our civilization to allow a human being to lie in prolonged agony which we should mercifully end in any other creature. . . . Believing this choice to be of social service in promoting wiser views on this question, I have preferred chloroform to cancer."

Gilman's courage (like her obituary) is focused on her death, not on her disease. Cancer was still untouchable as a subject. As long as breast cancer remained invisible inside the larger, formless terror, it could not become an adversary in the public imagination. Gilman, who had fought so hard for the recognition of a distinctly feminist consciousness, could not bring her radical perspective to bear on her own illness. She could defy the conventions of dying but not the conventional response to her disease. In the absence of a tangible target for her to address, resignation must have seemed a rational response and suicide a final bid for control of one's own suffering and death.

When Rachel Carson, the author of *Silent Spring*, died from breast cancer, the *New York Times* reported that she "had had cancer for some years," adding, in what was still an exception for the paper, that "she had been aware of her illness." This was well before doctors began to deal candidly with cancer patients, openly discussing their diagnosis and treatment with them. Surely it was Carson's own pioneering work raising our consciousness of the links between cancer and chemical pesticides that made this revelation both a pertinent and a respectful gesture. Even so, the newspaper could still not print the word "breast."

A year after Carson's death, the NCI, for the first time, listed breast cancer as a separate entry in its annual tally of deaths. By the 1970s, the disease was well out of the closet and into the realm of public debate. Yet newspapers remained reluctant to name it. Although it had been easy for women to reveal publicly that they were living with the disease (since the early days of Betty Ford and Happy Rockefeller in the 1970s), it remained much harder for obituaries to confirm that they were still dying from it. Women, in other words, could "have" breast cancer but were still deemed to die of the more undifferentiated disease "cancer."

This was the fate of Jacqueline Susann, who died in 1974 aged 53; her obituary played up the author's long-term survival after diagnosis, emphasizing breast cancer as a chronic disease rather than as a killer. Susann "died of cancer" but she had had "surgery for breast cancer in 1962 . . . and 10 years later began cobalt radiation treatments and chemotherapy when cancer was found in other areas."[4] This detailing of treatment over a period of years marked a new departure in reporting. The date of a woman's mastectomy was now included to serve as a marker for the onset of her protracted battle with the disease, demonstrating that breast cancer was no stealth killer; if death was predictable at least it behaved in an orderly (read "ladylike") manner. This is, of course, highly misleading. But even in its attenuated form, no parallel description of the course of a man's illness is anywhere to be found in the 1970s. No man died of prostate cancer: prostatectomies had absolutely not entered the public discourse.

Almost twenty years after Susann's death, when the poet Audre Lorde, one of the most vocal and eloquent of breast cancer activists, herself died of the disease, the *New York Times* attributed her death to liver cancer, rather than to breast cancer that had metastasized to her liver. This prolonged reticence must hark back to the days when obits drew a veil over domestic life and when it was men acting as heads of households who kept the home shrouded in secrecy.

Perhaps the death of Rose Kushner in 1990 prompted the first use of the words "breast cancer" in the boldface heading of an obituary. This would be entirely appropriate. Breast cancer had, after all, consumed the final decades of the *life* of Rose Kushner as well as causing her death. The publication of her obituary may mark the first formal recognition of breast cancer activism as a calling.

By the early 1990s in general, after the disease had become a regular feature of virtually every other newspaper column (news, science, personal health, society, even fashion), obituary editors finally took the plunge and made regular up-front disclosures of death from breast cancer (as happened at the death of May Sarton in 1995). And mastectomies themselves now enter the public domain; they even crop up occasionally in men's obituaries. The *New York Times* write-up of the screenwriter Robert Shaw told the story of his plans for a soap opera character on "Search for Tomorrow." He wrote that he had planned "one of the most tried-and-true plot devices in serials; a mastectomy." The long-serving actress who would undergo the surgery responded that "the mastectomy will fascinate my viewers because it will be my third."

Now that breast cancer has become almost a commonplace in obituary columns, we can see much more clearly how the disease cuts down women in their prime (only two of the six women I've mentioned in this chapter—Charlotte Perkins Gilman and May Sarton—actually made it to old age). Sadly, any review of a paper's obituary pages today will turn up a nonnegligible number of women in their forties and fifties, an age group for which breast cancer is the leading cause of death.

This has a galvanizing impact on the reader as well as a depressing one. It highlights the persistence of the disease as an unnatural cause of death, one that robs many women of a third of their lifespans. The roll call of premature deaths, accumulating with increasing frequency in our newspapers, is in itself a call to arms.

With the death of Kathy Acker at age 53 in December 1997, the battle to fight the disease has finally become integrated with the life story itself. Most obituaries of this American performance artist, bike girl, and novelist (*Blood and Guts in High School*) include some description of her final illness. The English *Guardian* devoted a considerable portion of its obituary to a retelling of Acker's reaction to her diagnosis (she had chosen to undergo a double mastectomy but refused chemotherapy).

> Okay, so I have always believed the men in the white coats had all the answers. But they didn't. It was like they had taken all the meaning from my body. I thought: "I will not die a meaningless death. I will find out the answers. I will make myself well or at least I will die in control of my body."

In a series of articles written for the British press over the year before she died, Acker documented her experience of breast cancer and her eventual rejection of conventional treatment. She believed that if she "remained in the hands of conventional medicine" she "would soon be dead, rather than diseased, meat." So her "search for a way to defeat cancer now became a search for life and death that were meaningful." This insistence on finding her own way through her ordeal, defining her own experience of disease, reflects the same defiance of orthodoxy that marks most of her other work. And even though her struggle was ultimately unsuccessful, her relentless engagement with the meaning of her illness (and with the relation of her beliefs to her body) forced itself into her obituaries. There it challenged the traditional view of death as just a final curtain or the abrupt interruption of a life which paid it no attention. Acker brings the life *with* and the death *from* breast cancer into a kind of alignment that obituaries have traditionally withheld from their readers.

Acker's voice is one of the more recent in a long succession of out-spoken women. Accustomed to lives as public figures while they were in good health, the women mentioned here had already proved them-selves capable of challenging whatever sexist barriers got in their way. So it is not surprising to find them rejecting recommended treatments (like Gilman and Acker) or sharing their experience of breast cancer with the public (like Lorde and Acker). Rachel Carson chose to keep her illness private. She feared that public exposure of her own breast cancer would compromise the reception of *Silent Spring*, which took an extremely controversial position linking the long-term use of man-made chemicals to cancer. As she wrote to a friend, "I have no wish to read of my ailments in literary gossip columns. Too much comfort to the chemical companies."[5] Jaqueline Susann did not publicly discuss her treatment either but she made her views plain enough in her fiction; one of her characters in the *Valley of the Dolls* chooses to kill herself rather than undergo a mastectomy.

Each of the women caught up in this struggle has expressed an atti-tude toward the sacrifice of her own life that has, bit by bit, moved us forward, toward a more uncompromising and unsentimental view of disease. It has taken almost a century for obituaries to acknowledge publicly that women do die, that cancer kills many of them, that breast cancer is a chronic disease of its own, of unknown origins and uncon-trollable outcomes, and that the treatments for it that we have been offered for decades are inadequate.

Of course, we knew many of these things before we saw them in print, but their appearance on the page has liberated them from the general hypocrisy that colors most obituaries and renders their sub-jects so lifeless. Seeing is believing. So, in a sense, the penetration of breast cancer into obituary columns might have a liberating effect on the form itself, as more obit writers, enlightened by their coverage of women, come to question the long-held assumptions that once gov-erned our views of the exemplary life and death. These turn out, like our understanding of the disease itself, not to be written in stone af-ter all.

NOTES

BIBLIOGRAPHY

INDEX

Notes

Introduction

1 There have been some interesting articles in academic journals (see, for example, Montini, "Resist and Redirect," and Reagan, "Engendering the Dread Disease") but for the most part historical interest in the disease remains medical in outlook.

2 The historical preference for the introverted individual account rather than the social history of disease finds a parallel in the literature on American hospitals. According to Charles Rosenberg, the social history of hospitals has been rather a latecomer in a field dominated by "chronicles of individual hospitals.... Such histories," he writes, "are written from a narrow internal perspective.... It is to be expected that we should have numerous histories of hospitals but no history of *the* hospital in America. To write about *the* hospital is to see it as a social institution, but to write about *a* hospital has normally been to chronicle its internal development" (Rosenberg, *The Care of Strangers,* 353–54).

3 For a succinct review of the many possible approaches to the history of diseases see Rosenberg, "Framing Disease," Introduction, in Rosenberg and Golden, *Framing Disease,* xiii–xxvi.

4 The special complexities of breast cancer have long been recognized by clinicians. The American pathologist James Ewing wrote in 1928: "From clinical and pathological studies, I have drawn the impression that, in dealing with mammary cancer, surgery meets with more peculiar difficulties and uncertainties than with almost any other form of disease. The anatomical types of the disease are so numerous, the variations in clinical course so wide, the paths of dissemination so free and diverse, the difficulties of determining the actual conditions so complex, and the sacrifice of tissue so great, as to render impossible in a majority of cases a reasonably accurate adjustment of means to an end." Cited in Reginald Murley, "Breast Cancer," 49.

5 Rosenberg and Golden, *Framing Disease,* xix.

6 In 1900, the death rate for Blacks was 27 per thousand in northern cities and 34 per thousand in southern cities. The comparable figure for whites in both areas was under 20 per thousand. Clement, "Managing on Their Own," 29.

7 Wright, *Life and Death in the United States,* Figs. 1–2, based on data from the *Statistical Abstract of the United States.* See also Ann Foote Cahn, ed., *Women in the U.S. Labor Force,* 29.

8   In 1900, there were only 10 states whose death registrations were included in the U.S. Census. These 10 states represented 26.2 percent of the total U.S. population. The actual number of recorded deaths from breast cancer was 991. It was not until 1933 that death registrations in the Census covered the entire U.S. population.

    Deaths from all cancers among Black women recorded in the 1900 census constituted under 7 percent of cancer deaths among women at a time when the Black female population was estimated to represent over 10 percent of the total U.S. female population. This may reflect some underreporting or misreporting of deaths (death certificates did not have to be signed by doctors until the 1930s), but if the figures are close to being accurate, they suggest that the mortality rates for Black women were at the time lower than for white. This is consistent with other findings. Four decades later, after significant improvements had been made in the gathering of national data, statistics show a similar pattern; deaths among Black women represented just 6 percent of the total number of breast cancer deaths among American women (887 out of 14,712). Census Reports Volume I, *Twelfth Census of the United States Population*, Part I, 1901, xciv, Washington, D.C.: United States Census Office; "Deaths from Cancer and Other Malignant Tumors: United States, 1939," *Vital Statistics—Special Reports* 12, No. 18 (March 17, 1941), 252. See also next note below.

9   By 1992, the mortality rates among Black women were more than 15 percent higher than for whites. Over the period 1950 to 1992, mortality rose by 53 percent among Black postmenopausal women, while it remained more or less constant among the equivalent white population. Although no one is really sure of the reason for this disturbing trend, many factors have been cited. These include (1) the higher proportions of African Americans living in close proximity to toxic waste sites, incinerators, and other locations that may expose them to carcinogenic substances; (2) the higher proportions of African Americans living in poverty with less access to quality (or any) health care or to vital health information; and (3) differences in the biology of tumors themselves. See Jodi A. Flaws, Craig J. Newschaffer, and Trudy L. Bush, "Breast Cancer Mortality in Black and in White Women," 1007–15.

Chapter 1

1   This is the Edwin Smith Surgical Papyrus, described in Cooper, "The History of the Radical Mastectomy," 36.

2   Numbers and Amundsen, *Caring and Curing*, 56. It's easy to imagine how the unpredictable behaviors of many breast cancers may have lent themselves to magical interpretations. The tendency of the disease to change its pace or direction at will, either to go into or come out of remission with no apparent warning, could be easily read as either a miraculous healing or a failed exorcism.

3   It has only been relatively recently that the church has formally acknowledged the change in beliefs. When the American Episcopal Church revised the Book of Common Prayer in 1979, the changes it introduced were described by one Episcopal commission: "Our attitudes towards sickness in the twentieth century have changed greatly from those of earlier periods. The grim view of illness as punish-

ment for sin . . . (is no longer) sound in the light of the advances of medical knowledge and techniques, particularly in the last fifty years, nor has such an approach any foundation in Scripture" (cited in ibid., 255–56).

4 Lewison, "Surgical Treatment of Breast Cancer," 904–53. In this particular telling, the text continues, "In the story of these skillful and courageous surgeons are prophecies of the past, the revelations of which have already cast their brilliance upon the present scene and give promise of adding luster to the triumphs of the future . . ." (904).

5 According to one commentator, a 17-year-old virgin mentioned in Eusebio's *Martyrbus Palestinae* also had her breasts cut off for confessing to her belief in the divinity of Christ before a magistrate. Eusebio makes the interesting point that *both* a young girl's breasts would have to be amputated to make sure that she would die; someone young and healthy could possibly survive the amputation of just one. Salvatore Romeo, *S. Agata V. M. e il suo culto*, 62.

6 Widowers, unlike widows, were not only expected to remarry but actively encouraged to do so, often by their dying wives. They remarried with much greater frequency than did widows. When on her deathbed in 1911, the dying wife of the British Prime Minister Ramsay Macdonald encouraged him "to seek, and soon, another woman who would 'mother' both him and the bairns." Pat Jalland, *Death in the Victorian Family*, 254–55.

7 In this sense, the fate of late-twentieth-century middle-aged women has vastly improved. Their opportunities to begin or return to education or employment when their childbearing and childrearing responsibilities decline are significantly greater than they had been a hundred years earlier.

8 Carroll Smith-Rosenberg and Charles Rosenberg, "The Female Animal," 13. The great German pathologist Virchow made the sexism of the prevailing medical view even more explicit. In his version, "woman is a pair of ovaries with a human being attached; whereas man is a human being furnished with a pair of testes." Ann Dally, *Women under the Knife*, 84. The standard explanation for the universal exclusion of women from major studies of disease has always been that disease in man sets the standard and that its expression in women is just a pale imitation of or deviation from that standard. But there is another explanation that is more consistent with the view of women's health as governed by their reproductive organs. This is the belief, or the unconscious residue of the belief, that women's bodies may not actually *contain* those other vital organs at all; or, to put it slightly less absurdly, that the womb itself is so much more powerful than any other organ in its capacity to do harm that all the others (heart, lungs, kidneys, and so on) may be safely ignored. It is worth pointing out that the dethroning of the uterus (through the legalization of birth control and abortion) did occur before biomedical research began to correct for the absence of women in research. It also preceded the recognition that women not only possessed a full complement of vital organs but also that the diseases to which they were prone behaved (and responded to treatment) in rather distinctive ways in female bodies.

9 The misplaced attribution of reproductive abnormality to symptoms of breast can-

cer survives today in the use of the term "milk arm." According to the breast surgeon and author Susan Love, this is the name given to lymphedema of the arm, the swelling that can occur following surgery in the lymph nodes. The name suggests that the cancer has somehow aggravated a pre-existing anomaly linking the arm to lactation (some women do have extra milk ducts and even nipples under the arm). But in this case, the painful condition is invariably the consequence of surgical intervention; it has nothing to do with the breast or with lactation. Susan Love with Karen Lindsey, *Dr. Susan Love's Breast Book*, 380. See n11 below.

10 George H. Napheys, *The Physical Life of Woman*, 300.

11 E. W. Tuson, *The Structure and Functions of the Female Breast*, 154. This was not a new idea. Leonardo da Vinci's sixteenth-century anatomical drawings illustrated the belief that veins extended from the uterus of a pregnant woman directly to her breasts, carrying blood from the uterus converted to milk for the anticipated baby.

12 Ibid., 153.

13 Smith-Rosenberg and Rosenberg, in "The Female Animal," 19, cite a Delaware physician who in 1873 described with almost ghoulish relish the grueling experience of cancer in a woman who had a history of practicing birth control: "about the fortieth year, the disease [cancer] grows as the energies fail—the cancerous fangs penetrating deeper and deeper until, after excruciating suffering, the writhing victim is yielded up to its terrible embrace."

14 "There is little doubt that pressure by the universal corset, directly on the breasts and indirectly on the pelvic organs, materially contributes to prepare the soil for future cancer in these regions." Herbert Snow, cited in Charles P. Childe, *Cancer and the Public*, 198.

15 Francis Power Cobbe, "The Little Health of Ladies," 281–82. Cobbe argued that the solution to this backwardness was for women to be allowed to train to become doctors themselves. Cobbe also wrote pioneering articles about Victorian wife-beating (what she called "wife torture") and campaigned for legislation to protect the lives and property of abused women.

16 See Emily Martin, *The Women in the Body*, Chapter 3, "Medical Metaphors of Women's Bodies: Menstruation and Menopause." Martin cites Walter Heape, a "militant antisuffragist and Cambridge zoologist" who described the consequences of menstruation as a process that left behind "a ragged wreck of tissue, torn glands, ruptured vessels, jagged edges of stroma, and masses of blood corpuscles, which it would seem hardly possible to heal satisfactorily without the aid of surgical treatment" (35).

17 Sir James Paget, quoted in Herbert Snow, *The Proclivity of Women to Cancerous Diseases*, 26.

18 Now that breast cancer is at home in the culture, it *has*, alas, been compromised by those same notions of blame and responsibility that still frame so much of the public discourse. It has become common not only to blame women for contracting breast cancer in the first place, by, for instance, choosing to have their babies late in life, eating the wrong diet, failing to exercise, and such. It has also become increasingly popular to make them responsible for curing themselves of the disease as well,

by adopting "right thinking," positive attitudes, and so on. This is a lamentable consequence of breast cancer's recent inclusion within the culture.

19 Barbara Ehrenreich and Deirdre English, *For Her Own Good*, 129.

20 The manuals have been widely cited to illustrate the way that medical theories worked to reinforce the oppression of women. The literature deftly reveals the connection between the medical arguments themselves and the social environment in which they were written. See *Women and Health in America*, an early standard, in particular the chapters by Carroll Smith-Rosenberg and Charles Rosenberg (cited above) and by Ann Douglas Wood. According to them, as women pressed more actively for greater access to the public arena, including admittance to education and the workplace, the theories themselves become more exigent, warning of the potential dangers to women as future mothers of "brain work," exertion, and fatigue.

21 Typical of the early lay guides is Peter J. Latz's *Manual of Health for Women: Plain Advice on Sickness and Health*. Published in 1906, it offers extensive coverage of vaginal conditions, from inflammation to vaginismus to cancer, but includes not a word on breast cancer. Where references to the breast do occur, they most commonly relate to lactation.

22 Typical among those excluding any reference to breasts are: *Practical Manual of Diseases of Women and Uterine Therapeutics* (Macnaughton Jones 1884); *A Textbook of Diseases of Women* (Penrose 1898), and *Diseases of Women* (Garriques 1900). The inclusion of a two-page chapter on menopause in the 530-page Penrose book does at least acknowledge that women may survive beyond their reproductive years but their quality of life does not sound promising. It warns that women often become "very fat at this period. The nervous derangement may be so severe as to result in insanity" (394).

23 Harry S. Crossen and Robert J. Crossen, *Diseases of Women*.

24 Harold Speert's *Obstetrics and Gynecology in America*, 129, describes the series produced by Thomas. Six years after the last of the Thomas editions appeared (1891), the first of six editions of *The Diseases of Women: A Handbook for Students and Practitioners* was published. Written by two surgeons, J. Bland-Sutton and Arthur E. Giles, this too failed to include any discussion of the breast, even in its last edition (1907) with 542 pages of text.

25 Illustrated frontispieces to J. H. Kellogg, *Ladies Guide in Health and Disease*.

26 Deborah McGregor, *The Birth of American Gynecology*, 190.

27 Comyns Berkeley, *Diseases of Women*, 535.

Chapter 2

1 Sir Astley Paston Cooper (1768–1841) was a British surgeon who published two famous books on the breast. *Illustrations of the Diseases of the Breast*, published in 1829, gave the first clear diagnostic account of fibroadenoma and a classic account of chronic cystic mastitis. The second, *The Anatomy and Diseases of the Breast*, published in 1845, provided an early comprehensive description of the structures of the breast.

2 Before the twentieth century, most medical treatises on the breast in English were

written by British surgeons such as Thomas Bryant, author of *Diseases of the Breast* (1887) and W. Roger Williams, author of *Monograph on Diseases of the Breast*. The Williams textbook, first published in London in 1894, was reissued the next year in New York. This was a transcontinental tradition that continued into the next century. The first edition of the surgeon W. Sampson Handley's *Cancer of the Breast and Its Treatment* was published in London in 1906; the second edition, in New York in 1922. One of the earliest American surgeons to participate in the pedagogical development of breast cancer studies was a surgeon named William Rodman, who had been a student of the surgeon Samuel Gross in Philadelphia. Gross (1805–84) made important contributions to the development of pathological anatomy and was one of the founders of the American Medical Association. He was also the subject of an 1875 surgical tableau painted by Thomas Eakins. His pupil, Rodman, wrote his first monograph, *Diseases of the Breast with Special Reference to Cancer* in 1908.

3 There were, of course, exceptions. The English writer Fanny Burney (1752–1840) agreed to undergo a mastectomy, but it was performed in her own home, not in a hospital, and she was attended by seven doctors (one of them Napoleon's own surgeon) and a nurse, as well as by her own domestic staff.

4 Emily Gosse (1806–57) was the wife of the naturalist Philip Gosse and the mother of the writer Edmund Gosse (1849–1928, author of *Father and Son*). For an extremely detailed history of her grim ordeal, see L. R. Croft, "Edmund Gosse and the 'New and Fantastic Cure' for Breast Cancer," 143–59.

5 Although Paget (1814–99) was himself a surgeon, he took a much more circumspect view of the usefulness of operative procedures than did many of his colleagues. "We have to ask ourselves whether it is probable that the operation will add to the length or comfort of life, enough to justify incurring the risk for its own consequences . . . we may, I think, dismiss all hope that the operation will be a final remedy for the disease." Paget carefully distinguished between women whose cancers and personal circumstances suggested that they might benefit from the surgery and those who would not. In Edward F. Lewison, "The Surgical Treatment of Breast Cancer," 919.

6 Luke Demaitre, "Medieval Notions of Cancer," 636. Hippocrates thought it was better not to treat some cancers, noting that "I have not been able to cure one woman of a single cancer in spite of frequent efforts with all my powers" (ibid., 633).

7 Ann Dally, *Women under the Knife*, 21–31. In 1852, Sims published his popular treatise "On the Treatment of Vesico-Vaginal Fistula." He moved to Europe in 1861 where he became the physician to Princess Eugénie; Clara Erskine Clement, *Charlotte Cushman*, 90.

8 *Medical and Surgical History of the War of the Rebellion (1861–65)*, 3 volumes, prepared under the direction of Joseph K. Barnes, Surgeon General (Washington, D.C.: Government Printing Office, 1870–1888).

9 Harvey Cushing, for example, left Hopkins in 1912 for the Peter Bent Brigham Hospital in Boston where he "introduced a duplicate of the Baltimore program," notes A. McGhee Harvey, in *The Influence of William Stewart Halsted's Concepts of Surgical Training*, 50. Other Halsted-trained residents included George Heuer and

Mont Reid, who set up a Halsted-type residency program at the Cincinnati General Hospital, and Roy McClure who set up a similar program at the Ford Hospital in Detroit. A tabulation of surgeons trained either by Halsted or by one of his resident surgeons lists 37 professors of surgery, 14 clinical professors, 18 associate professors as well as many others in less exalted academic positions, and 99 surgeons in private practice. According to Noland Carter, who put this table together, "It is doubtful if any one man in medicine or surgery has ever influenced a greater number of teachers and disciples and through them an additional vast host of medical students." Emile Holman, "A Surgical Philosopher's Credo," 369.

10 He *had* considered the possibility of spread via the bloodstream but concluded that "although it undoubtedly occurs, I am not sure that I have observed, from breast cancer, metastasis which seemed definitely to have been conveyed by way of the blood vessels." William S. Halsted, "The Results of Radical Operations for the Cure of Cancer of the Breast."

11 George Heuer, "Dr. Halsted."

12 A survey carried out in 1969 in England reported that only 21 percent of surgeons there were still performing radical mastectomies. A parallel survey carried out two years later in Ohio revealed a corresponding figure among that state's surgeons of 63 percent. See Robert E. Hermann and Stanley O. Hoerr, "Ohio Breast Cancer Surgery, 1960–1969."

13 Edward F. Scanlon, "Evolution of Breast Cancer Treatment."

14 Mortality rates from radical mastectomies had dropped significantly following the introduction of Lister's antiseptic treatment of wounds in the mid-nineteenth century. By the late 1870s, a decade before Halsted took up his position at Johns Hopkins, the operative mortality had already fallen from 21.3 percent to 10.5 percent. De Moulin, *Short History of Breast Cancer.*

15 Arpad Gerster, *The Rules of Aseptic and Antiseptic Surgery,* 119.

16 The mortality rate was derived from a study of 416 surgical patients. R. B. Greenough, C. G. Simmons, and J. D. Barney, "End Results," 20. None of these studies is strictly comparable with any other; each clinic used different criteria to determine the selection of "operable" cancers, and their surgical cases comprised a unique (if unknown) distribution of cancers of different size and extent of disease. Generally agreed classifications and staging systems were not commonly adopted until well after Halsted's death.

17 Halsted himself was not convinced that this extension of his basic operation (that is, the additional removal of superclavicular lymph nodes) improved the cure rate and so eliminated it from many of his later surgeries. Nor did he attempt the removal of mammary lymph nodes located under the chest wall, whose existence and possible significance had been pointed out to him by the surgeon Harvey Cushing. (See Oliver Cope, *The Breast.*) But some of his students did go down this path, removing ever more muscle, tissue, and lymph nodes to the point where the surgery bordered on "humanectomy . . . the contemporary consummation of somatic reduction . . . limited only by the ability of the human remnant to survive" (Lewison, *Surgical Treatment of Breast Cancer,* 931).

18 Michael Baum, "Surgery and Radiotherapy in Breast Cancer."

19 Hugh Young, *A Surgeon's Autobiography*, 62.

20 In 1926, M. Greenwood reported on his six-year study of 651 women with untreated breast cancer. Only 60 were still alive at the end of this period. M. Greenwood, *Natural Duration of Cancer*. A year later, Ernest Daland published his study of 100 women who had either refused or were ineligible for surgery; their average survival was 40.5 months following the onset of symptoms. In most of these studies there is, of course, no way of knowing how long disease was present before a woman sought a doctor's advice. Ernest Daland, "Untreated Cancer of the Breast."

21 H. J. G. Bloom, W. W. Richardson, and E. J. Harries, "Natural History of Untreated Breast Cancer."

22 Some researchers have argued that inevitable biases in the studies of untreated patients may make it difficult to use the results as a baseline against which to measure the effectiveness of treatment. The high proportion of women with very advanced tumors, for example, suggests that the study populations tend to include those with extremely poor prognoses. This has the effect of lowering the average survival period for those with untreated disease. See Michael Baum, "Natural History of Breast Cancer," 4.

23 Halsted, *Surgical Papers*, 15.

24 There has been a general reluctance to look closely at Halsted's personal life, to examine his strange and reclusive behavior, his long-term addiction to cocaine (see Heuer, "Dr. Halsted"; Arthur I. Holleb, "Halsted Revisited"; Penfield, "Halsted of Johns Hopkins") or his possible homosexuality (Colp, "Notes on Dr. William S. Halsted"), none of which was thought likely to enhance the status of the emergent surgical profession. Most of the accounts of his life were written by former students, still practicing surgeons at the time.

   Halsted had become addicted to cocaine by using the drug on himself to study its potential as an anesthetic. He knew he was addicted and entered treatment hospitals more than once. Both William Welch and William Osler, Halsted's equally prominent colleagues, who had arrived at Johns Hopkins before him, were aware of his habit and of his attempts to cure himself of it, which left him addicted to morphine in place of cocaine. Both nevertheless kept his secret, recommending him for appointment as surgeon-in-chief at the Johns Hopkins Hospital. Osler knew that Halsted continued to use drugs, seeing him six months after his appointment "in a severe chill . . . the first intimation I had that he was still taking morphia," but he did not intervene. Colp has written that at the moment Halsted "reached the apogee of his career in surgery, he had to recognise that he needed morphine to sustain him in his surgical work." Ralph Colp, "Notes on Dr. William S. Halsted," 879.

   Not one of Halsted's colleagues or later commentators ever expressed (at least in print) any concern for the impact of his addiction on his patients, whether in face-to-face consultations or, of much greater consequence, in the operating theater. Nor, as far as I know, has anyone ever speculated on the possible connection between Halsted's long-term drug use and the evolution of his surgical technique.

25 Harvey Cushing, "William Stewart Halsted 1852–1922," 461, 464.

26 Colp, "Notes on Dr. William S. Halsted," 886 n 36.

27 Ibid., 883.

28 Cope, *The Breast: Its Problems*, 58.

29 This does not mean that medicines applied to the skin could not also be lethal; they often were.

30 The removal of healthy ovaries was called "Battey's operation," named for Robert Battey, the surgeon from Georgia who introduced it. It was the most famous gynecological procedure of the time, performed enthusiastically by surgeons on both sides of the Atlantic between the early 1870s and the end of the nineteenth century. See Lawrence D. Longo, "The Rise and Fall of Battey's Operation." For a broader history of "sexual" surgery performed by men on women see Ann Dally, *Women under the Knife*.

31 Amputations carried out in Civil War field hospitals just a few decades earlier had taken a terrible toll; one in every three leg amputations, for instance, ended in death.

32 James Patterson, *Dread Disease*, 101.

33 The English surgeon D'Arcy Power believed that Mitchell Banks failed to receive the recognition he deserved because he took little trouble to publicize his results. He published his work locally, in the *Liverpool and Manchester Reports*, which had a very limited circulation of less than 500, while Halsted, according to Power, had access to "a well-organized medical press" and a large reading public (D'Arcy Power, "The History of the Amputation of the Breast to 1904," 55). Willy Meyer presented his own operation for breast cancer before the New York Academy of Medicine in the same year that Halsted presented his surgical results before the Clinical Society of Maryland (1894). Their solutions appear to have been arrived at independently of one another and were virtually identical with a few minor exceptions. Meyer advocated the removal of the minor as well as major pectoral muscle, an amendment that Halsted later incorporated into his own operation.

The elevation of Halsted to the position of standard-bearer certainly fanned the flames of international rivalries among surgeons. Edward Lewison, a surgeon at Johns Hopkins and one of Halsted's most idolatrous admirers, confessed, when describing Halsted's radical mastectomy, that "the spirit of Chauvinism burns bright within me. . . ." He wrote that Halsted's operation "established a paragon of surgical precision which had no precedent in the history of the treatment of malignant disease." Lewison, "The Surgical Treatment of Breast Cancer," 930.

34 Nabothian cysts, for example, mucous cysts of the cervix, are named after Martin Naboth (1675–1721); Bartolin glands, lining the vagina, are named after the seventeenth-century Caspar Bartolin (1655–1738). Harold Speert's *Obstetric and Gynecologic Milestones: Essays in Eponymy* includes a great many other examples.

The idea of a woman's body as exotic, uncharted territory is an old poetic conceit. The seventeenth-century poet John Donne adopted the explorer's outlook in approaching his lover's body—"Oh my America, my new found land"—in the elegy "To His Mistress Going to Bed." When the poet Emily Dickinson took up the same theme two hundred years later, she turned it to very different ends. Addressing Hernando de Soto, a sixteenth-century Spanish explorer of the present-day United States, she wrote:

Soto! Explore thyself!
Therein thyself shalt find
The "Undiscovered Continent"
No Settler had the Mind.

35 Patterson, *Dread Disease*, 22.

36 This separation between theory and practice had also characterized the adoption of Listerism in the United States. American surgeons remained suspicious of and resistant to the underlying germ theory that justified the use of antiseptic and aseptic practices in the operating theater. Even when the evidence of declining operative mortality rates associated with Listerism was so convincing that they had to apply them in their own practices, surgeons, for the most part, remained indifferent to the theory that justified their use. Lily L. Saint, "American Listerism: A Practical Reflection."

37 Letter of Francis Sim to Wealthy Hathaway, from Nebraska City, December 6, 1879; letter of John W. Clark to Wealthy Hathaway, from Otoe County, Nebraska, January 30, 1880. Sim Family Correspondence, Nebraska State Historical Society.

38 Letter of John W. Clark to his mother, from Nebraska City, April 9, 1880. Sim Family Correspondence, Nebraska State Historical Society.

39 Lewison, "The Surgical Treatment of Breast Cancer," 930. And see Chapter 8, note 29.

40 Both Paul Starr's *The Social Transformation of American Medicine* and Roy Porter's *The Greatest Benefit to Mankind* feature the Eakins painting on their covers.

41 Bridget L. Goodbody, " 'The Present Opprobrium of Surgery,' " 47. See also Margaret Supplee Smith, "The Agnew Clinic." Smith analyzes what she calls the "medical patriarchy" revealed in this and Eakins' other large medical canvas, also in Philadelphia, "The Gross Clinic," painted in 1875. "That the only two instances of unclothed women in Eakins' art are the artist's model and the doctor's patient is a telling comment on the opportunities for Victorian women, in life and art" (177).

42 Thomas Agnew, *Principles and Practice of Surgery*, 710–12.

43 Bernard Fisher, "Surgery of Primary Breast Cancer," 3.

44 Myra Morgenstern, "Role of Mammography in the Detection of Breast Cancer," 277.

45 There have been hundreds of retrospective studies carried out since the late 1890s evaluating the results of radical mastectomies (see Carl M. Mansfield, *Early breast cancer*) but there are simply too many uncontrolled variables in all these studies to make any comparisons meaningful. Many of them contain too few patients to meet modern criteria for statistical significance. The patients in each group are likely to be too different, to reflect different criteria of operability, a different distribution of age and stage of disease, different hormonal status, different cancer histories (some with recurring disease, metastasis, or a history of earlier treatment), and so on. Modern clinical trials have attempted to reduce if not to eliminate this wide variability by imposing much stricter controls on all criteria and by designing trials to run prospectively rather than retrospectively. The relatively greater consistency of the results makes it possible to make more meaningful comparison between studies, although, of course, difficulties remain.

46 Grantley W. Taylor and Richard H. Wallace, "Carcinoma of the Breast," 836.

47 Every retrospective study relied upon its own definitions of operability or "incurability." Portman, for instance, writing in 1950, put the estimate of incurability much higher than Taylor and Wallace, at "about 45 per cent" (U. V. Portmann, "Cancer of the Breast," 515).

48 R. McWhirter, "Discussion," 122. McWhirter first began treating his patients with simple mastectomy and radiotherapy as early as 1941, at the Royal Infirmary in Edinburgh. George Crile, Jr., who appears in this book's Chapter 4, was very much influenced by McWhirter's ideas and by the evidence he was able to bring to his arguments.

49 About 1,200 women died of breast cancer in New York City in 1939, at the end of the fifty-year series of survival statistics shown on page 74. Allowing for a conservative ratio of newly diagnosed cases to deaths of 2.5:1 (it is currently more than 4:1) gives an estimate of new incidences of breast cancer in 1939 of about 3,000.

50 In 1933, there were 1,690 deaths from breast cancer in New York State and 847 in New York City. In the City, less than a third of these deaths occurred in a hospital; in rural areas the proportion was even lower. Many of these women had probably received some form of treatment in a hospital and had been discharged. But many of them probably died without having been treated at all. (*Monthly Vital Statistics Review*, New York State Department of Health; Neva Deardorff and Marta Fraenkel, *Hospital Discharge Study*, 191.) This WPA-sponsored study, which analyzed over half a million patients discharged from hospitals in 1933, included only 226 breast cancer deaths, or 6 percent of the total number of cancer deaths occurring in any hospital covered by the survey. Breast cancer deaths, in fact, accounted for about 10 percent of all cancer deaths in New York City. See also Hoffman, *The Statistical Experience Data.*

51 Of 668 new cases of breast cancers referred to surgeons at the Presbyterian Hospital in New York between 1935 and 1942, 173 (25 percent) were not treated by radical mastectomy. 107 were deemed to be inoperable because their disease was considered to be too advanced; a further 36 were classified as "constitutionally inoperable" (too ill from other causes or too old to risk surgery). Ten women refused to undergo a radical mastectomy point blank. Three women had lesions that had been mistakenly diagnosed as malignant and one woman was referred elsewhere because of a lack of accommodations. All but 37 of these patients had some alternative form of therapy, either more conservative surgery or radiation; the rest (495) had radical mastectomies. C. D. Haagenson, *Diseases of the Breast*, p. 631.

52 Several epidemiological studies (that looked at, e.g., the geographical distribution of cancer within the United States or within countries in Western Europe) were undertaken earlier in the century but they all had to rely on mortality statistics rather than on any data describing the incidence of disease. See, for example, Frederick Hoffman, *The Mortality from Cancer Throughout the World*, and Mary Gover, *Cancer Mortality in the United States, 3. Geographic Variation . . .*

53 Deardorff and Fraenkel, *Hospital Discharge Study*, footnote 2, 175. By the time of this study (1942), the rule of thumb was well established. An article published in

1927 under the name of the American Society for the Control of Cancer suggests, "in the absence of better figures, it appears not an exaggeration to assume that the number of cases of cancer which exist at any place at any time is about three times the number of deaths which occur there in the course of a year" (198).

54 National estimates today are made from statistics collected by the National Cancer Institute's SEER program (Surveillance, Epidemiology, and End Results) and by the U.S. Bureau of the Census. In the early 1970s, the SEER program was expanded to include residents in nine areas in the United States: Atlanta, Detroit, the San Francisco–Oakland area, the Seattle–Puget Sound area, and the states of Connecticut, New Mexico, Hawaii, Iowa, and Utah. Many of the more recent studies documenting, for example, geographic variations in mammography screening or in breast cancer treatments depend on data describing the treatment of Medicare patients, that is, treatment sponsored by public expenditure. The data base, like the treatment, has also been underwritten by public funds and exists within the public domain. This distinguishes it from the semi-private statistics regularly entered as evidence in ongoing discussions of medical research found in the pages of professional journals.

Chapter 3

1 Frederick Hoffman, *Some Final Results of the San Francisco Cancer Survey,* 9 (for 1922 death rate); Washington, D.C.: United States Department of Health and Human Services, Public Health Service, *Monthly Vital Statistics Report* 14 (July 15, 1966): 15 (for 1964 figures). For most of the early years of the century, death rates were based upon the United States population as a whole—men and women combined—rather than on the population of women alone. If only women are included, the rate doubles. The overall rate of 13.7 for 1964, when disaggregated by gender, yields a rate of death of 26.6 women (per 100,000 women) and 0.2 men (per 100,000 men).

2 "No one can deny that radical surgery often entails, in addition to an appreciable operative mortality, a really hideous mutilation" (Geoffrey Keynes, "Conservative Treatment of Cancer of the Breast"). The surgeon Geoffrey Keynes (brother of Maynard) was one of the earliest opponents of the routine performance of radical mastectomies in England. Advocating the use of more conservative surgery as early as the 1920s, he was almost universally vilified by the surgical community (see Joan Austoker, "The 'Treatment of Choice.' ").

3 For early American studies recommending the use of "simple" rather than radical mastectomies (together with radiation), see, for example, E. J. Grace and W. J. Moitrier, "Simple Mastectomy with X-ray," 701–4. European physicians responded much more favorably and much earlier to the possible benefits of radiation, with or without surgery. By the 1950s, evidence began to appear suggesting the presence of cancer cells in the bloodstream. This contradicted prevailing theories based on cancer spreading in a mass in an orderly and predictable fashion along lymphatic pathways.

4 Joyce Hemlow et al., eds., *The Journals and Letters of Fanny Burney,* volume 6:

596–616; Julia Epstein, "Writing the Unspeakable"; John Wiltshire, "Early Nineteenth-Century Pathography," 9–23; ibid., 16; ibid., 13.

5   The patient's name and those of her relatives have been changed at the request of the Alan Mason Chesney Medical Archives.

6   Julia Epstein, "Writing the Unspeakable."

7   A study of a group of 519 cases of breast cancer over the period 1917–18 revealed that the average time between the appearance of the first symptom of disease and admission to the hospital for surgery was 12.4 months (Simmons and Daland, "Cancer: Delay," 15).

8   Joseph Bloodgood was Halsted's fourth resident surgeon. Halsted's suggestion that he undertake more systematic investigation of tissues removed at operation led to the establishment of the department's first specialty: surgical pathology (Harvey, "Influence," 51). Bloodgood was one of the first pathologists in the country to adopt frozen section techniques for the analysis of tissues during an operation. He was instrumental in developing the technique and in promoting its use. It was not until the 1920s and 1930s that it became a routine feature of cancer surgery (James Wright, "Development of the Frozen Section").

9   Among a list of rules issued to agents and underwriters by the Preferred Accident Company in 1905 was one stating that "Health policies will not be issued to women." (*The Western Underwriter, the National Underwriter Company*, Cincinnati, February 16, 1905, 19).

10   To be eligible for a new policy offered to women for the first time in 1905 applicants had to be "women between the ages of 18 and 45 . . . who are regularly engaged in occupations from which they derive a regular income and upon which they are dependent for support. . . . This does not include housekeepers, housewives (or) domestics." (*Continental Agent's Record*, CNA Archives, New York, December 1905.)

11   Fidelity and Casualty started life as the Knickerbocker Company in 1874 and is still trading as part of the CNA group of companies.

12   *The Western Underwriter*, (n. ix), June 22, 1905, 16.

13   Ibid., July 27, 13.

14   Unless otherwise noted, all the letters come from the William S. Halsted Collection, Alan Mason Chesney Medical Archives of the Johns Hopkins Medical Institutions.

15   See Penfield, "Halsted of Johns Hopkins," 2214–18.

16   Lowy, *Between Bench and Bedside*, 91.

17   Murphy, "Studies in X-Ray Effects"; Murphy and Morton, "Effects of X-Rays on the Resistance to Cancer"; Murphy, Means, and Aub, "Clinical Calorimetry."

18   Mont Reid became Halsted's surgical intern upon graduating from Johns Hopkins Medical School in 1912. A year after he treated Barbara Mueller, he was appointed resident surgeon (Harvey, "Influence," 58).

19   See Chapter 2, note 17.

20   William S. Halsted, "The Swelling of the Arm after Operations for Cancer of the Breast—Elephantiasis chirurgica—Its Cause and Prevention," in *Surgical Papers*, volume 2, 96.

21 "Special Report: Treatment of Primary Breast Cancer," *New England Journal of Medicine* 301, no. 6 (August 9, 1979), 340. Twelve years after this recommendation, more than half of the women diagnosed with in situ breast cancer and almost 50 percent of women diagnosed with Stage I disease were being treated with lumpectomy. *National Cancer Institute Journal* 87, no. 5 (March 1, 1995): 339.

22 Edward F. Scanlon, "The Evolution of Breast Cancer Treatment," 1280–82. According to Dr. Steven Come, an oncologist at the Beth Israel Deaconess Medical Center, "with regard to survival rates for metastatic disease, there is little debate that it is virtually always ultimately fatal. . . . Duration of survival might be longer as we have more therapy and supportive care but even with that we haven't done much at all. . . . There may be a very small fraction of metastatic disease patients for whom ultimate survival has been altered (through bone marrow transplants) but all others will ultimately succumb, if they don't die of something else first" (conversation March 30, 1998). The recent decrease in breast cancer mortality in the 1990s is more a reflection of earlier detection and adjuvant therapies than any progress in overcoming metastatic disease itself.

A provocative article written twenty years ago by Maurice Fox ("On the Diagnosis and Treatment of Breast Cancer") suggested that breast cancer consisted of at least two separate diseases, "one with a rapidly fatal outcome and the other with an outcome only modestly different from that of a group of women of similar ages without evidence of the disease. Although nearly all patients with breast cancer are treated, those suffering a rapidly fatal outcome show a mortality not significantly different from untreated patients in the nineteenth-century" (493).

Chapter 4

1 *New York Times*, March 29, 1959, 52.

2 For an evaluation of this trial, see Bernard Fisher, R. G. Ravdin, R. K. Ausman, et al., "Surgical Adjuvant Chemotherapy."

3 Walter Ross, *Crusade*, 97.

4 Letter of Rachel Carson to George Crile, Jr., February 17, 1963. See page 140 for the full text of this letter.

5 This is of course a distortion of the historical perspective and betrays the inevitable bias of the present toward the past. Compared to our intimacy with the recent past, particularly the past that overlaps with our own lifetimes, our familiarity with the *zeitgeist* of any earlier period is much more limited. However hard we try, it remains impossible to reconstruct the sensibility of an earlier generation with anything like the same subtlety or comprehensiveness. Particularly when we have outgrown their belief systems (scientific as well as cultural), we find it hard to pay proper attention to the social repercussions of what we now recognize as outdated or discredited ideas.

6 Mary A. McCay, *Rachel Carson*, 14. So ingrained was the belief that women could not be scientists that a review in the 1990s of important books written by women in the 1960s claimed, almost thirty years after the publication of *Silent Spring*, that its

author "was not a scientist of any kind." (McCay, 13, citing Robert Fulford, "When Jane Jacobs Took on the World," *New York Times Book Review,* February 16, 1992, 28.)

7 Dr. Jerome Urban, Memorial Sloan Kettering, New York, quoted in Philip Nobile, "King Cancer," 205.

8 Freeman, *Always, Rachel,* letter of March 28, 1962.

9 Myrtle Williamson, *One Out of Four,* 50.

10 "Any Dose Dangerous," *Washington Post,* June 5, 1960, from the *Silent Spring* files in The Rachel Carson Papers, Beinecke Library Yale University.

11 From an article clipped by Carson from *Medical News,* May 11, 1960, in the *Silent Spring* files, The Rachel Carson Papers, Beinecke Library Yale University.

12 *Always, Rachel: The Letters of Rachel Carson and Dorothy Freeman, 1952–1964,* edited by Martha Freeman.

13 Ibid., 405. Carson maintained this secrecy until her death. Just a few months before she died, she declined an offer to speak at the University of Pennsylvania, citing "arthritis" as the cause (letter from Loren Eiseley, February 11, 1964, The Rachel Carson Papers, Beinecke Library, Yale University).

14 Donald Okun, "What to Tell Cancer Patients?" Sixteen years after Oken's 1961 study, in 1977, another research team used an almost identical questionnaire to see how attitudes toward disclosure might have changed over the intervening period (Dennis H. Novack, Robin Plumer, Raymond L. Smith, et al. "Changes in Physicians' Attitudes Toward Telling the Cancer Patient"). They found an almost complete reversal of attitudes, with 97 percent of the physicians now indicating a preference for telling the patient his/her true diagnosis.

15 Ibid., 1125.

16 "Should Doctors Tell the Truth to a Cancer Patient?," *Ladies' Home Journal,* May 1961, 109.

17 Donald Okun, "What to Tell Cancer Patients?," 1127.

18 For contributions to the early debates on disclosure see M. G. Seelig, "Should Cancer Victims Be Told the Truth?"; C. C. Lund, "Doctor, Patient and the Truth"; William D. Kelly and Stanley R. Friesen, "Do Cancer Patients Want to Be Told?"

19 F. Davis, "Uncertainty in Medical Prognosis, Clinical and Functional."

20 Jim McIntosh, "The Routine Management of Uncertainty in Communication with Cancer Patients," 114–15. McIntosh observed and recorded the interactions between doctors and patients in an English cancer ward for a year in the mid-1970s.

21 Some surgeons believed that cutting into a tumor could itself encourage a cancer to spread by disturbing otherwise confined cancer cells, providing them with additional avenues of escape. If this were true, then even a biopsy might put a patient at risk by promoting metastases. Opening her up a second time would then double that risk. Although no one really believed this after the 1950s, it did provide additional justification for consolidating two surgeries into one. See James R. Wright, Jr., "The 1917 New York Biopsy Controversy."

22 Tom Beauchamp and Ruth R. Faden, "History of Informed Consent," 1235.

23 One of the landmark legal decisions in the evolution of the doctrine of informed consent (*Natanson v. Kline*, 1960) was initiated by a breast cancer patient. Irma Natanson sued her radiologist, John R. Kline, for failing to warn her of the dangers of cobalt therapy which she received following a mastectomy in Kansas in 1955. See Jay Katz, *Silent World of Doctor and Patient*, 65–71.

24 This chronology has been pieced together from four sources: Linda Lear, *Rachel Carson: Witness for Nature*; The Rachel Carson Papers, Beinecke Library, Yale University; *Always, Rachel: The Letters of Rachel Carson and Dorothy Freeman, 1952–1964*, Martha Freeman, ed.; Papers of George Crile, Jr. M.D., The Cleveland Clinic Foundation Archives.

   The letters include references to more than a dozen physicians consulted by Carson during the course of her illness, in addition to George Crile, Jr. Except for Crile, all of these doctors were working in the Washington area. Fred R. Sanderson (1893–1979), who performed Carson's radical mastectomy in 1960, was a general surgeon who specialized in abdominal surgery. He practiced in Washington for 50 years, many of them as chief surgeon at Georgetown University Hospital. Ralph Caulk (1909–89), the radiologist recommended by Crile, had been medical director of the cancer detection clinic at Garfield Hospital in the early 1950s and became president of the medical and dental staff after the Garfield joined with other institutions to become the Washington Hospital Center.

   In the letters reproduced below, I have added a few words in brackets to clarify the occasional medical term. A few longer discussions of aspects of Carson's medical treatment have been included in the notes.

25 Lear, *Rachel Carson*, 185.

26 Lear, *Rachel Carson*, 367; and letter from Rachel Carson to Marjorie Spock and Polly Richards, April 12, 1960. The Rachel Carson Papers, Beinecke Library, Yale University.

27 Rachel Carson to Paul Brooks, December 27, 1960. The Rachel Carson Papers, Beinecke Library, Yale University.

28 Letter to Ralph Caulk, July 5, 1962 (Crile Papers, Cleveland Clinic).

29 This procedure had been around since the end of the nineteenth century. See George Beatson, "On the Treatment of Inoperable Cancer of the Mammae," 162–65.

30 In 1957, following the death of her niece Marjorie Christie, Carson, then approaching 50 herself, took on full-time responsibility for Marjorie's 5-year-old son Roger. She also continued to support her mother, Maria Carson, who lived with her until her death in 1958.

31 Freeman, *Always, Rachel*, letters of January 3 and 4, 1961, 326, 327. Carson's experience is confirmed by contemporary data, which give a 50 to 60 percent response rate in a hormonal patient. Today she would be classified as a perimenopausal patient, someone with irregular periods on the cusp of menopause. Women in this group are the most difficult to treat with hormones. The fact that she responded at all did open up the possibility of using other hormone treatments down the line. Even today, hormone therapy is used whenever feasible since it is less toxic and just

as good as chemotherapy in terms of the quality of remissions it can provide. The response to radiation doesn't occur instantaneously; it takes at least three or four weeks to see the full extent of the shrinkage it induces. The process lethally injures cells but that injury is not expressed until the cells come to divide. In other words, the initial exposure plants a time bomb in cells but their death will not be manifest until they come to separate.

32 Freeman, *Always, Rachel*, letter of March 25, 1961, 365–66.

33 Ibid., letter of March 28, 1962, 400.

34 Lear, *Rachel Carson*, 320.

35 Freeman, *Always, Rachel*, letter of April 1, 1962, 401.

36 Ibid., letter of April 10, 1962, 403–4.

37 Lear, *Rachel Carson*, 409.

38 Ibid., 443.

39 Irradiation to the chest wall and lymphatic chains on the left can be associated with a slightly greater risk of heart attacks but the gain in tumor control is thought to outweigh this long-term risk.

40 Laetrile was a substance derived from apricot pits that was marketed as a cancer drug throughout the 1970s. Despite the fact that it was never shown to provide any benefits, failed to win FDA approval, and was banned in many states, it had huge contraband sales and was smuggled across the border from labs in Mexico in great quantities. It was taken up as a "freedom of choice" issue by members of the right-wing John Birch Society who saw in the government's refusal to legalize it a conspiracy between physicians and pharmaceutical companies seeking to profit from conventional—and ineffective—cancer treatments.

41 "Answer on Krebiozen—It's Useless," *Life*, October 4, 1963, 50.

42 Letter from Ralph M. Caulk to George Crile, Jr. April 11, 1963. Crile Papers.

43 Adrenalectomy is the removal of the adrenal glands. Hypophysectomy is the removal of the pituitary gland. Both are forms of hormonal ablation, that is, the surgical removal of hormone-producing organs that are considered as second-line treatments following sterilization. Both came into general use in the 1950s (see Rolf Luft and Herbert Olivecrona, "Experience with Hypophysectomy in Man). The pituitary manufactures ACTH (adreno-cortical-stimulating hormone) which stimulates the adrenal glands to make cortisone. The adrenal glands, however, also produce androgen, which the liver and fatty tissue convert to estrogen. The removal or disabling of the pituitary, then, is a secondary attempt to eliminate estrogens from the body. This can be achieved by a variety of means. The one Crile has suggested involved the use of yttrium-90, an isotope that produces a short-range radioactive particle that can be used to burn the pituitary and shut down the adrenal glands. It's no longer necessary to rely on this procedure, or on any type of surgery, to achieve the same end. There now are drugs that can be used to block the conversion of adrenal androgens to estrogen. These can be administered after a breast cancer patient has been sterilized.

44 Dr. Andrew C. Ivy had been involved with Krebiozen since 1949 when he first injected patients with the substance after experimenting with it on just four or five

animals and even fewer human beings, including himself. The director of the Krebiozen Research Foundation, Ivy was brought to trial in 1963, alongside other beneficiaries of the drug's sales, for violations of FDA regulations and fraud. They were all acquitted. James F. Holland, "The Krebiozen Story."

45 Freeman, *Always, Rachel,* letter of September 18, 1963, 469.

46 Ibid., letter of November 3, 1963, 489–90.

47 Ibid., letter of November 20, 1963, 495.

48 Ibid., letter of December 12, 1963, 501.

49 Ibid., letter of January 9, 1964, 514–15.

Chapter 5

1 Wright, *Life and Death,* Fig. 1–2 and Table 2–1.

2 Women have just recently begun to become familiar with some of the more common distinctions in the varieties of breast cancer, for instance, between ductal and lobular carcinoma (the first in the breast ducts, the second in the lobes) and between carcinoma in situ and invasive carcinoma (the first contained within, say, the ducts or lobes, the second, proliferating in tissue outside them, with access to the bloodstream). Joseph Bloodgood, the Johns Hopkins pathologist who carried out a biopsy of Barbara Mueller's cancer in 1917 (see Chapter 3), investigated the behaviors of early-stage breast cancers, what he called "border-line breast tumors" as early as the 1920s and 1930s. More unusual, special types of invasive breast cancers—for instance, "tubular," "medullary," and "mucinous"—were first adumbrated in the 1940s.

3 Frederick L. Hoffman, "The Menace of Cancer." Frederick Hoffman (1865–1946) was a tireless and, some have said, compulsive collector of cancer data. Among other recommendations he made for the new society in 1913 were proposals to carry out epidemiological research, some of which he later undertook himself. He advocated the study of geographical distributions of cancers, including local areas with high rates of cancer deaths (what we now call cancer clusters). He also recommended "a thoroughly scientific investigation" into "the occupational incidence of cancer" as well as into the impact of diet. Many of his ideas remained underdeveloped for half a century.

4 The Society's decision to change its name, dropping the word "Control" and adopting the more generic American Cancer Society, coincided with its first foray into the funding of biomedical research.

5 *Mortality from Cancer and Other Malignant Tumors in the Registration Area of the United States 1914.* Bureau of the Census, Department of Commerce. Washington, D.C.: Government Printing Office, 1916.

6 Schereschewsky, "The Course of Cancer Mortality," 22 and 67. The results were based on data from the ten original Registration states collecting cancer mortality statistics. These were the six states in New England plus Indiana, Michigan, New Jersey, and New York. Their combined population grew from about 20 million in 1900 to about 27 million, or roughly 25 percent of the United States population, in 1920.

7   For the population as a whole (including both men and women), breast cancer claimed the lives of 4.7 of every 100,000 Americans in 1900 and 12.6 in 1950. The actual numbers of deaths, according to the Bureau of the Census, rose from about 3,780 in 1900 to almost 19,000 in 1950. See Chapter 8, note 31.

While deaths from breast cancer rose steadily, overall mortality among American women (amalgamating deaths from all causes) fell dramatically, from 16.5 (per 1,000 women) in 1900 to half that level (8.2) in 1950. For a variety of reasons—in particular, the survival of more children to adulthood—the American population was aging. Between 1900 and 1950, the percentage of people living to 65 or older doubled, rising from 4.1 percent of all Americans in 1900 to 8.2 percent in 1950. This change in the age distribution of the population clearly contributed to the rise in both the numbers of women dying and the unadjusted death rate for breast cancer. So did continuous improvements in the efficiency and accuracy of death registrations. Although breast cancer was easier to diagnose than many other, more hidden cancers, deaths from metastatic disease (to the lungs, bones, or brain, or other sites), were often misattributed to other causes. As the accuracy in reporting increased over the course of the century, the number of deaths attributed to breast cancer rose. But it seems unlikely that these biases in the early statistics can explain all of the dramatic rise in the numbers and rates of death over the first half of the century. After all, the more recent age-adjusted rates of the 1970s and 1980s, which correct for many of these statistical shortcomings, still show increasing mortality rates for breast cancer, even if these are more modest, suggesting that the underlying secular trend cannot be wholly explained by reference to changes in the age distribution of the population or to improvements in data collection. (Donald J. Bogue, *The Population of the United States*, 113; J. W. Schereschewsky, *The Course of Cancer Mortality*, 75; Federal Security Agency, "Trend of Cancer Mortality in the United States 1900–1945," 13.)

8   The absence of reliable incidence rates before the 1970s made it impossible to compare, with any accuracy, the numbers of women diagnosed with the disease in the second half of the century with those diagnosed in the first half.

9   Marchand, *Advertising the American Dream*, 6.

10   Ibid., 18; 368n39, 344, 22. Kotex introduced a "Nurse Ellen Buckland" who signed her name on the advertising copy but then softened its image with the introduction of the friendlier "Mary Pauline Callender." Marchand gives a long list of other invented women whose stories enlivened the advertising of every kind of domestic product. It may be that these early testimonials played some role in establishing the later cultural mania for confessions of personal shame. The Kotex campaign was masterminded by the firm of Lord and Thomas. Twenty years later, the financial resources of its president, Albert Lasker, combined with the political skills of his wife Mary, would come to transform the American Cancer Society into a major player in the field of cancer research.

11   Adolph Niemoeller, *The Complete Guide to Bust Culture*. The first edition of this book appeared in 1939. Niemoeller had also written an earlier book called *Superfluous Hair and Its Removal*. To his credit, he did warn his readers of the dangers

of quack remedies, the astringents designed to reduce breast size and fatty ointments sold as breast "foods" intended to enlarge breasts by supplying "nourish-
ment for the tissues" (78).

12 Adolph Niemoeller, *The Complete Guide to Bust Culture*, 17.

13 William L. Rodman, "Care of the Breast," 5.

14 Adolph F. Niemoeller, *The Complete Guide to Bust Culture*, 13.

15 The American Society for the Control of Cancer, "What Every Woman Should Do
    about Cancer," 1929. New York: The American Society for the Control of Cancer.

16 Benjamin R. Shore, "Education of the Public," 57. These figures are consistent
    with the findings of a study carried out at the Massachusetts General Hospital over
    the 13-year period 1917–30 (Channing Simmons, "Delay in Treatment"). Evaluat-
    ing the delay between the first sign of a suspicious lump and its removal at surgery,
    the study found a decrease in the so-called "average duration of disease" from 11.4
    months in 1917–18 to 9.3 months in 1930.

17 Donald E. Shaughnessy, "The Story of the American Cancer Society" (Ph.D. diss.,
    Columbia University, New York, 1957), 191.

18 The first cancer prevention clinic was opened in 1937 by Dr. Elise Strang L'Esper-
    ance, working at the New York Infirmary for Women and Children in New York. It
    provided complete physical exams to determine the possible presence of cancer in
    any part of the body, relying where necessary on the use of lab tests and diagnostic
    x-rays. This uncovered cancers in about 10 percent of all the cases seen between
    May 1937 and January 1940 and a fair proportion of these were found early (Elise
    Strang L'Esperance, "The Cancer Prevention Clinic," *Quarterly Review*, American
    Society for the Control of Cancer, April 1940). The Strang Clinic still exists today
    as part of Memorial Sloan-Kettering Cancer Center.

19 Shaughnessy, "Story of the American Cancer Society," 194. Efforts to establish the
    WFA in Massachusetts were abandoned because of "nervousness by the State Med-
    ical Society and the State Department of Health" (196).

20 Harry C. Saltzstein, "The Average Treatment of Cancer," 466.

21 The women might have been inspired by the passage in 1921 of the Sheppard-
    Towner Act. This empowered the federal government to grant funds (matching
    state contributions) to support prenatal and child-health centers that had been set
    up and staffed by female physicians and lay health workers. The AMA opposed the
    legislation, arguing that federal aid was "unAmerican" and that the program should
    not be administered by a lay organization, the Children's Bureau. In 1929, Congress
    failed to renew it. (Regina M. Morantz-Sanchez, *Sympathy and Science*, 301–2.)

22 Shaughnessy, "Story of the American Cancer Society," 198; and Editorial, *JAMA*
    135, no. 15 (1947): 991.

23 Walter Ross, *Crusade*, 211. In the years leading up to the Second World War, the
    AMA was equally effective in blocking legislative attempts to introduce compulsory
    medical insurance.

24 Ella Hoffman Rigney, "The Women's Field Army," 23.

25 The Surgeon General, Thomas Parran, also claimed that the WFA had been an im-
    portant influence in the passage of the 1937 National Cancer Act. (General Federa-

tion of Women's Clubs, *Official Report of the Second Triennial Convention May 10–17, 1938*; Washington, D.C.: General Federation of Women's Clubs Headquarters, 1938), 41.

26 *Time*, March 22, 1937, 49–56.

27 American Society for the Control of Cancer, 1926.

28 P. Brooke Bland, "Cancer in Women," 460.

29 Patterson, *Dread Disease*, 67.

30 John E. Leach and Guy F. Robbins, "Delay in the Diagnosis of Cancer," 5.

31 Russell Ferguson, "When Cancer Is Not Guilty," 893.

32 Stuart W. Harrington, "Results of Surgical Treatment of Unilateral Carcinoma," 1007.

33 Ross, *Crusade*, 96–97.

34 This was not the ACS's first venture into the world of film. It produced its first (silent) film as early as 1921. In 1929, it produced another film ("The Great Peril") that was shot on a shoestring budget in apartments and offices loaned by ACS members, with volunteer actors performing all roles. This told a cautionary tale of a woman taken in by cancer quacks. Before she is rescued by her future son-in-law (soon to become a doctor, of course), she enters a so-called sanitarium where the quack specialist tells her, "We do not believe in operations, Madam, we are *scientists*." (*Campaign Notes*, June 1929, 4–5). The "March of Time" produced the first sound film, "Conquering Cancer," in 1937. The first film aimed at women was a 15-minute sound film, "Choose to Live," made in conjunction with the U.S. Public Health Service in 1940.

35 "Medical Motion Pictures," *JAMA* 143, no. 7 (1950): 673.

36 Maurice Black and Francis D. Speer, "Biologic Variability," 1560.

37 "Variations in biologic behavior within this disease are of far greater importance in determining survival than speed of diagnosis or surgical intervention." Ibid., 1563. Black and Speer estimated that the curative effect of radical mastectomy "probably does not exceed 10 per cent." They also argued that the "use of ultraradical surgical attempts to cure breast cancer is not consistent with the biology of the disease."

38 Carl M. Mansfield, *Early Breast Cancer*, 64. For early studies evaluating radiation treatment see Geoffrey Keynes, "Treatment of primary carcinoma of the breast"; Geoffrey Keynes, "Place of radium" and M. Lenz, "Tumor dosage and results in roentgen therapy," 67–74. See also R. McWhirter, "The Value of Simple Mastectomy."

39 Myra Morgenstern, "The Role of Mammography," 305.

40 Ibid., 276.

41 Ibid., 293.

42 See Ellen Leopold, "Not Every Picture Tells a Story."

43 The education work of the American Cancer Society was at first concentrated in the east coast and in urban areas. Although many campaigns operated to some extent in almost every state, the ASC did not become a truly national organization until after the Second World War.

44 Marilyn Yalom, *A History of the Breast*, 137–38.

45 Marcia Angell, *Science on Trial*, Chapter 2. Although there is little information on the historical pattern of implant use, records from one county in Minnesota (home of the Mayo Clinic) suggest the shape of its growth. There, the practice of breast enlargement grew quickly from 1964, when there were 3.5 implant recipients for every 100,000 women in the population, to 1979 when the number had risen to 95 per 100,000. Its growth has continued unabated. Despite the ban on silicone implants introduced in 1992 (when an estimated one to two million American women already had them), breast augmentation remained, two years later, the third most popular cosmetic operation in the United States.

46 At the same time, the availability of breast implants may have offset some of the terrors of radical mastectomies, which remained, in the 1960s, the only form of treatment for two-thirds of American women. The use of breast implants for reconstruction after breast cancery surgery did increase from 10 percent of all the breast augmentation procedures in 1964 to 30 per cent in 1991. (Angell, *Science on Trial*, 47).

47 There were other factors contributing to a decline in the death rate from reproductive cancers, including the huge increase in the number of hysterectomies performed for other reasons. See next chapter. By 1961, 30 per cent of American women had had at least one Pap smear. (Ross, *Crusade*, 90). Over the fifty years between 1940 and 1990, the death rate from uterine cancer dropped from 28.5 per 100,000 to 5.2. (Wright, *Life and Death in the U.S.*, Figure 4–5).

48 The refinement of mammography (improvement in film quality, magnification, etc), has revived the notion of the almost instantaneous occurrence of origin and detection. The increasingly common discovery of precancerous signs, so small that they hardly have any real mass at all, reinforces this notion.

49 Mary Lasker, the powerhouse behind the postwar growth of the American Cancer Society, placed articles in the *Reader's Digest* through a friend who was the medical editor there. In 1949, an article headlined "Some Facts of Life-and-Death Interest to You" ended with a one-line appeal for funds that brought in $84,000. (Ross, *The American Cancer Society*, 37).

50 Clarence C. Little, "The Conquest of Cancer," *Good Housekeeping*, December 1936, p. 108.

51 Isaac F. Marcosson, "The Cured Cancer Club," *Hygeia*, August 1939, 695.

52 By 1946, the number of women in employment had dropped by three million from its wartime peak. But according to Sheila Tobias and Lisa Anderson, in "What Really Happened to Rosie the Riveter," there were really two Rosie the Riveters, not one. The first was a working-class girl already in a low-skilled job as a waitress or laundress before the war began. (By 1940, in fact, about 30 percent of American women were already working full-time.) The war allowed her to move into better-paying employment and perhaps even to join a union. When peace returned and she lost that job, she didn't retire to suburban domesticity but returned instead to another low-skill low-wage job. The second Rosie was the one who more closely fit the stereotype. With no previous experience or expectation of employment, her wartime work acclimated her to a totally different life. At the end of the war, she

(along with 85 per cent of all women working) wanted to stay on the job and was sorry to be forced to step down (356–57).

53   Breasts of course play a role in promoting the unholy alliance between sexism and consumerism that Friedan spells out in great detail: "Manufacturers put out brassieres with false bosoms of foam rubber for little girls of ten." Betty Friedan, *Feminine Mystique*, 16. The self-destructiveness of sexism was also highlighted: "women dying of cancer refused a drug which research had proved might save their lives: its side effects were said to be unfeminine" (17).

Chapter 6

1   Friedan, *Feminine Mystique*, 268.

2   E. Neuman, *Insight* 8, *Washington Times*, February 9, 1992: 6–11, 24–26.

3   Breast cancer was not mentioned at all in the first edition of *Our Bodies, Ourselves*, published as a pamphlet in 1971. In later editions, the subject was covered under broader subject headings. In 1976 (Third Edition), it appeared in "Taking Care of Ourselves" and in 1984 in a chapter called "Some Common and Uncommon Health and Medical Problems." Even the most recent 1998 edition combines its breast cancer coverage with other topics in a chapter called "Selected Medical Practices, Problems and Medical Care" within Part Five: "Knowledge Is Power."

4   David J. Garrow, *Liberty and Sexuality*, 281. As early as 1933, for instance, two American doctors each published books advocating a change in the laws against abortion. One even cited "the right of the woman to her own body."

5   The Internet has become a very valuable tool for newly diagnosed women. There is a surfeit of hard information at sites such as that run by the National Cancer Institute (http://cancernet.nci.nih.gov). There are also several breast cancer discussion groups online which put women with breast cancer histories directly in touch with one another. This can greatly expand their understanding of all aspects of the disease, personal and political. The easy availability of information on, for example, alternative and experimental as well as orthodox treatments may, in turn, alter the nature of many women's consultations with their own doctors.

6   Three years earlier, the refusal of a New York hospitals commissioner to allow a doctor to fit a diaphragm for a diabetic mother of three got similar national newspaper coverage. (Garrow, *Liberty and Sexuality*, 287–88.)

7   Frederick S. Jaffe, Barbara L. Lindheim, and Philip R. Lee, *Abortion Politics*, 167.

8   Garrow, *Liberty and Sexuality*, 301, and 796 n 62. In addition to these articles in popular magazines, Garrow also cites related articles appearing during the same time frame in the *Washington Post, Western Reserve Law Review, American Bar Association Journal*, and *Civil Liberties in New York*.

9   See references to Rose Kushner, Rosamond Campion, Helga Sandburg Crile, and others, next chapter.

10   See note 3 above.

11   Barbara Hinkson Craig and David M. O'Brien, *Abortion and American Politics*, Table 4.1, 111.

12   *The New York Times Index*, Volume 85.

13 Leslie J. Reagan, *When Abortion Was a Crime*, 220.
14 Theresa Montini, "Resist and Redirect."
15 These briefs were filed in *Webster v. Reproductive Health Services*, brought before the Supreme Court in 1989. (Craig and O'Brien, *Abortion and American Politics*, 204.)
16 Ibid., 77.
17 Garrow, *Liberty and Sexuality*, 507.
18 J. Douglas Butler and David F. Walbert, editors, "Decisions of the United States Supreme Court in January 1973 with Respect to the Texas and Georgia Abortion Statutes," *Abortion, Medicine and the Law*, Appendix 1, 394–95. Supreme Court decisions cited the roots of the right of privacy "in the First Amendment (*Stanley v. Georgia*, 394 U.S. 557, 564 (1969); in the Fourth and Fifth Amendments, *Terry v. Ohio*, 392 U.S. 1, 8–9 (1968), *Katz v. United States*, 389 U.S. 347, 350 (1967) . . . in the penumbras of the Bill of Rights, *Griswold v. Connecticut*, 381 U.S. 479, 484–485 (1965); in the Ninth Amendment . . . or in the concept of liberty guaranteed by the first section of the Fourteenth Amendment."
19 Many feminists objected to the use of the privacy argument in *Roe v. Wade*. The legal scholar Catharine MacKinnon preferred to see the issue defended on grounds of equality. That the burdens of reproduction fell almost entirely on women, she argued, was itself a symptom of pervasive inequality. The real problem was finding ways to control women's sexual availability in general, to protect them from unwanted sex as well as from unwanted pregnancies. To redress the inequality between men and women required the active intervention of the state, not its passive acquiescence in privacy arguments. See Ruth Gavison, "Feminism and the Public/Private Distinction," 30–31. This article gives a thorough airing to feminist debates on the issue.
20 Reagan, *When Abortion Was a Crime*, 235–38. The case was brought by civil liberties lawyers Sybille Fritzsche and Susan Grossman in 1970 as a constitutional challenge to the Illinois criminal abortion law. It combined, in one class action suit, both feminist interests and the medical interests of doctors.
21 Among other important contributions, support groups play a critical role in mediating women's response to the barrage of media pronouncements. For example, the release in the popular press, in April 1999, of the early results of clinical trials on bone marrow transplants for breast cancer patients has caused widespread alarm among many women. Linda Falstein, a member of a Boston group of cancer patients who have all had transplants, said that her group experience made it much easier for her to cope with the distress caused by these provisional findings. "If I didn't know these other people in the group, who had their transplants ten or twelve years ago, I wouldn't be able to read and interpret this news with the proper skepticism. It has made an enormous difference" (conversation with author).
22 The first "radical" hysterectomy was performed in 1895, not long after the introduction of radical mastectomies. Ann Dally, *Women under the Knife*, 141.
23 Dr. Peter Barglow, staff psychiatrist at Michael Reese Hospital in Chicago, quoted in Deborah Larned, "The Epidemic in Unnecessary Hysterectomy," 206.
24 Ibid., 200.

25 See Ivan K. Strausz, *You Don't Need a Hysterectomy*, 41–44.
26 Larned, "The Epidemic in Unnecessary Hysterectomy," 204.
27 Crile, *What Women Should Know*, 51.
28 Stanley West, *The Hysterectomy Hoax*, 23.
29 Ibid., 12.
30 Craig and O'Brien, *Abortion and American Politics*, 26.

Chapter 7

1 Typical of early articles written by male doctors was Francis Carter Wood's "What Every Woman Should Know about Cancer" published in the February 1919 issue of *Women's Home Companion*. Similar articles appeared in the *Delineator*, the *Woman's Magazine*, and the *Designer*, which featured, in its March 1919 issue, an article by Dr. Eugene Lyman Fisk. Probably the first book written for the lay public was published in 1906 by a British physician, C. P. Childe. The word "cancer" appeared not in its title—*The Control of a Scourge*—but in its subtitle. It was not until its 1926 edition that the book's title could be changed to *Cancer and the Public*. Walter Ross, *Crusade*, 18. Joseph Bloodgood, the Johns Hopkins pathologist, was also an early contributor to breast cancer education campaigns for early detection. His pamphlet *What Every Woman Should Know about the Breast*, written in 1914 for the American Medical Association, was the first of a great many articles addressed to women themselves. See also Joseph Bloodgood, "The Greatest Scourge in the World."
2 For example, "The Cured Cancer Club," an article that appeared in the August 1939 issue of *Hygeia*, was reprinted in the September issue of the *Reader's Digest*.
3 Paul Starr, *Social Transformation of American Medicine*, 309.
4 Marion W. Flexner, "Cancer—I've Had It"; Gretta Palmer, "Face Your Danger in Time."
5 The American Society for the Control of Cancer, "The Story of Mrs. Harrison," 1914.
6 Ibid.
7 Babe Didrikson Zaharias, as told to Harry Paxton, *This Life I've Led*.
8 James L. Ford, "One Woman in Ten," 37.
9 *Ladies' Home Journal*, February 1962, 130.
10 Sheila Rowbotham, *A Century of Women*, 378–79.
11 Bernard Fisher has pointed out that women like Rosamund Campion, who rejected radical surgery and sought out physicians willing to consider alternatives, played a role, not just in changing clinical practice but in establishing the reputations of the unorthodox clinicians who were willing to listen to them. "These women," Fisher remarked, "may claim responsibility for the immortality of those pioneers!" Bernard Fisher, "Revolution in Breast Cancer Surgery," 657.
12 As Craig Henderson, a cancer researcher at the University of California Medical School in San Francisco, confirms of this small band of pioneers, "these people were really reviled. It's hard to appreciate just how passionately people felt and how they expressed their anger in the literature towards these men who now, of course, have been proven largely to be correct." Interview with author, March 28, 1994.

13 William Nolan, "How Doctors Are Unfair to Women," 50.

14 P. Strax, L. Venet, and S. Shapiro, "Value of Mammography," 686–89.

15 Bernard Fisher, "Revolution in Breast Cancer Surgery," 659.

16 The NSABP had been set up by Fisher and others in 1958. Its first trials tested the effectiveness of chemotherapeutic agents (like thiotepa) as a treatment for breast cancer. The next generation of trials designed to test the efficacy of radical surgery was carried out in two separate stages. The first stage (the B-04 trial), begun in 1971, compared the results of radical mastectomy with those of simple mastectomy (removal of the breast only) plus radiation. These showed no differences in the pattern of long-term survival between the two groups (see Fisher, "Revolution in Breast Cancer Surgery," 655–66). Encouraged by these results, the follow-up study pushed the hypothesis further, introducing treatment options based on even less invasive surgery. Recruiting its first patients in 1976, the B-06 trial had three treatment arms rather than two. Newly diagnosed women were randomly assigned to treatment either by lumpectomy, by lumpectomy plus radiation, or by simple mastectomy. *All* the women in this trial had their underarm lymph nodes removed compared with only those women undergoing radical mastectomies in the B-04 trial. For a discussion of the history of axillary dissection, see Ellen Leopold, "The Breast Cancer Surgery You Rarely Hear About," 30–31. The results of the B-06 protocol, like the earlier study, showed no important differences in survival among the different treatment groups. The landmark report, which generated front-page news in March 1985 in the *Los Angeles Times* and the *New York Times*, appeared in Fisher et al., "Five Year Results"; typical of the newspaper coverage of the earlier trials was Harold Schmeck's "Study seeks to determine best treatment for breast cancer," *New York Times*, April 8, 1973, 28.

17 Letter from Rose Kushner to Flora, Nan, et al., October 8, 1974. Rose Kushner Papers, Schlesinger Library, Radcliffe College. Eighteen months later, Kushner wrote to Hugh Hefner, soliciting funds for her Breast Cancer Advisory Service as soon as it received tax-exempt status as a charity. "*Playboy* and similar men's magazines," she wrote, "[have] instilled the notion that no woman is complete without two, preferably ample, mammary glands. Because of this image, *Playboy*, in my opinion, would be doing a valuable and commendable deed by helping a Breast Cancer Advisory Service begin." No funds were forthcoming although the magazine did offer to publish a fundraising letter if Kushner submitted one. She did, but the editor found her first sentence "a shade too melodramatic for the Forum." She submitted a redraft that pandered much more to the sympathies of her male audience. (Letters to *Playboy* of June 24, August 27, and September 15, 1975.)

18 Jane E. Brody, "Parley Scores the Denial of Jobs to Persons Who Have Had Cancer Treatment," *New York Times*, November 28, 1974, 12.

19 *New York Times*, December 4, 1972, 53.

20 Letter from Rose Kushner to Pat Sweating, *Ms.*, October 2, 1974. Letter from Rose Kushner to Flora, Nan, et al., October 8, 1974; letter from Rose Kushner to Doris Black, *Reader's Digest*, October 8, 1974.

21 Rosamond Campion's memoir, *The Invisible Worm*, published three years earlier (1972), remained a highly personal retelling of the author's own experience. Shortly

after her book was published, she did say in an interview "that neither men nor surgeons, nor a 103-year-old tradition of removing the entire breast if a lump is cancerous, could tell me what to do" (*New York Times*, December 12, 1972).

22 Rose Kushner, *Breast Cancer*, 346.

23 The Metropolitan Life Insurance Company carried out a study of the charges submitted in claims for a modified radical mastectomy carried out in 1988. Published in 1990, the year Kushner died, the investigation revealed total costs that ranged from $4,100 in Iowa to $7,870 (almost twice as high) in New York. Included in these totals were physician charges that rose from $1,340 in Iowa to $3,280 (two and a half times higher) in New York. (Metropolitan Life, "Modified Radical Mastectomies: Average Charges, 1988," *Statistical Bulletin* 71:4, October-December 1990, 29.) Even at their highest, physician charges constituted less than half of the total. This explains the drive, in the 1990s, to shorten the hospital stay associated with mastectomies. Women were being sent home so early after surgery that their health was being put in jeopardy. It took national legislation to put a stop to this practice.

24 For suggesting, in a newspaper interview, a link between fees and surgical practice and for dismissing the radical mastectomy as "archaic," Crile was summoned before the Ethics Committee of the Cleveland Academy of Medicine (AMA) and had his wrist slapped. They felt his comments to the press had been "reprehensible. The Committee was disturbed over your obvious lack of concern for the patients who have had a radical mastectomy performed and the impact that your comments have on these women . . . your comments have already had a deleterious effect on the relationship patients have with their surgeons . . . in permitting another obstacle to be erected between the confidence and understanding so necessary for success in an operative procedure" (George Crile, Jr., "The Surgeon's Dilemma," *Harper's*, May 1975: 33).

25 Kushner, *Breast Cancer*, xii.

26 Draft introduction to *Why Me?*, 1979 re-issue of *Breast Cancer*. Rose Kushner Papers, Schlesinger Library.

27 Win Ann Winkler, in a letter responding to a review of Kushner's *Breast Cancer*, *New York Times*, October 26, 1975, VII, 57.

28 See, for instance, Betty Rollin, *First You Cry*, and Helga Sandburg (later Crile), "Let a Joy Keep You."

29 Being Hitchcock, however, he couldn't resist twisting the knife, quite literally. The only prop he requested other than a desk and two chairs was a letter opener. He interrupted the actor portraying the doctor, the young William Shatner, to ask him to begin playing with it, while talking to his patient about her impending surgery.

30 Telephone interview with Bill Bell, April 15, 1998. Two other characters on "The Young and the Restless" (Mary Williams and Katherine Chancellor) have also had breast cancer scares. More than 15 years before this story was broadcast in the late 1950s, the trail-blazing Agnes Nixon, soap opera writer and executive, wrote a story into "As the World Turns" about a woman undergoing a Pap smear. Nixon got clearance for the plot but she was forbidden to use the words "uterus," "cancer," or "hysterectomy" in the dialogue.

31 On the movie screen it is a wholly different story. In Hollywood, women die regu-

larly from all kinds of cancer. Susan Sarandon in "Step Mom" is just the most recent in a long line of terminally afflicted cancer heroines that stretches back through Allie McGraw in "Love Story" to Bette Davis in "Dark Victory." Men, on the other hand, seem to have largely escaped this cinematic fate.

Chapter 8

1 Hugh Gallagher, *FDR's Splendid Deception*, 30.

2 Ibid., 149.

3 Shaughnessy, *Story of the American Cancer Society*, 173.

4 Although no one in the early 1950s was calling attention to the lack of funds earmarked specifically for breast cancer research, there were some who did point out the relative scarcity of research funds allocated to cancer altogether. In an article in the February 1950 issue of *McCall's* ("The Cancer in Our Breast"), the journalist John Gunther, "thinking of all the women—and men—suffering from cancer in this country," began to wonder "why indeed we do not do more about it. In 1948 over a billion dollars were spent on horse racing and another billion on jewelry and I do not know how many more billions on alcohol, nightclubs and cigarettes. But all that Congress would appropriate for cancer research was a piker's $20,725,000." This was less than half the money raised by the March of Dimes in the same year.

5 Breast cancer has, of course, proved to be a much more difficult scientific problem to solve than was polio. Vaccines cannot be effective where the target cells are heterogeneous and have the capacity to develop resistance (if they survive the initial exposure to a vaccine). Cancer is much more of a "moving target" than an infectious agent and has a greater capacity to mutate.

6 Gallagher, *FDR's Splendid Deception*, 149. In 1948, 1,895 Americans died of polio, a mortality rate of 1.3 per 100,000 population. In the same year, about 19,000 American women died of breast cancer, a mortality rate of 26.9 per 100,000 population (figures from "Poliomyelitis Annual Statistical Review," The National Foundation, New York, 1960; and Harrington, "Results of Surgical Treatment," 1007). The $203 million in direct subsidies to defray medical costs was intended to make possible "the best available care for all those who could not meet the costs themselves without undue hardship." The money was distributed among all 3,100 local chapters. ("The Story Behind the Polio Vaccine," The National Foundation for Infantile Paralysis, New York, 1956).

7 Robert Proctor, *Cancer Wars*, 8, 12–13, and 102, 110.

8 Kushner's long-term legacy, however, has been profound, if still undervalued. Rita Arditti, one of the founders of the Women's Community Cancer Project in Cambridge, Mass., remembers that when she herself was first diagnosed in 1974, she "was in a fog. There was nothing to read and I just stumbled along. . . . When I read *Why Me?* in 1982, I felt that Kushner validated the choices I had made earlier. Like her, I had asked to have the 'two-step' procedure but had to fight for it. When I had a recurrence in my lungs in 1989 I called her. She answered the phone herself and gave me clear and helpful information. I was devastated when I learned she had a recurrence and when she died. I do not think she has been recognized enough for

the pioneer that she was" (personal communication with the author November 5, 1998).

9 Jimmy Carter had at least been able to appoint Rose Kushner to the National Cancer Advisory Board in 1976.

10 Cited in Montini, "Gender and Emotion," 15.

11 Tamar Lewin, "Nancy Reagan Defends Her Decision to Have Mastectomy," *New York Times*, March 5, 1988, Late City Final Edition, I, 6.

12 Gina Kolata, "Mastectomy Seen as Extreme for Small Tumor," *New York Times*, Late City Final Edition, October 18, 1987, I, Part 1, 32.

13 Ann Nattinger, Raymond Hoffman, Alicia Howell-Pelz, and James Goodwin, "Effect of Nancy Reagan's Mastectomy." The effect was most noticeable in the Central and Southern regions of the country and in counties with lower levels of education and income.

14 Anne Hawkins, *Reconstructing Illness*, 14. Hawkins uses the word "pathography" to describe a narrative of illness. She divides the genre roughly into three groups. The first, the didactic or testimonial pathography, shares an experience of illness with the reader, providing an emotional commentary as a complement to the medical one, and offering suggestions, along the way, both practical and emotional, that might be of use to someone else in a similar situation. The second, the angry pathography, serves more as a cautionary tale, opening the reader's eyes to the inadequacy, indifference, or even cruelty of the medical system and its personnel. The third type describes the author's experience of alternative treatments (using substances such as laetrile or sharks' cartilage, or processes such as visualization). Writing in the early 1990s, she found that most breast cancer accounts fall into the first category, testimonials that blend the personal with the practical. If she had written fifteen or twenty years earlier she might have found the second category much more heavily represented. Hawkins, 4–15.

15 See the narratives in Sylvia Dunnavant, ed., *Celebrating Life: African American Women Speak Out About Breast Cancer*.

16 One study that followed a group of 930 patients for up to 40 years postoperatively found 25 women whose metastases *first appeared* ten or more years after their radical mastectomies. In six of this group of 25, the appearance of metastasis was very late indeed, not showing up until 20 to 30 years later. Deaths from metastatic disease, therefore, might occur 30 or 40 years after diagnosis. (Edwin B. Buchanan, "A Century of Breast Cancer Surgery," 375.)

17 British memoirs seem to be less squeamish about and more concerned with the prospects of dying. The work of Gillian Rose (*Love's Work*), the writer-photographer Jo Spence, and more recently, of Ruth Picardie, Matt Seaton, and Justine Picardie (*Before I Say Goodbye*), all directly confront death with a directness and lack of sentimentality, characteristics that are, with the rare exception of books like Christina Middlebrook's *Seeing the Crab*, distinctly un-American.

18 The case of tamoxifen (sold as Nolvadex) illustrates the dangers involved in a pharmaceutical company's gaining direct access to a drug's consumers through the media. The drug has been successfully used for over twenty years as an adjuvant ther-

apy for women with metastatic breast cancer. When a recent NCI-sponsored study indicated that it might also be effective as a way to decrease the incidence or delay the onset of breast cancer among those at increased risk, Zeneca tried to win FDA approval to describe it as a drug that could *prevent* the disease. Thanks to intervention by women's health activists, the label approves only the claim that the scientific evidence supports, i.e., that the use of tamoxifen could contribute to a "short-term reduction in the incidence of breast cancer for women at increased risk." Nevertheless, by the time news of the FDA's approval reached the newspapers, it had acquired the attributes of a "miracle drug," hailed as a "scientific breakthrough" in the *prevention* of breast cancer. Zeneca lobbyists had done their job.

19 The side effects of tamoxifen, for example, include the risk of endometrial cancer, strokes, blood clots, and liver and eye damage.

20 Halsted argued that "to attempt to close the breast wound more or less regularly by any plastic method is hazardous, and, in my opinion, to be vigorously discountenanced." William S. Halsted, "Cancer of the Breast," 79. In the place of plastic repair or reconstruction, Halsted argued for the use of skin grafts to cover up what is called the "mastectomy defect."

21 It was in 1979 that the NIH Consensus Development Panel formally recommended the change in standard treatment from the Halsted radical mastectomy to what the panel called a "total" mastectomy, i.e., a procedure that preserved the pectoral muscles. The panel also, on this occasion, recommended the use of a two-step procedure, separating the diagnostic biopsy from primary treatment. Rose Kushner was a member of this panel. "Special Report: Treatment of Primary Breast Cancer," *New England Journal of Medicine* 301, no. 6 (August 9, 1979): 340.

22 A tissue expander is a device that can be inserted at the time of a mastectomy or later. It allows the area to be progressively filled with a solution that gently stretches the skin and tissue to make it possible to insert a more permanent implant later.

23 TRAM stands for transverse rectus abdominis myocutaneous. The TRAM procedure uses a flap of skin and muscle taken from a woman's stomach to recreate a breast. The potential for stomach-flattening, for many women, is an added bonus of the surgery; abdominal muscular impairment is a potential drawback.

24 Scott L. Spear and Alexander Majidian, "Immediate Breast Reconstruction," 56.

25 Estimates based on the pattern of breast implant use in Olmstead County, Minnesota. See Marcia Angell, *Science on Trial*, 47.

26 Bernadine P. Healy, "Breast Implants Rise Again," 639–40.

27 Philip P. Trabulsy, James P. Anthony, and Stephen J. Mathes, "Changing Trends in Postmastectomy Breast Reconstruction."

28 "Harvesting" refers to the preparation or removal of tissue from the patient's "donor site" (typically, from her stomach or back) for use in the reconstruction of her breast. To save time in the operating theater, the process of "harvesting" a woman's stomach flap may be carried on by a plastic surgeon simultaneously with the performance of a mastectomy by another surgeon.

29 The surgeon's enthusiasm can be shared with colleagues, if not with patients. "I enjoy doing TRAM flaps," writes a plastic surgeon from Missouri in an editorial for

Plastic and Reconstructive Surgery. "It is an operation that expresses the essence of plastic surgery, incorporating a fundamental appreciation for flap physiology and a flair for aesthetic creation and simultaneously satisfying the general surgery-spawned plastic surgeon's thirst for an invigorating operative catharsis. No timid incisions here." C. Lin Puckett, "Selling the TRAM," 153. Puckett then reins in this enthusiasm to compare the reliable benefits of implants with the serious risks of the TRAM flap procedure.

30   There has, recently, been some revival of interest in the importance of local and regional as well as systemic control of the disease. An editorial in the *New England Journal of Medicine* ("Stopping Metastases at Their Source") addresses the role of radiation therapy in patients treated with chemotherapy. It considers the argument that "chemotherapy can eliminate distant micrometastases but is less effective against local and regional disease. These persistent sites of disease, according to this hypothesis, are the source of subsequent fatal metastases" (October 2, 1997, 996).

31   This is my own estimate of twentieth-century breast cancer deaths. It has been pieced together from two main sources, both issued by the Department of Commerce, Bureau of the Census (Washington, D.C: Government Printing Office); Figures for the years 1900-1936 were derived from Mortality Statistics; for 1937-95, from Volume II of the annual series *Vital Statistics of the United States.* For the last six years of the 1990s, I have used the estimates supplied by the Center for Disease Control and the American Cancer Society. My estimated total for the century is 2,160,600.

32   *Sojourner: The Women's Forum,* September 1989. Susan Shapiro, who later died of the disease, called for "an organization—of women, for women—that will encompass political action, direct service, and education." The goals she sought—putting breast cancer on the political agenda, lobbying for research that promotes prevention rather than treatment, demanding the regulation and/or elimination of potentially harmful chemicals, improving women's access to and information about health care—all remain central concerns of the group she helped to found, the Women's Community Cancer Project in Cambridge, Massachusetts. At roughly the same time in San Francisco, members of a support group for women with metastatic disease (including Elenore Pred and Susan Claymon) set up Breast Cancer Action together with Belle Shayer. BCA has published a bimonthly newsletter ever since and, in 1995, hired Barbara Brenner to be its first full-time staff person (and executive editor). Of the eleven women in the support group that spawned BCA, only one survives and she is very ill.

33   Project LEAD is an intensive four-day course designed by the NBCC for breast cancer activists to familiarize them with the basic scientific concepts relevant to breast cancer research. This includes an introduction to, for instance, the biology and genetics of cancer. Similar programs are also underway at the Department of Defense's breast cancer research project. Those who participate are expected to improve consumer participation in breast cancer research, whether in their own local communities or at the state or federal level.

34 For a discussion of the additional burdens on and risks to the uninsured, see Hardisty and Leopold, "Cancer and Poverty."

35 Samuel Epstein and David Steinman, *The Breast Cancer Prevention Program*, 307.

The Last Word

1 Virginia Woolf, *A Room of One's Own*, 50. Woolf's sister, the painter Vanessa Bell, died of breast cancer in 1961.

2 I should add that because the story has been traced primarily through the *New York Times*, it offers a largely white representation of cancer.

3 Cited in Leslie J. Reagan, "Engendering the Dread Disease."

4 *New York Times*, September 23, 1974, 38.

5 Letter from Rachel Carson to Marjorie Spock and Polly Richards, April 12, 1960, from Rachel Carson Papers / Beinecke Library, Yale University.

Bibliography

Agnew, Thomas. *Principles and Practice of Surgery.* Philadelphia: Lippincott, 1883.

American Society for the Control of Cancer. *The American Society for Cancer Control: Its Objects and Methods.* New York: American Society for the Control of Cancer, 1926.

———. "The Story of Mrs. Harrison." Circular 4, July 1914–January 1916. 11 pages.

———. "The Total Number of Cases of Cancer." *Boston Medical & Surgical Journal* 196, no. 5 (1927).

———. "What Every Woman Should Do about Cancer." New York: American Society for the Control of Cancer, 1929.

Angell, Marcia. *Science on Trial.* New York: W. W. Norton, 1996.

Austoker, Joan. "The 'Treatment of Choice': Breast Cancer Surgery 1860–1985." *The Bulletin for the Society of the Social History of Medicine* 37 (December 1985): 100–107.

Baum, Michael. "Natural History of Breast Cancer." In *Primary Management of Breast Cancer: Alternatives to Mastectomy,* edited by J. S. Tobias and M. J. Peckham. London: Edward Arnold, 1985, 3–21.

———. "Surgery and Radiotherapy in Breast Cancer." *Seminars in Oncology* 1, no. 2 (1974): 101–8.

Beatson, George. "On the Treatment of Inoperable Cancer of the Mammae." *The Lancet* 2 (1896): 104–65.

Beauchamp, Tom L., and Ruth R. Faden. "History of Informed Consent." In *Encyclopedia of Bioethics,* vol. 3, 2d ed., edited by Warren Thomas Reich. New York: Macmillan Library Reference, Simon & Schuster Macmillan, 1995, 1232–41.

Berkeley, Comyns. *Diseases of Women by Ten Teachers.* New York: Longmans, Green, 1922.

Black, Maurice M., and Francis D. Speer. "Biologic Variability of Breast Carcinoma in Relation to Diagnosis and Therapy." *New York State Journal of Medicine,* July 1, 1953: 1560–63.

Bland, P. Brooke. "Cancer in Women." *Hygeia* (May 1930): 460.

Bland-Sutton, J. and Giles, Arthur E. *The Diseases of Women: A Handbook for Students and Practitioners.* Philadelphia: W. B. Saunders, 1897.

———. *The Diseases of Women: A Handbook for Students and Practitioners.* Philadelphia: W. B. Saunders, 1909.

Bloodgood, Joseph C. "The Greatest Scourge in the World." *Good Housekeeping* 88 (1929): 56–206.

Bloom, H.J. G., W. W. Richardson, and E. J. Harries. "Natural History of Untreated Breast Cancer (1805–1933): Comparison of Untreated and Treated Cases According to Histological Grade of Malignancy." *British Medical Journal* (July 28, 1962): 213–21.

Bogue, Donald J. *The Population of the United States.* Glencoe: The Free Press, 1959.

Brooks, Paul. *The House of Life: Rachel Carson at Work with Selections from Her Writings Published and Unpublished.* Boston: Houghton Mifflin, 1972.

Bryant, Thomas. *Diseases of the Breast.* London: Cassell, 1887.

Buchanan, Edwin B. "A Century of Breast Cancer Surgery." *Cancer Investigation* 14, no. 4 (1996): 371–77.

Butler, J. Douglas, and Walbert, David F., eds. *Abortion, Medicine and the Law,* 5th ed. New York: Facts on File Publications, 1986.

Cahn, Ann Foote, ed. *Women in the U.S. Labor Force.* New York: Praeger, 1979.

Campion, Rosamond. *The Invisible Worm.* New York: Macmillan, 1972.

Cheyne, W. Watson. *Antiseptic Surgery.* London: Smith, Elder, 1882.

Childe, Charles P. *Cancer and the Public.* New York: E. P. Dutton, 1925.

Clement, Clara Erskine. *Charlotte Cushman.* Boston: James R. Osgood, 1882.

Clement, Priscilla F. "Managing on Their Own: Ailing Black Women in Philadelphia and Charleston, 1870 to 1918." In *Wings of Gauze: Women of Color and the Experience of Health and Illness,* edited by Barbara Bair and Susan E. Cayleff. Detroit: Wayne State University Press, 1993.

Cobbe, Frances Power. "The Little Health of Ladies." *The Contemporary Review* 31 (January 1878): 276–96.

Colp, Ralph. "Notes on Dr. William S. Halsted." *Bulletin of the New York Academy of Medicine,* 2nd Ser., 60, no. 9 (1984): 876–87.

Cooper, Sir Astley Paston. *The Anatomy and Diseases of the Breast.* Philadelphia: Lea & Blanchard, 1845.

———. *Illustrations of the Diseases of the Breast.* London: Longman, Rees, Orme, Brown and Green, 1829.

Cooper, William A. "The History of the Radical Mastectomy." *Annals of Medical History* III, 3rd Series. New York: Paul B. Hoeber, 1941.

Cope, Oliver. *The Breast: Its Problems—Benign and Malignant—and How to Deal with Them.* Boston: Houghton Mifflin, 1977.

Craig, Barbara Hinkson, and David M. O'Brien. *Abortion and American Politics.* Chatham, N.J.: Chatham House, 1993.

Crile, George, Jr. *Cancer and Common Sense.* New York: Viking Press, 1955.

———. "The Surgeon's Dilemma." *Harper's* (May 1975): 30–38.

———. *What Women Should Know About the Breast Cancer Controversy.* New York: Macmillan, 1973.

Croft, L. R. "Edmund Gosse and the 'New and Fantastic Cure' for Breast Cancer." *Medical History* 38 (1994): 143–59.

Crossen, Harry S., and Robert J Crossen. *Diseases of Women.* 9th ed. St. Louis: C. V. Mosby, 1941.

Cushing, Harvey. "William Stewart Halsted 1852–1922." *Science* 56 (1922): 461–64.

Daland, Ernest M. "Untreated Cancer of the Breast." *Surgery, Gynecology and Obstetrics* 44 (1927): 264–68.

Dally, Ann. *Women under the Knife: A History of Surgery.* New York: Routledge, 1991.

Davis, F. "Uncertainty in Medical Prognosis, Clinical and Functional." In *Medical Care,* edited by W. R. Scott and E. H. Volkart. New York: Wiley, 1966, 311–21.

Deardorff, Neva, and Marta Fraenkel. *Hospitalized Illness in New York City: Hospital Discharge Study,* vol. 2. New York: Welfare Council of New York City, 1942.

Demaitre, Luke. "Medieval Notions of Cancer: Malignancy and Metaphor." *Bulletin of the History of Medicine* 72 (1998): 609–37.

De Moulin, Daniel. *A Short History of Breast Cancer.* Boston: Martinus Nijoff, 1983.

Dixon, Edward H. *Woman and her Diseases from the Cradle to the Grave.* 10th ed. New York: A. Ranney, 1857.

Dunnavant, Sylvia, ed. *Celebrating Life: African American Women Speak Out About Breast Cancer.* Dallas: USFI, Inc., 1995.

Ehrenreich, Barbara, and Deirdre English. *For Her Own Good: 150 Years of the Experts' Advice to Women.* New York: Doubleday, 1989.

Epstein, Julia. "Writing the Unspeakable: Fanny Burney's Mastectomy and the Fictive Body." *Representations* 16 (Fall 1986): 131–66.

Epstein, Samuel S., and David Steinman. *The Breast Cancer Prevention Program.* New York: Macmillan, 1997.

Ewen, Stuart. *Captains of Consciousness: Advertising and the Social Roots of the Consumer Culture.* New York: McGraw-Hill, 1977.

Federal Security Agency, "Trend of Cancer Mortality in the United States 1900–1945," *Vital Statistics Special Reports* 32, no. 1 (December 28, 1949): 13.

Ferguson, Russell S. "When Cancer Is NOT Guilty." *Hygeia* (October 1939): 893.

Fisher, B., R. G. Ravdin, R. K. Ausman, et al. "Surgical Adjuvant Chemotherapy in Cancer of the Breast; Results of a Decade of Cooperative Investigations." *Annals of Surgery* 168 (1968): 337–56.

Fisher, Bernard. "The Revolution in Breast Cancer Surgery: Science of Anecdotalism?" *World Journal of Surgery* 9 (1985): 655–66.

———. "Surgery of Primary Breast Cancer." In *Breast Cancer 1: Advances in Research and Treatment: Current Approaches to Therapy,* edited by William L. McGuire. New York: Plenum Medical, 1977, 1–42.

Fisher, Bernard, M. Bauer, R. Margolese, et al. "Five-Year Results of a Randomized Clinical Trial Comparing Total Mastectomy and Segmental Mastectomy with or without Radiation in the Treatment of Breast Cancer." *New England Journal of Medicine* 312 (March 14, 1985): 665–73.

Flaws, Jodi A., Craig J. Newschaffer, and Trudy L. Bush. "Breast Cancer Mortality in Black and in White Women: A Historical Perspective." *Journal of Women's Health* 7 (October 1998): 1007–15.

Flexner, Marion W. "Cancer—I've Had It." *Ladies' Home Journal* (May 1947): 57–150.

Ford, James L. "One Woman in Ten." *The Bookman* 63, no. 1 (1926): 37–43.

Fox, Maurice S. "On the Diagnosis and Treatment of Breast Cancer." *Journal of the American Medical Association* 241, no. 5 (1979): 489–94.

Freeman, Martha, ed. *Always, Rachel: The Letters of Rachel Carson and Dorothy Freeman, 1952–1964.* Boston: Beacon Press, 1995.

Friedan, Betty. *The Feminine Mystique.* New York: W. W. Norton, 1963.

Gallagher, Hugh. *FDR's Splendid Deception.* New York: Dodd, Mead, 1985.

Garriques, Henry J. *Diseases of Women.* 3rd ed. Philadelphia: W. B. Saunders, 1900.

Garrow, David J. *Liberty and Sexuality: The Right to Privacy and the Making of* Roe v. Wade. New York: Macmillan, 1994.

Gavison, Ruth. "Feminism and the Public/Private Distinction." *Stanford Law Review* 45 (November 1992): 1–45.

Gerster, Arpad. *The Rules of Aseptic and Antiseptic Surgery; A Practical Treatise for the Use of Students and the General Practitioner.* New York: D. Appleton, 1888.

Goodbody, Bridget L. " 'The Present Opprobrium of Surgery'—The Agnew Clinic and Nineteenth Century Representations of Cancerous Female Breasts." *American Art* 8, no. 1 (1994): 32–51.

Gordon-Taylor, Gordon, and R. McWhirter. "Discussion: The Treatment of Cancer of the Breast." *Proceedings of the Royal Society of Medicine* 41, Section of Surgery, (1948): 118–29.

Gover, Mary. *Cancer Mortality in the United States, 3. Geographic Variation in Recorded Cancer Mortality for Detailed Sites, for an Average of the Years 1930–1932. Public Health Bulletin* no. 257. Washington, D.C.: Government Printing Office, 1940.

Grace, E. J., and W. J. Moitrier. "Simple Mastectomy with X-ray in Treatment of Cancer of the Breast." *New York State Journal of Medicine* 36 (1936): 701–4.

Greenough, Robert B., Channing C. Simmons, and J. Dellinger Barney. "End Results of 376 Primary Operations for Carcinoma of the Breast at the Massachusetts General Hospital between January 1, 1894, and January 1, 1904." *Annals of Surgery* 46, no. 1 (1907): 20–27.

Greenwood, M. *A Report on the Natural Duration of Cancer.* Report on public health and medical subjects, no. 33. Ministry of Health, London: HMSO, 1926.

Haagenson, C. D. *Diseases of the Breast.* Philadelphia: W. B. Saunders, 1957.

Halsted, William S. "The Results of Radical Operations for the Cure of Cancer of the Breast." *Annals of Surgery* 46, no. 1 (1907): 1–19.

———. *Surgical Papers,* Vol. 2. Baltimore: Johns Hopkins Press, 1924.

Handley, W. Sampson. *Cancer of the Breast and Its Treatment.* London: John Murray, 1906.

Hardisty, Jean V., and Ellen Leopold. "Cancer and Poverty: Double Jeopardy for Women." In *Myths about the Powerless: Contesting Social Inequalities,* edited by M. Brinton Lykes, Ali Banuazizi, Ramsay Liem, and Michael Morris. Philadelphia: Temple University Press, 1996: 219–36.

Harrington, Stuart W. "Results of Surgical Treatment of Unilateral Carcinoma of Breast in Women." *Journal of the American Medical Association* 148, no. 12 (1952): 1007–11.

Hartmann, Susan M. *The Home Front and Beyond: American Women in the 1940s.* Boston: Twayne Publishers, 1982.

Harvey, A. McGhee. "The Influence of William Stewart Halsted's Concepts of Surgical Training." In *Research and Discovery in Medicine: Contributions from Johns Hopkins.* Baltimore: Johns Hopkins University Press, 1981.

Hawkins, Anne. *Reconstructing Illness: Studies in Pathography.* West Lafayette, Ind.: Purdue University Press, 1993.

Healy, Bernadine P. "Breast Implants Rise Again." Editorial, *Journal of Women's Health* 7, no. 6 (August 1998): 639–40.

Hemlow, Joyce, with Curtis D. Cecil and Althea Douglas, eds. *The Journals and Letters of Fanny Burney (Madame d'Arblay),* vol. 6. Oxford: Oxford University Press, 1975, 596–616.

Hermann, Robert E., and Stanley O. Hoerr. "Ohio Breast Cancer Surgery, 1960–1969." *American Journal of Surgery* 122 (1971): 765–69.

Heuer, George W. "Dr Halsted." Supplement to *Bulletin of Johns Hopkins Hospital* 90, no. 2 (February 1952): 1–105.

Hoffman, Frederick L. "The Menace of Cancer." *American Gynecological Society* 38 (1913): 400–52.

———. *The Mortality from Cancer Throughout the World.* Newark: The Prudential Press, 1915.

———. *Some Final Results of the San Francisco Cancer Survey.* Newark, N.J.: The Prudential Press, 1929.

———. *The Statistical Experience: Data of the Johns Hopkins Hospital, Baltimore, Md., 1892–1911.* Baltimore, Md.: Johns Hopkins Press, 1913.

James F. Holland, "The Krebiozen Story: Is Cancer Quackery Dead?" *Journal of the American Medical Association* 200, no. 3 (1967): 125–30.

Holleb, Arthur I. "Halsted Revisited." *Bulletin of the American College of Surgeons* 71, no. 9 (1986): 21–24.

Holman, Emile. "A Surgical Philosopher's Credo: Excerpts from the Writings of William Stewart Halsted." *Surgery, Gynecology & Obstetrics* 101 (July–December 1955): 369–76.

Jaffe, Frederick S., Barbara L. Lindheim, and Philip R. Lee. *Abortion Politics: Private Morality and Public Policy.* New York: McGraw-Hill, 1981.

Jalland, Pat. *Death in the Victorian Family.* Oxford: Oxford University Press, 1996.

Jones, H. McNaughton. *Practical Manual of Diseases of Women and Uterine Therapeutics.* New York: Appleton, 1884.

Jordanova, Ludmilla. *Sexual Visions: Images of Gender in Science and Medicine between the Eighteenth and Twentieth Centuries.* Madison: University of Wisconsin Press, 1989.

———. "The Social Construction of Medical Knowledge." *Social History of Medicine* 7 (1995): 361–81.

Katz, Jay. *The Silent World of Doctor and Patient.* New York: The Free Press, 1984.

Kellogg, J. H. *Ladies Guide in Health and Disease: Girlhood, Maidenhood, Wifehood, Motherhood.* Battle Creek, Mich.: Modern Medicine Publishing, 1882.

Kelly, William D., and Stanley R. Friesen. "Do Cancer Patients Want to Be Told?" *Surgery* 27, no. 6 (1950): 822–26.

Keynes, Geoffrey. "Conservative treatment of cancer of the breast." *The British Medical Journal* (October 2, 1937): 643–47.

———. "The place of radium in the treatment of cancer of the breast." *Annals of Surgery* 106 (October 1937): 619–30.

———. "Treatment of primary carcinoma of the breast with radium." *Acta Radiologica* 10, no. 2 (1929): 393–401.

Kushner, Rose. *Breast Cancer: A Personal History and an Investigative Report.* New York: Harcourt Brace Jovanovich, 1975.

Larned, Deborah. "The Epidemic in Unnecessary Hysterectomy." *Seizing Our Bodies: The Politics of Women's Health,* ed. Claudia Dreifus. New York: Vintage Books, 1977. First published as "The Greening of the Womb," *New Times Magazine,* December 1974.

Latz, Peter J. *Manual of Health for Women: Plain Advice in Sickness and Health.* Chicago: J. S. Hyland, 1906.

Leach, John E., and Guy F. Robbins. "Delay in the Diagnosis of Cancer." *Journal of the American Medical Association* 135, no. 1 (1947): 5–8.

Lear, Linda. *Rachel Carson: Witness for Nature.* New York: Henry Holt, 1997.

Leavitt, Judith, ed. *Women and Health in America: Historical Readings.* Madison: University of Wisconsin Press, 1984.

Lenz, M. "Tumor dosage and results in roentgen therapy of cancer of the breast." *American Journal of Roentgenology and Radium Therapy* 56 (July 1946): 67–74.

Leopold, Ellen. "The Breast Cancer Surgery You Rarely Hear About." *Sojourner: The Women's Forum* (July 1995): 30–31.

———. "Not Every Picture Tells a Story." *Women's Community Cancer Project Newsletter,* Cambridge, Mass. (Summer 1998).

L'Esperance, Elise Strang. "The Cancer Prevention Clinic." *Quarterly Review,* American Society for the Control of Cancer (April 1940).

Lewison, Edward F. "The Surgical Treatment of Breast Cancer: An Historical and Collective Review." *Surgery* 34 (November 1953): 904–53.

Longo, Lawrence D. "The Rise and Fall of Battey's Operation: A Fashion in Surgery." *Bulletin of the History of Medicine* 53 (Summer 1979): 244–67.

Love, Susan, with Karen Lindsey. *Dr. Susan Love's Breast Book.* 2nd ed. Reading, Mass.: Addison-Wesley, 1995.

Löwy, Ilana. *Between Bench and Bedside: Science, Healing, and Interleukin-2 in a Cancer Ward.* Cambridge, Mass.: Harvard University Press, 1996.

Luft, Rolf, and Herbert Olivecrona. "Experience with Hypophysectomy in Man." *Journal of Neurosurgery* 10 (1953): 301–16.

Lund, C. C. "Doctor, Patient and the Truth." *Annals of Internal Medicine* 24 (1946): 955–59.

MacPhee, Rosalind. *Picasso's Woman: A Breast Cancer Story.* New York: Kodansha, 1996.

Mansfield, Carl M. *Early breast cancer: its history and results of treatment. Experimental biology and medicine.* Vol. 5. Basel: Karger, 1976.

Marchand, Roland. *Advertising the American Dream: Making Way for Modernity, 1920–1940.* Berkeley: University of California Press, 1986.

Martin, Emily. *The Woman in the Body.* Boston: Beacon Press, 1987.

Matas, Rudolph, M.D. "Surgical Operations in the Antiseptic Era." In *Surgery in America: From the Colonial Era to the Twentieth Century, Selected Writings,* edited by A. Scott Earle. Philadelphia: W. B. Saunders, 1965, 196–207.

Mayer, Musa. *Examining Myself: One Woman's Story of Breast Cancer Treatment and Recovery.* Boston: Faber & Faber, 1993.

McCay, Mary A. *Rachel Carson.* New York: Twayne Publishers, 1993.

McGregor, Deborah. *From Midwives to Medicine: The Birth of American Gynecology.* New Brunswick: Rutgers University Press, 1998.

McIntosh, Jim. "The Routine Management of Uncertainty in Communication with Cancer Patients." In *Relationships between Doctors and Patients,* edited by Alan Davis. Farnborough, Eng: Saxon House, 1978, 106–31.

McWhirter, R. "Discussion: The Treatment of Cancer of the Breast." *Proceedings of the Royal Society of Medicine* (December 3, 1947): 122.

———. "The Value of Simple Mastectomy and Radiotherapy in the Treatment of Cancer of the Breast." In "Carcinoma of the Breast Symposium," *The British Journal of Radiology* 21 (December 1948): 599–610.

Metropolitan Life. "Modified Radical Mastectomies: Average Charges, 1988." *Statistical Bulletin* 71 (October–December 1990): 26–32.

Middlebrook, Christina. *Seeing the Crab: A Memoir of Dying.* New York: Basic Books, 1996.

Montini, Theresa. "Gender and Emotion in the Advocacy for Breast Cancer Informed Consent Legislation." *Gender & Society* 10, no. 1 (1996): 9–23.

———. "Resist and Redirect: Physicians Respond to Breast Cancer Informed Consent Legislation." *Women & Health* 26, no. 1 (1997): 85–105.

Morantz-Sanchez, Regina Markell. *Sympathy and Science: Women Physicians in American Medicine.* New York: Oxford University Press, 1985.

Morgenstern, Myra. "The Role of Mammography in the Detection of Breast Cancer." In Lester Breslow, *A History of Cancer Control in the United States 1946–1971,* History of Cancer Control Project, UCLA School of Public Health. DHEW publication. NIH no. 78, Book One, Chapter 5. Bethesda, Md.: Department of Health, Education and Welfare, 1977.

Morris, David B. *Illness and Culture in the Postmodern Age.* Berkeley: University of California Press, 1998.

Murphy, James B. "Studies in X-Ray Effects on Cancer Immunity." Abstract. *New York Medical Journal* 106 (1917): 480.

Murphy, James B., J. H. Means, and J. C. Aub. "Clinical Calorimetry. Twenty-Third Paper. The Effect of Roentgen-Ray and Radium Therapy on the Metabolism of a Patient with Lymphatic Leukemia." *Archives of Internal Medicine* 19 (1917): 890–907.

Murphy, James B., and John J. Morton. "The Effects of X-Rays on the Resistance to Cancer in Mice." *Science* 42, no. 1093 (1915): 842–43.

Napheys, George H. *The Physical Life of Woman: Advice to the Maiden, Wife and Mother.* Philadelphia: George Maclean, 1870.

Nattinger, Ann, Raymond Hoffman, Alicia Howell-Pelz, and James Goodwin. "Effects of Nancy Reagan's Mastectomy on Choice of Surgery for Breast Cancer by U.S. Women." *Journal of the American Medical Association* 279, no. 10 (1998): 762–66.

The New York Times Index: A Book of Record. Volume 84, New York: New York Times Company, 1997.

Niemoeller, Adolph F. *The Complete Guide to Bust Culture*. New York: Harvest House, 1944.

Nobile, Philip. "King Cancer." *Esquire* (June 1973): 103–224.

Nolan, William. "How Doctors are Unfair to Women." *McCall's* (August 1973): 50.

Novack, Dennis H., Robin Plumer, Raymond L. Smith, et al. "Changes in Physicians' Attitudes Toward Telling the Cancer Patient." *Journal of the American Medical Association* 241, no. 9 (1979): 897–900.

Numbers, Ronald L., and Darrel W. Amundsen. *Caring and Curing: Health and Medicine in the Western Religious Traditions*. Baltimore, Md.: Johns Hopkins University Press, 1998.

Oken, Donald. "What to Tell Cancer Patients? A Study of Medical Attitudes." *Journal of the American Medical Association* 175, no. 13 (1961): 1120–28.

Palmer, Gretta. "Face Your Danger in Time." *Ladies' Home Journal* (July 1947): 143–53.

Patterson, James. *The Dread Disease: Cancer and Modern American Culture*. Cambridge, Mass.: Harvard University Press, 1987.

Penfield, Wilder. "Halsted of Johns Hopkins: The Man and His Problem as Described in the Secret Records of William Osler." *Journal of the American Medical Association* 210, no. 12 (1969): 2214–18.

Penrose, Charles B. *A Text-Book of Diseases of Women*. 2d ed. Philadelphia: W. B. Saunders, 1898.

Peters, Vera. "Wedge Resection and Irradiation." *Journal of the American Medical Association* 200, no. 2 (1967): 144–53.

Picardie, Ruth, with Matt Seaton and Justine Picardie. *Before I Say Goodbye*. London: Penguin, 1998.

Porter, Roy. *The Greatest Benefit to Mankind: A Medical History of Humanity*. New York: W. W. Norton, 1997.

Portmann, U. V. "Cancer of the Breast: Classification of Cases, Criteria of Incurability and Treatment." *Journal of the American Medical Association* 144, no. 7 (1950): 513–16.

Power, D'Arcy. "The History of the Amputation of the Breast to 1904." *The Liverpool Medico-Chirurgical Journal* 42, Part I (1934): 20–56.

Proctor, Robert. *Cancer Wars: How Politics Shapes What We Know and Don't Know about Cancer*. New York: Basic Books, 1995.

Puckett, C. Lin. "Selling the TRAM." Editorial, *Plastic and Reconstructive Surgery* 99, no. 7 (July 1996): 153–54.

Reagan, Leslie J. "Engendering the Dread Disease: Women, Men and Cancer." *American Journal of Public Health* 87, no. 11 (1997): 1779–87.

———. *When Abortion Was a Crime: Women, Medicine, and Law in the United States, 1867–1973*. Berkeley: University of California Press, 1997.

Rigney, Ella Hoffman. "The Women's Field Army Throughout the Country." *Quarterly Review* (April 1941): 23–36.

Rodman, William L. "Care of the Breast." Prevention of Cancer Series, Pamphlet no. 5, Chicago: American Medical Association, 1925.

———. *Diseases of the Breast with Special Reference to Cancer*. Philadelphia: P. Blakiston's Son & Co., 1908.

Rollin, Betty. *First You Cry.* Philadelphia: Lippincott, 1976.

Romeo, Salvatore. *S. Agata V. M. e il suo culto.* Catania: Libraio della R. Casa, 1922.

Rose, Gillian. *Love's Work.* London: Vintage, 1997.

Rosenberg, Charles E. *The Care of Strangers: The Rise of America's Hospital System.* New York: Basic Books, 1987.

———. "Framing Disease: Illness, Society, and History." In *Framing Disease: Studies in Cultural History,* edited by Charles E. Rosenberg and Janet Golden. New Brunswick: Rutgers University Press, 1992.

Ross, Walter. *Crusade: The Official History of the American Cancer Society.* New York: Arbor House, 1987.

Rowbotham, Shcila. *A Century of Women: The History of Women in Britain and the United States.* London: Viking, 1997.

Saint, Lily L. "American Listerism: A Practical Reflection." Mt. Sinai Hospital, Department of Surgery, 1997.

Saltzstein, Harry C. "The Average Treatment of Cancer: Report of a Survey of Facilities Available in the Average American City, with Especial Reference to Early Care." *Journal of the American Medical Association* 91, no. 7 (1928): 465–70.

Sandburg, Helga. "Let a Joy Keep You." *McCall's* (November 1974).

Scanlon, Edward F. "The Evolution of Breast Cancer Treatment." *Journal of the American Medical Association* 266, no. 9 (1991): 1280–82.

Schereschewsky, Joseph. "The Course of Cancer Mortality in the Ten Original Registration States for the 21-Year Period, 1900–1920." *Public Health Bulletin* no. 155. Washington, D.C.: Government Printing Office, 1925.

Seelig, M. G. "Should Cancer Victims Be Told the Truth?" *Journal of the Missouri State Medical Association* 40, no. 2 (1943): 33–35.

Shapiro, Susan. "Cancer as a Feminist Issue." *Sojourner: The Women's Forum* (September 1989): 18–19.

Shaughnessy, Donald E. "The Story of the American Cancer Society." Ph.D. diss., Columbia University, New York, 1957.

Shore, Benjamin R. "The Education of the Public." *Quarterly Review,* no. 3 (1936).

Shorter, Edward. *Doctors and Their Patients: A Social History.* New Brunswick, N.J.: Transaction Publishers, 1991.

———. *A History of Women's Bodies.* Harmondsworth, Middlesex: Penguin Books, 1982.

Simmons, Channing C., and Ernest M. Daland. "Cancer: Delay in Its Surgical Treatment." *Boston Medical and Surgical Journal* 190, no. 1 (1924): 15–19.

Simmons, Channing C., Ernest M. Daland, and Richard H. Wallace. "Delay in the Treatment of Cancer." *New England Journal of Medicine* 208, no. 21 (1933): 1097–1100.

Smith, Margaret Supplee. "The Agnew Clinic: 'Not Cheerful for Ladies to Look At.'" *Prospects* 11 (1986): 161–98.

Smith-Rosenberg, Carroll, and Charles Rosenberg. "The Female Animal: Medical and Biological Views of Woman and Her Role in Nineteenth-Century America." In *Women and Health in America: Historical Readings,* edited by Judith W. Leavitt. Madison: The University of Wisconsin Press, 1984, 12–27.

Snow, Herbert. *The Proclivity of Women to Cancerous Diseases.* London: J. & A. Churchill, 1891.

Spear, Scott L., and Alexander Majidian. "Immediate Breast Reconstruction in Two Stages Using Textured, Integrated-Valve Tissue Expanders and Breast Implants: A Retrospective Review of 171 Consecutive Breast Reconstructions from 1989 to 1996." *Plastic and Reconstructive Surgery* 10, no. 1 (1998): 53–63.

Speert, Harold. *Obstetric and Gynecologic Milestones: Essays in Eponymy.* New York: Macmillan, 1958.

———. *Obstetrics and Gynecology in America: A History.* Chicago: The American College of Obstetricians and Gynecologists, 1980.

Spence, Jo. *Putting Myself in the Picture: A Political, Personal, and Photographic Autobiography.* London: Camden Press, 1986.

Starr, Paul. *The Social Transformation of American Medicine.* New York: Basic Books, 1982.

Strausz, Ivan K. *You Don't Need a Hysterectomy: New and Effective Ways of Avoiding Major Surgery.* Reading, Mass.: Addison-Wesley, 1993.

Strax, Philip, Louis Venet, and Sam Shapiro. "Value of Mammography in Reduction of Mortality from Breast Cancer in Mass Screening." *American Journal of Roentgenology* 117, no. 3 (1973): 686–89.

Taylor, Grantley W., and Richard H. Wallace. "Carcinoma of the Breast: Fifty Years Experience at the Massachusetts General Hospital." *Annals of Surgery* 132, no. 4 (1950): 833–38.

Thomas, T. Gaillard. *A Practical Treatise on the Diseases of Women.* Philadelphia: Lea, 1868–91.

Tobias, Sheila, and Lisa Anderson. "What Really Happened to Rosie the Riveter: Demobilization and the Female Labor Force, 1944–47." In *Women's America: Refocusing the Past*, edited by Linda K. Kerber and Jane DeH. Mathews. New York: Oxford University Press, 1982, 354–73.

Trabulsy, Philip P., James P. Anthony, and Stephen J. Mathes. "Changing Trends in Postmastectomy Breast Reconstruction." *Plastic and Reconstructive Surgery* 93, no. 7 (June 1994): 1418–27.

Tuson, E. W. *The Structure and Functions of the Female Breast as They Relate to Its Health, Derangement and Disease.* London: John Churchill, 1846.

West, Stanley. *The Hysterectomy Hoax.* New York: Doubleday, 1994.

Williams, W. Roger. *Monograph on Diseases of the Breast.* London: John Bale & Sons, 1894.

Williamson, Myrtle. *One Out of Four: A Personal Experience with Cancer.* Richmond, Va.: John Knox Press, 1960.

Wiltshire, John. "Early Nineteenth-Century Pathography: The Case of Frances Burney." *Literature and History*, 2d ser., 2 (Autumn 1993): 9–23.

Wood, Ann Douglas. "'The Fashionable Diseases': Women's Complaints and Their Treatment in Nineteenth-Century America." In *Women and Health in America*, edited by Judith W Leavitt, 222–38. Madison: The University of Wisconsin Press, 1984.

Woolf, Virginia. *A Room of One's Own.* San Diego: Harcourt Brace, 1989.

Wright, James R. "The Development of the Frozen Section, the Evolution of Surgical

Biopsy and the Origins of Surgical Pathology." *Bulletin of the History of Medicine* 59 (1985): 295–326.

———. "The 1917 New York Biopsy: A Question of Surgical Incision and the Promotion of Metastases." *Bulletin of the History of Medicine* 62 (1988): 546–62.

Wright, Russell O. *Life and Death in the United States*. Jefferson, N.C.: McFarland, 1997.

Yalom, Marilyn. *A History of the Breast*. New York: Alfred A. Knopf, 1997.

Young, Hugh H. *A Surgeon's Autobiography*. New York: Harcourt Brace, 1940.

Zaharias, Babe Didrikson. *This Life I've Led*. London: Robert Hale, 1956.

Index

abortion reform: as legal rather than medical issue, 197, 201–2; media coverage of, 192–93, 196–97; professional involvement in campaigns promoting, 197–98; as public issue, 213; relationship to breast cancer advocacy, 193–94. *See also Roe v. Wade*

Acker, Kathy, 281–82

advertising: by drug companies in the 1990s, 260–61; impact on cancer campaigns in the interwar period, 158; Kotex campaign, 303n10

African American experience of breast cancer, 19–20, 252, 255

Agatha, Saint, 30

Agnew, David, 70, 71

American Cancer Society, 13, 247, 273; co-sponsor of "Tactic," 238; co-sponsors breast cancer detection centers with NCI, 229–30; fails to support informed consent legislation, 273; sponsors breast self-exam film, 113, 175; works to end workplace discrimination, 231

American Medical Association (AMA), 145, 171, 192, 193; opposes bill to establish NCI, 168, 304n21

American Society for the Control of Cancer (after 1945 *see* American Cancer Society), 12, 158, 165, 168, 170, 171, 244; class bias of campaigns, 163; early emphasis on control rather than prevention, 155–56; early pamphlet on breast cancer, 162; influence on government cancer policy, 156–57; members appointed by FDR to National Advisory Panel, 245–46; origins of, 155. *See also* Women's Field Army

Arditti, Rita, 312n8

Bell, Bill, 311n29

birth control, 189, 190, 195–96; early expressions of support for, 192; early media coverage of, 193; natural links with abortion reform, 194; Supreme Court decisions legalizing, 193

Biskind, Morton, 138–39

handling of, 122–25; Mueller's experience of, 93; Rachel Carson's experience of, 127, 130–31, 171

Patterson, James, 1

Pearson, Cindy, 261

Perkins, Frances, 248

physicians: response to women's symptoms, 42–43; attitude toward volunteers in Women's Field Army, 167. *See also* doctor/patient relationship; patient disclosure

Planned Parenthood, 198

polio (infantile paralysis): FDR's response to, 243–44; national perception of, 243

postmastectomy surgery. *See* breast implants; breast reconstruction

prevention, 79, 80, 246, 267, 269, 274, 314n18; distinction between cancer control and, 155–56, 182; first clinics devoted to, 166; as flexible concept, 182; hope of cure as substitute for, 174; privatized, 258, 259

privacy, ambiguity of concept, 202–3; as deterrent to evolution of breast cancer advocacy, 203–5. *See also Roe v. Wade*

Proctor, Robert, 247

radiation, 111, 118, 120; Barbara Mueller's interest in, 96–98; first introduced, 177; Rachel Carson's experience of, 132, 134, 135, 138, 139, 140, 143, 144, 148, 300n31

radical mastectomy: ambivalent feel-

ings evoked by, 61–62; consequences for doctor/patient relationship, 57–62; as fixed procedure in the context of social change, 110; impact of, 66–70, 71–72; misrepresentation of results, 72–77; William Stewart Halsted's experience with, 54–55; William Stewart Halsted's version of, 51

Reagan, Nancy, experience of breast cancer, 251–53

representation of breast disease, 34, 70

representation of the breast, 30, 41

reproduction: diminished role in women's lives, 188–89; mistaken association with breast cancer, 36; and nineteenth century theories of disease, 33–34; sexual politics of, 195–97

Rinehart, Mary Roberts, 217, 218

Roe v. Wade, privacy argument cited in, 202

Rollin, Betty, 4, 238, 254

Roosevelt, Eleanor, 168

Roosevelt, Franklin Delano: appoints ASCC directors to national cancer advisory panel, 245–46; response to polio, 243–44, 246

Saint, Lily, 294

Sandburg, Helga (Mrs. George Crile, Jr.), 117, 238

Sanderson, Fred R., 127, 130, 300n24